Yearbook of Anesthesiology-7

Editorial Board

VP Kumra MD DAc FICA
Past President and Advisor
Indian College of Anaesthesiologists
Ex-Vice President
Indian Society of Anaesthesiologists (National)
Emeritus Consultant and Advisor
Department of Anaesthesiology Pain and Perioperative Medicine
Sir Ganga Ram Hospital
New Delhi, India
ved_kumra@yahoo.com

B Radhakrishnan MD MPhil FICA
President
Indian College of Anaesthesiologists
Ex-President
Indian Society of Anaesthesiologists (National)
Principal
Academy of Medical Sciences
Kannur, Kerala, India
brktvm@yahoo.com

Jayashree Sood MD FFARCS PGDHHM FICA
CEO
Indian College of Anaesthesiologists
Professor and Chairperson
Department of Anaesthesiology Pain and Perioperative Medicine
Honorary Joint Secretary
Board of Management
Sir Ganga Ram Hospital
New Delhi, India
jayashreesood@hotmail.com

Baljit Singh MD
CEO
Indian College of Anaesthesiologist
Director Professor
GB Pant Institute of Postgraduate Medical Education and Research
New Delhi, India
drbaljitsingh@gmail.com

Yearbook of Anesthesiology-7

Editors

Raminder Sehgal MD DA FICA
Ex–Director Professor
Maulana Azad Medical College
New Delhi, India
Ex–Senior Consultant
Sir Ganga Ram Hospital
New Delhi, India
ramindersehgal@hotmail.com

Anjan Trikha MD FICA
Professor
All India Institute of Medical Sciences
New Delhi, India
anjantrikha@gmail.com

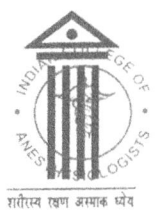

Indian College of Anaesthesiologists
Whole Constituent of
Indian Society of Anaesthesiologists
(Member of the World Federation of
Societies of Anaesthesiologists)

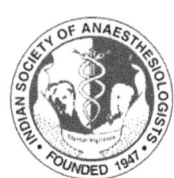

Foreword
SM Basu

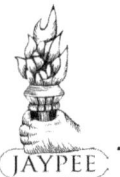

JAYPEE **The Health Sciences Publisher**
New Delhi | London | Panama

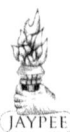 **Jaypee Brothers Medical Publishers (P) Ltd**

Headquarters
Jaypee Brothers Medical Publishers (P) Ltd.
4838/24, Ansari Road, Daryaganj
New Delhi 110 002, India
Phone: +91-11-43574357
Fax: +91-11-43574314
E-mail: jaypee@jaypeebrothers.com

Overseas Offices

JP Medical Ltd.
83, Victoria Street, London
SW1H 0HW (UK)
Phone: +44-20 3170 8910
Fax: +44(0)20 3008 6180
E-mail: info@jpmedpub.com

Jaypee-Highlights Medical Publishers Inc.
City of Knowledge, Bld. 235, Clayton
Panama City, Panama
Phone: +1 507-301-0496
Fax: +1 507-301-0499
E-mail: cservice@jphmedical.com

Jaypee Brothers Medical Publishers (P) Ltd.
17/1-B, Babar Road, Block-B, Shyamali
Mohammadpur, Dhaka-1207
Bangladesh
Mobile: +08801912003485
E-mail: jaypeedhaka@gmail.com

Jaypee Brothers Medical Publishers (P) Ltd.
Bhotahity, Kathmandu, Nepal
Phone: +977-9741283608
E-mail: kathmandu@jaypeebrothers.com

Website: www.jaypeebrothers.com
Website: www.jaypeedigital.com

© 2018, Jaypee Brothers Medical Publishers

The views and opinions expressed in this book are solely those of the original contributor(s)/author(s) and do not necessarily represent those of editor(s) of the book.

All rights reserved. No part of this publication may be reproduced, stored or transmitted in any form or by any means, electronic, mechanical, photocopying, recording or otherwise, without the prior permission in writing of the publishers.

All brand names and product names used in this book are trade names, service marks, trademarks or registered trademarks of their respective owners. The publisher is not associated with any product or vendor mentioned in this book.

Medical knowledge and practice change constantly. This book is designed to provide accurate, authoritative information about the subject matter in question. However, readers are advised to check the most current information available on procedures included and check information from the manufacturer of each product to be administered, to verify the recommended dose, formula, method and duration of administration, adverse effects and contraindications. It is the responsibility of the practitioner to take all appropriate safety precautions. Neither the publisher nor the author(s)/editor(s) assume any liability for any injury and/or damage to persons or property arising from or related to use of material in this book.

This book is sold on the understanding that the publisher is not engaged in providing professional medical services. If such advice or services are required, the services of a competent medical professional should be sought.

Every effort has been made where necessary to contact holders of copyright to obtain permission to reproduce copyright material. If any have been inadvertently overlooked, the publisher will be pleased to make the necessary arrangements at the first opportunity. The CD/DVD-ROM (if any) provided in the sealed envelope with this book is complimentary and free of cost. **Not meant for sale.**

Inquiries for bulk sales may be solicited at: jaypee@jaypeebrothers.com

Yearbook of Anesthesiology-7

First Edition: **2018**

ISBN: 978-93-5270-297-8

Printed at:

Contributors

Shivani Aggarwal
Department of Cardiac Anesthesia
Cardiothoracic Centre (CTC)
All India Institute of Medical Sciences
New Delhi, India
drshivani.del@gmail.com

Sharmila Ahuja MD
Ex-Professor
Department of Anesthesiology and
Critical Care, University College of
Medical Sciences and GTB Hospital
New Delhi, India
sharmilaahuja@gmail.com

SP Ambesh MD FICA FAMS CCST (UK)
Professor of Anesthesiology
Consultant In-Charge ICU and Head
Department of Emergency Medicine
Sanjay Gandhi Postgraduate Institute of
Medical Sciences
Lucknow, Uttar Pradesh, India
ambeshsp@hotmail.com

Sanjeev Aneja MD DNB FFARCS
Clinical Fellowship in Liver Transplant
Anesthesia (University of Toronto)
Senior Consultant in Anesthesia and
Intensive Care
Apollo Hospital, New Delhi, India
sanjeevaneja@hotmail.com

Dipika Bansal MD DM
Associate Professor
Department of Anesthesia and
Intensive Care
Postgraduate Institute of Medical
Education and Research
Chandigarh, India
dedeep97@gmail.com

Pooja Bhangui MD
Associate Consultant
Division of Liver Transplant Anesthesia
and Intensive Care
Medanta—the Medicity
Gurgaon, Haryana, India
drpooja81@gmail.com

Nidhi Bhatia MD
Associate Professor
Department of Anesthesia and
Intensive Care
PGIMER, Chandigarh, India
nidhi.bhatia75@gmail.com

Anuradha Borle
Assistant Professor
Department of Anesthesia
All India Institute of Medical Sciences
New Delhi, India
andromeda85l@gmail.com

Suman D Chaudhry
MD FFARCSI FRCA (Assoc)
Consultant Anesthetist Wrightington
Wigan and Leigh NHS Foundation
Trust and Rotherham NHS Foundation
Trust, United Kingdom, London
sumchaudhry@gmail.com

Prabhat Choudhary MD
Consultant
Department of Anesthesiology, Pain
and Perioperative Medicine
Sir Ganga Ram Hospital
Old Rajinder Nagar, New Delhi, India
drprabhat_sgrh@rediffmail.com

Amitabh Dutta MD PGD-HR
Senior Consultant
Department of Anesthesiology, Pain
and Perioperative Medicine
Professor of Anesthesiology, GRIPMER

Member, Ethics Committee and Science (Protocol) Committee
Sir Ganga Ram Hospital and Ganga Ram Institute for Medical Education and Research (GRIPMER)
Old Rajinder Nagar, New Delhi, India
duttaamitabh@yahoo.co.in

Babita Ghai MD DNB MAMS
Professor
Department of Anesthesia and Intensive Care
Postgraduate Institute of Medical Education and Research
Chandigarh, India
ghaibabita1@gmail.com

Anju Grewal MD
Professor
Department of Anesthesiology
Dayanand Medical College and Hospital
Ludhiana, Punjab, India
Chief Editor
Journal of Anesthesiology Clinical Pharmacology
dranjugrewal@gmail.com

Anju Gupta MD DNB
Assistant Professor
Department of Anesthesiology
Chacha Nehru Bal Chikitsalya
New Delhi, India
dranjugupta@rediffmail.com

Nishkarsh Gupta MD DNB
Associate Professor
Department of Onco-Anesthesiology and Palliative Medicine
DRBRAIRCH
All India Institute of Medical Sciences
New Delhi, India
drnishkarsh@rediffmail.com

Basavaraj Herekar MD
Assistant Professor
Department of Anesthesiology
Kasturba Medical College
Manipal, Karnataka, India
herekarbasavaraj@rediffmail.com

Krishna HM MD DNB
Professor
Department of Anesthesiology
Kasturba Medical College
Manipal, Karnataka, India
hmkrishna20032002@yahoo.com

Ashok Jadon
MD DNB MNAMS FIPM FIPP FAMS
Chief Consultant and HOD
Department of Anesthesia
In-charge Pain Relief Service
Tata Motors Hospital
Jamshedpur, Jharkhand, India
jadona@rediffmail.com

Poonam Malhotra Kapoor
MD DNB MNAMS FIACTA (Hony) FTEE (Hony) FISCU (Hony)
Professor
Department of Cardiac Anesthesia
Cardiothoracic Center (CTC)
All India Institute of Medical Sciences
New Delhi, India
drpoonamaiims@gmail.com

Anil Karlekar MD
Executive Director, Anesthesiology
Director, Clinical Affairs
Fortis Escorts Heart Institute
Okhla Road, New Delhi, India
karlekar@gmail.com

Dilip Kumar Kulkarni
Senior Professor
In-charge Neuroanesthesiology
Department of Anesthesiology and Intensive Care
Associate Dean
Nizam's Institute of Medical Sciences
Hyderabad, Telangana, India
dilipkum@gmail.com

Lakshmi Kumar MD
Professor and Head
Department of Anesthesiology and Critical Care
Amrita Institute of Medical Sciences
Kochi, Kerala, India
lakshmi.k.238@gmail.com

Contributors

Pramod Kumar MD
Dean Medical Sciences
Teerthanker Mahaveer University
Moradabad, Uttar Pradesh, India
pkumar_pain@rediffmail.com

Yatin Mehta
MD MNAMS FRCA FAMS FICCM FIACTA FTEE
Chairman, Medanta Institute of Critical Care and Anesthesiology
Medanta-The Medicity
Gurgaon, Haryana, India
yatinmehta@hotmail.com

Priya R Menon MBBS MD PDCC
Facharzt Anästhesie EDAIC DESA EACTA
Diploma in Transesophageal Echocardiography
Honorary Fellowship IACTA
Consultant
Abteilung der Kardioanästhesie und Intensive Medizin
Herzzentrum Leipzig
Leipzig, Germany
drpriyamenon@gmail.com

Medha Mohta MD MAMS
Director Professor
Department of Anesthesiology and Critical Care, University College of Medical Sciences and GTB Hospital
New Delhi, India
medhamohta@gmail.com

Monish Nakra
Colonel and Senior Advisor
(Anesthesiology and Critical Care)
Army Hospital (Research and Referral)
New Delhi, India
monishnakra@gmail.com

Keerthi Nandakumar MD DNB
Senior Resident
Department of Anesthesiology and Critical Care
Amrita Institute of Medical Sciences
Kochi, Karala, India
keerthipnandakumar@gmail.com

Murali Pandurangan MD FRCA EDIC
Specialist Anesthetist
Medcare Hospital LLC
Dubai, UAE
drmuralip@hotmail.com

Akshaya Rai MD DNB PDCC
Clinical Associate
Department of Pediatric Cardiac Anesthesia
Kokilaben Dhirubhai Ambani Hospital
Mumbai, Maharashtra, India
aksvrai@yahoo.co.in

Amit Rai MD DNB MNAMS PDC (Paed Anaesth)
Associate Professor (AFMC, Pune) and Pediatric Anesthesiologist
Command Hospital
Pune, Maharashtra, India
drraiamit@gmail.com

Chand Sahai DA MD
Senior Consultant
Department of Anesthesiology, Pain and Perioperative Medicine
Sir Ganga Ram Hospital
Old Rajinder Nagar, New Delhi, India
chandsahai@gmail.com

Deepti Saigal MD
Assistant Professor
Department of Anesthesiology
Safdarjung Hospital and Vardhaman Mahavir Medical College
New Delhi, India
deeptisaigal21@gmail.com

Rashmi Salhotra MD
Associate Professor
Department of Anesthesiology and Critical Care
University College of Medical Sciences and GTB Hospital
New Delhi, India
rashmichabra33@gmail.com

Susmita Sarangi MD
Specialist
Deen Dayal Upadhyay Hospital
Hari Nagar, New Delhi, India
drpsarangi@yahoo.com

Ashok Kumar Saxena
Professor and Head
Department of Anesthesiology
Critical Care and Pain Medicine
University College of Medical Sciences
and GTB Hospital
New Delhi, India
profashoksaxena@gmail.com

Bimla Sharma MD FICA
Senior Consultant
Department of Anesthesiology, Pain
and Perioperative Medicine
Sir Ganga Ram Hospital
Old Rajinder Nagar, New Delhi, India
bimsharma@rediffmail.com

Kavita Rani Sharma MD
Director Professor
Department of Anesthesiology and
Intensive Care
Maulana Azad Medical College
New Delhi, India
drkavitadn@gmail.com, drkavitadn@hotmail.com

Gunjan Singh MD DNB
Fellow (Paediatric Anesthesiology)
All India Institute of Medical Sciences
New Delhi, India
gunjanafmc@gmail.com

Preet Mohinder Singh MD DNB
Assistant Professor
Department of Anesthesia
All India Institute of Medical Sciences
New Delhi, India
preetrajpal@gmail.com

Dipali Taneja DNB
Specialist
Deen Dayal Upadhyay Hospital
Hari Nagar, New Delhi, India
taneja.sandeep13@gmail.com

Deepak K Tempe MD FRCA FAMS
Director Professor
Department of Anesthesiology
GB Pant Institute of Postgraduate
Medical Education and Research
New Delhi, India
Former Dean, Maulana Azad Medical
College, New Delhi, India
tempedeepak@hotmail.com

Asha Tyagi MD DNB MNAMS
Director Professor
Department of Anesthesiology and
Critical Care
University College of Medical Sciences
and GTB Hospital
New Delhi, India
drashatyagi@gmail.com

Elsa Varghese DA MD
Fellowship Pediatric Anesthesia (USA)
Former Professor
Department of Anesthesiology
Kasturba Medical College
Manipal, Karnataka, India
Senior Consultant Anesthesiologist
MIOT International Hospital
Chennai, Madras, India
elsakmc@gmail.com

Vijay Vohra MD FRCA
Chairman
Division of Liver Transplant Anesthesia
and Intensive Care
Medanta—the Medicity
Gurgaon, Haryana, India
vijay.vohra@medanta.org

LN Yaddanapudi MD
Professor
Department of Anesthesia and
Intensive Care
PGIMER, Chandigarh, India
narayana.yaddanapudi@gmail.com

Foreword

The Indian College of Anaesthesiologists (ICA) was established with the mission of achieving academic excellence in the field of anaesthesiology.

Apropos to its promise, as the initial venture, the college started the publication of the *Yearbook of Anesthesiology* in 2011, within three years of its establishment (in November 2008). Bringing out a standard book is no mean achievement. Definite set of principles was laid down for its publication with the first volume and this has been followed down the lane to the present volume.

In each volume, newer topics of current interest were incorporated. Renowned anaesthesiologists (senior consultants or teachers), having vast experience of work with updated knowledge in the particular field have been given the task of particular chapter. Each chapter has been designed to include the recent updated knowledge in the field. Together, the authors have shared their wisdom to prepare comprehensive but concise chapters after collecting materials from different sources. Chapters have been written maintaining the clarity yet comprehensive in updated information with a modest size so that they are helpful for postgraduate students, consultants and teachers alike.

Editors have been chosen who have excellent credentials of such vital work having past experience of accepting the great responsibility so that the principles as well as the format do not change. It is needless to say that present editors Professor Raminder Sehgal and Professor Anjan Trikha do not need any introduction in this country about their credibility.

Unfortunately, the pioneer editor of the Yearbook, Dr Umesh Chandra, FFARCS passed away in the month of July this year. He alone shouldered the responsibility of editing the volume 1 and co-edited volumes 2 and 3, setting a new era in anesthetic literature in our country. While paying homage, let us pray for eternal peace of the departed soul.

While congratulating the editorial team for the commendable work, we must acknowledge the constructive suggestions and guidance received from Dr Manorama Mittal, Dr VP Kumra, Dr Jayshree Sood, Dr Baljit Singh and very importantly the President of the College Dr B Radhakrishnan.

The publishing house Jaypee Brothers Medical Publishers, New Delhi, India should receive applause for their immaculate work.

Taking care of the academic field, the college is steering ahead in bringing out the Yearbook every year which are being well appreciated by our fraternity. The College is presenting the 7th volume of the Yearbook without compromising the quality, incorporation of newer information or punctuality of publication. Let the Yearbook bear the annual testimony of academic credential of the Indian College of Anaesthesiologists.

SM Basu MD (Cal) DA (Lond.) MR CA (Eng.) FICA
Emeritus Professor, ESI Institute of Pain Management, Kolkata
Ex-Professor and Head, Calcutta National Medical College, Kolkata
Ex-Editor, Indian Journal of Anaesthesia
Ex- President, Indian Society of Anaesthesiologists (National)

Preface

The present *Yearbook of Anesthesiology* is the seventh in the series brought out under the auspices of the Indian College of Anaesthesiologists—the academic wing of the Indian Society of Anaesthesiologists. Year after year, every new edition has met with an unanticipated response. The popularity of the book is evident from the increasing number of the titles published every year. The feedback received from different parts of the country has made us realize that the volumes of the yearbook are more popular between two distinct groups; postgraduate students who are studying for their exams and practicing anesthesiologists, especially in non-metro cities who look forward to this annual update. Keeping these in mind we choose the topics in all the three subspecialties of anesthesiology—regional and general anesthesia, intensive care and pain. In addition, on popular demand we have added a chapter on statistics and made a beginning by discussing ethical issues related to conflict of interest in anesthesiology.

Among the anesthesia chapters a few important ones, which we as editors thought needed to be revisited, are on pre-oxygenation, clinical applications of pulmonary function tests, management of local anesthetic systemic toxicity, anesthesia for liver transplantation and causes and management of perioperative atrial fibrillation. The information given by the authors is a mix of classical concepts and the present knowledge and practice. Another chapter highlights the pharmacokinetics, pharmacodynamics and use of remifentanil for alleviation of labor pains. This ultrashort acting opioid is likely to be available in India in the near future and both students and the practicing anesthesiologists would find this chapter very useful. Also of interest is the chapter on perioperative medication errors which is an important cause of perioperative morbidity and mortality. Video laryngoscope is gaining immense popularity in the country and is likely to be standard airway management device in the future. A chapter on this device highlights its advantages and its usefulness in management of difficult airway.

Amongst the specialty anesthesia, there are chapters on anesthetic management of congenital tracheoesophageal fistula and extremely premature infant; intracranial pressure and brain relaxation; laryngotracheal stenosis and prognostication after cardiac arrest and myocardial protection during cardiac surgery, all penned by experts in their respective field. Two chapters are related to the process of hemostasis and perioperative fibrinogen supplementation. While ICU management of patients with sepsis is discussed often, we have devoted one chapter to the anesthetic management of such patients.

In the field of intensive care, the readers are likely to find the chapters on extracorporeal membrane oxygenation; pain, delirium and agitation very informative with updated information on these topics. The chapters on neuropathic pain and management of chronic back pain highlight the present treatment modalities as per the latest evidence-based practice guidelines.

Similar to the earlier two volumes the section on the 'Journal Scan' carries experts' opinion on certain landmark articles published during the last year, which are likely to change clinical practice.

We would like to express our gratitude to all contributors for sparing their precious time for contributing to this yearbook without any kind of financial rewards. Our special thanks are also due for the staff of M/s Jaypee Brothers Medical Publishers (P) Ltd., New Delhi, India, for their support.

Both of us as editors of the past four titles try our best to list recent topics that are likely to be useful to our anesthesiology community. So far, we think we have achieved what this book was envisaged to do. In this regard we would welcome opinions, suggestions and criticism regarding our efforts, as we strongly believe that without these we will not be able to improve the future content of the books.

Raminder Sehgal
Anjan Trikha

Contents

1. Conflict-of-Interest in Anesthesiology 1
   Amitabh Dutta, Prabhat Choudhary
2. Understanding Hemostasis: The Knowns and the Unknowns 16
   Anil Karlekar
3. Moving away from Null Hypothesis Significance Testing 36
   LN Yaddanapudi
4. Remifentanil for Labor Analgesia 43
   Preet Mohinder Singh, Anuradha Borle
5. Low Flow Anesthesia: Revisited and Reiterated 52
   Asha Tyagi, Rashmi Salhotra
6. Local Anesthetic Systemic Toxicity 63
   Nishkarsh Gupta, Anju Gupta
7. Videolaryngoscopy: Current Perspectives 76
   Chand Sahai, Bimla Sharma
8. Preoxygenation: Physiological Basis, Techniques, Benefits and Potential Risks 90
   Kavita Rani Sharma
9. Pulmonary Function Tests and their Clinical Applications 103
   Susmita Sarangi, Dipali Taneja
10. Neuropathic Pain 122
    Pramod Kumar
11. Management of Chronic Low Back Pain: An Overview 129
    Babita Ghai, Dipika Bansal
12. Intracranial Pressure versus Brain Relaxation 142
    Dilip Kumar Kulkarni
13. Sepsis and the Anesthesiologist 152
    Krishna HM, Basavaraj Herekar
14. Congenital Tracheoesophageal Fistula: Anesthetic Considerations and Management 159
    Sharmila Ahuja, Medha Mohta
15. Extremely Premature Infants and Anesthesia 168
    Elsa Varghese
16. ECMO: Need of the Hour 179
    Poonam Malhotra Kapoor, Shivani Aggarwal
17. Anesthesia for Laryngotracheal Stenosis 190
    Amit Rai, Gunjan Singh
18. Perioperative Fibrinogen Supplementation: Safety and Efficacy 204
    Anju Grewal, Nidhi Bhatia

19. **Pain, Agitation and Delirium in Adult Intensive Care Unit** — 210
    SP Ambesh

20. **Perioperative Atrial Fibrillation:
    A Perioperative Physician's Outlook** — 226
    Priya R Menon, Akshaya Rai

21. **Perioperative Medication Errors** — 241
    Lakshmi Kumar, Keerthi Nandakumar

22. **Prognostication after Cardiac Arrest** — 252
    Suman D Chaudhry, Murali Pandurangan

23. **Anesthesia for Liver Transplantation** — 267
    Vijay Vohra, Pooja Bhangui

24. **Myocardial Protection during Cardiac Surgery:
    An Overview of Cardioplegia** — 285
    Deepak K Tempe, Deepti Saigal

25. **Journal Scans:** — 306
    1. *Sanjeev Aneja* — 306
    2. *Ashok Jadon* — 310
    3. *Yatin Mehta* — 314
    4. *Monish Nakra* — 318
    5. *Ashok Kumar Saxena* — 321

Index — 325

CHAPTER 1

Conflict-of-Interest in Anesthesiology

Amitabh Dutta, Prabhat Choudhary

Whose bread I eat his song I sing

A German Proverb

KEY POINTS

- COI is ubiquitous in medical healthcare and anesthesiology.
- It represents a conflict between the primary interest (assigned work) and secondary interest (other gains).
- COI influence decision-making, induces bias, and sometimes 'harm' the patient/research participants.
- COI negatively affects objectivity of science and public confidence and trust in medical system.
- Secondary interests could be financial—easy to detect and estimate, or nonfinancial which are difficult to fathom.
- COI emanates out of misuse of individual 'authority' but 'institutional' misgivings also contribute to COI.
- COI needs to be identified and evaluated sensitively.
- Disclosure of the COI is key to management of COI.
- Institutions should establish policies against for COI matters, such as declare COI, diffuse (mitigate) COI effects or disassociate (drop out) from COI.

INTRODUCTION

Conflict-of-Interest (COI) is omnipresent in medical science and the field of *Anesthesiology* is no exception.[1,2] Though COI issues are known for a century and well entrenched in healthcare, its common understanding and awareness in *Anesthesiology* is severely limited.[3] Like in Medicine, COI impacts almost every aspect of *Anesthesiology:* i.e. clinical practice; academics and research domains. So, in order to avoid conduct reprimand and legal retribution arising out of lack of awareness or ignorance, it is high time that we wake up to applied implications of COI and embrace it in a wholesome manner.

Per se, *Anesthesiology* is a complex applied clinical specialty that amalgamates mechanistic, automation, and electronics to the most important element of clinical practice, i.e. the patients.[4] In practice, therefore, there are as many interfaces of *Anesthesiology* as one can imagine and that each has the potential to be adversely affected by COI situations. COI has the ability to dampen fluidity of anesthesia healthcare delivery; block research and development of the specialty; sublimate patients' trust; and most importantly, break specialty-public bridges (public awareness, confidence, and trust) even before they are formed. Therefore, it is of utmost importance that we look up to COI matters in *Anesthesiology* before it complicates our existential status (amongst other medical specialties) and isolate us further.

Conflict-of-Interest: Definition

Conflict-of-Interest '*is a set of circumstances that create a risk that professional judgment or action regarding a primary interest will be unduly influenced by a secondary interest.*'[5] In simpler terms, COI is a situation in which personal considerations or interests, primarily financial, has a potential to induce bias in professional decision-making that adversely affects objectivity. The core ethical element that connects different stakeholders (Box 1) with activities enshrined in a typical healthcare gamut (clinics, research, academics) is 'trust'.[6] Further, objective reflection of clinical practice; justification of the treatment cost; research conduct and evidence creation; application of new evidence/recent advances; and disseminating awareness about health and treatment options is central to creation and sustenance of trust in the general public (Flowchart 1). The generation of COI by extraordinary pursuit of secondary interest, especially which result in deficit of primary service, fuel public mistrust and attracts greater regulation by relevant authority (departmental, institutional, sub-specialty, organization, government, state).

Therefore, howsoever subtle the COI possibility for a given set of circumstances may be, the seeking behavior of sensitive public and the media do not fail to identify misgivings in healthcare delivery; usually maintains a low threshold for over-the-board outcry; and are always quick to seek legal opinion and policy regulation upgrade. In context of anesthesiology, since the naïve and unaware public has a general lack of knowledge of the specialty and its clinical care delivery proceeds, they are overly suspicious to the slightest change in anticipated course of care.[7]

DECONSTRUCTING CONFLICT-OF-INTEREST

Conflict-of-Interest in itself is a generic term applied inflexibly and inconsistently in context of medical healthcare. COI is a concept that situates a possibility

Box 1: Stakeholders in conflict-of-interest in healthcare		
Individual	**Institution**	**Public**
• Clinical practitioner • Research investigator • Academic professor • Medical administrator	• Medical school • Research organization • Medical school • Health advocacy groups • Bio-scientific Journals • Grant Commission	• Society at large • General public • Patients/research participants • Law experts • Opinion makers • Media/journals • Educationist • Non-profit organization

Flowchart 1: Taxonomy of medical practice and research.

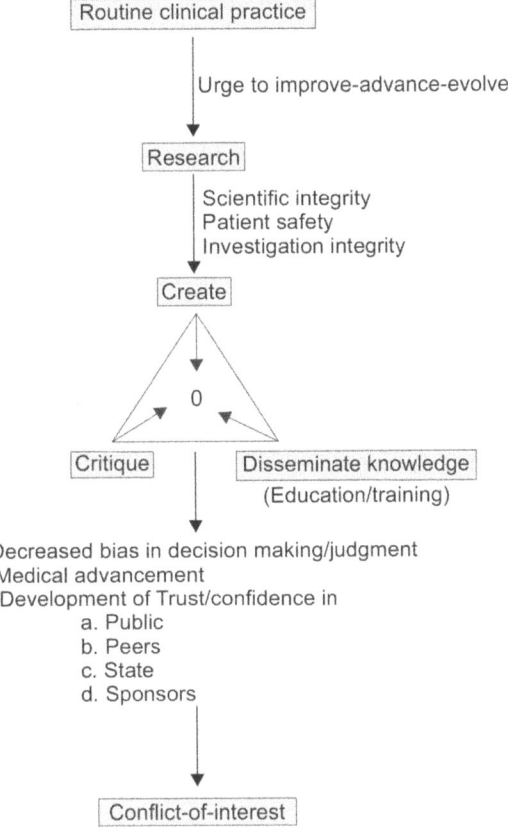

that a particular set of circumstances may undermine the *primary interest* by secondary financial/non-financial interest. COI typically follows a potential → apparent → actual continuum, is subject to evaluation and adjudication of context it relates to, and its severity is defined by the overall harm to the recipient stakeholder. Although COI may involve both individual professionals and/or institution, it usually emanates out of the use of positional authority to eke out personal secondary gains from the assigned primary work for which he/she is being paid or employed for. COI can be broadly categorized into 'tangible' (that involves direct or indirect financial gains and pecuniary relationships) and 'intangible' (involving academics/research activity leading to name, fame, and influence) (Box 2).[8] Evaluation of COI situations is based on identifying and relating the primary interest to the secondary consideration and then analyzing 'conflict' between the two.

Primary Interest in healthcare context signifies the purpose of a scheduled/emergent medical professional activity. The service for patient's health and wellness; promoting research and protecting integrity; and sustaining quality of medical education and training are the main aspects of primary interest. Thus, the primary work of a medical professional can be based on the expected goals/

end-point (promoting practice and research); obligation (towards patients); and rights (protecting and realizing patient's constitutional interest).

Secondary Interest, a common byproduct of a relatively non-altruistic professional mindset, is touted to be the most important element of a COI situation. Unlike truly altruistic individual who are more focused and dedicated to their specific work, others may have concurrent lateral thoughts and possibilities. Not uncommonly, these possibilities translate into self/other (secondary) interests. It is their lower threshold for leaning towards secondary interests while being involved in the primary core work that gives rise to 'undue influence' on their judgment and decision-making. The fallout of the above may be represented by apparent bias, awkward decisions, and sometimes, harm to the patients. When a multitasking conflicted professional pursues both primary and the secondary interest perpetually, it becomes a COI. When the secondary proposition with expected returns accrue greater significance, and demands greater time and commitment than the primary interest, there is a chance that decision-making may be unduly influenced (e.g. bias). The secondary interest may be financial or non-financial.[9] Typically, a secondary interest invests in and targets financial gain and then there are other interests that do not involve money. The financial COI constitutes payments that are paid to investigators from sources other than his/her own institution in form of direct payments, share in equity, facilitation of intellectual property rights, or consulting fees. The payment to investigators on

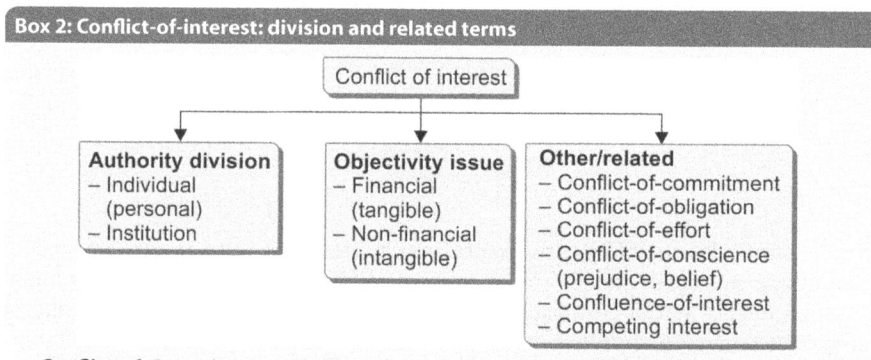

Box 2: Conflict-of-interest: division and related terms

Conflict of interest

Authority division	Objectivity issue	Other/related
– Individual (personal) – Institution	– Financial (tangible) – Non-financial (intangible)	– Conflict-of-commitment – Conflict-of-obligation – Conflict-of-effort – Conflict-of-conscience (prejudice, belief) – Confluence-of-interest – Competing interest

- **Conflict-of-Commitment, Conflict-of-Effort, and Conflict-of-Obligation:** are more or less synonymous. They occur when the time expenditure on unrelated activity competes with the time of assigned primary work. (e.g. clinics time conflicted by teaching, personal work like-child's homework, reading novels, or busy on social media)
- **Conflict-of-Conscience:** as a term signifies that personal belief and prejudice influence objectivity, which may result in deviation from standard of care and practice guidelines (e.g. when SOC is balanced GA for non-cardiac cases; giving opioid- heavy or low-dose opioids as an essential component of balanced GA; amounts to deviation and *conflict-of-conscience*)
- **Confluence-of-Interest:** There has been number of attempts to change the terminology *Conflict-of-Interest* to *Confluence-of-Interest* to justify the interactions of multiple interests with better clarity. (Cappola AR, FitzGerald GA. Confluence, not conflict of interest: name change necessary. JAMA 2015; 314: 1791-92)
- **Competing Interests:** is another term that is more forthcoming and reflects that there may be presence of more than two primary interests which have potential to compete with each other. In *competing interests* scenario, combination may be primary-secondary, primary- primary (two primary interests), primary- secondary- secondary (two or more secondary interests).

account of lectures, academic teaching, seminar, panel discussion, even when funded from outside sources is not considered COI if it is from a 'not-for-profit' entity or a public agency.[10] The COI policies are specifically designed to analyze and to enforce sanctity on secondary financial interest, not because other interests are less important or irrelevant, but because they are more amenable to objective quantification. Sometimes the financial secondary interests are acceptable to an extent and are even valid provided they do not have any undue influence on the related primary interest. Although it is almost impossible to exclude secondary interest from a set of circumstances, social science investigations suggest that even miniscule returns (gift, favor, acknowledgment) which does not cloud primary interest as such, can lead to behavioral changes without the professional being aware of it.[11] This, over a period of time, can lead to individual professional developing a habit of seeking secondary interests and creating neo-COI situations.

Conflict is an essential part of COI and reflects a circumstance wherein tension is created between the primary and the secondary interest during the course of service delivery. Conflict is neither a reality for every situation nor does it always reflect that primary interest is undermined by secondary interest. Rather it suggests a situation where there is a possibility or a risk that the professional decision-making may possibly get tilted more towards secondary interest than the primary interest. Even clear presence of a conflict is not indicative of whether it will distort professional judgment or ultimately harm the patient.

HISTORY OF EVOLUTION OF CONFLICT-OF-INTEREST IN MEDICINE AND ANESTHESIOLOGY

Ernest Hemingway, the noted noble laureate, in his literary classic *'For Whom The Bell Tolls'* (1940), deciphered complex conflicts (-of-interest!) within his characters that led to dereliction from their assigned primary duty of blowing up a fascist-controlled bridge during Spanish civil war of 1937.[12] Little did he know that almost eight decades later, JAMA Surgery would draw inexplicable comparison with the literary epic for explaining controversy around the use of vena-cava filters in the article entitled 'For Whom The Benefit Tolls'.[13] The first seeds of COI can be traced back a century ago when individuals and institutions collaborated with industries for research, education and practice. In 1920s Eli Lily, with researchers of University of Toronto manufactured insulin in quantities enough for clinical use and President Woodrow Wilson requested National Academy of Science to raise money from companies for academic research. However, the real conundrum of COI circumstances in healthcare delivery as we know today started in the 1950s when an out-of-the-box rethink was utilized to defend tobacco industries that were almost on the brink of banishment by scientific evidence that smoking causes lung cancer. John Hill, considered the 'father of inventing COI', when invited to navigate the tobacco industry out from troubled waters, stormed into the very fabric of medical practice and healthcare research by engineering a COI inventory designed to systematically run down the contemporaneous scientific evidence.[14] Interestingly, by not actually resorting to direct disapproval or denial of what scientific consensus asserted and tormented tobacco industry, he raked up controversy around the validity of prevailing evidence by cultivating a carefully designed strategy that appeared to be in consonance with public health and supported scientific research. Hill and Knowlton Co., as a part of their service to a consortium of tobacco industry which was reeling under reactive backlash from restive consumers and public, rode on the shoulders of cynical, skeptical, and critical scientists who reveled in questioning the hypothesis, methodological conduct, and the generated evidence that tobacco kills.[15] In a matter of decade (1950 → 60), the service conglomerate were able to manipulate and control scientific research, media communication, legal framework, and even the contemporary polity to induce confusion, create doubt, and also, fuel hedonistic smoking rituals. Probably, this was the first instance where financial COI forayed into purist institutions. The COI due to money pumped in by tobacco industry cultivated general public health advocacy and diluted direct tobacco-lung cancer link. They effectively used financial might and public relations to suppress any opposing viewpoint like, isolated outcry, 'new' evidence, motivated litigations, and random opinions. More surprisingly, the COI was able to shift responsibility of decision-making on ill-effects of smoking to the discretion of smokers by instituting statutory warnings on the cigarette packs.[16]

The world moved on, and now it was the turn of pharmaceuticals. Introduced by the US congress, the Bayh-Dole Act of 1980[17] not only radically changed the conservative attitude of the Government who retained the rights to the outcome of research and discovery, they empowered Universities and investigators to take control of decisions regarding the applications of their research, even those funded by the federal Government. The faculty members were allowed to patent the discoveries and also to direct transfer of technology. A new era of University-industry shared relationship had already begun. But over the period of time, the liberal times had its own share of downsides, primarily relating to unintended generation of newer COI situations, including the prescription behavior of physicians, publication practices, and research motivation and choices.

The US Public Health Service, in order to adapt to ongoing changes of the research environment, responded to related emerging issues by introducing regulations under the heading of "Responsibility of Applicants for Promoting Objectivity in Research" (1995).[18] The regulations covered three essential aspects: *First*, the Institutions are required to develop internal policies and procedures to manage COI. *Second*, the investigators are required to disclose 'significant financial interests' to their Institution. And *finally*, the Institutions must inform the federal authorities of any situation where COI exhibited a potential to affect research. These rules have been recently redefined by Human and Health Services USA.[19]

In *Anesthesiology*, as early as in 1997, the American Association of Anesthesiologists (ASA) were considering discussions around conflict-of-interest, competing interests, and sponsored research issues.[20] All the major journals now have their own COI policies to govern conduct and publication of sponsored research. There is also a policy of disclosure to cover competing interests and industry collaboration issues. To create greater awareness and reinforcement of objective clinical practice, training and research, structured talks around professionalism and COI had begun to emerge in the first decade of 21st century.[21,22]

GENERAL TYPES AND FUNCTIONAL CLASSIFICATION OF CONFLICT-OF-INTEREST

Conflict-of-Interest can be personal, professional, prejudice, or financial. While financial COIs are dealt extensively,[23] the other three which are classified under 'individual' COI need elaboration. The following types of COI situations are common (Box 3):

Self-dealing is when a professional controls an organization and makes it enter into a business interaction with self or with another organization that directly/indirectly benefits him. Thus, the professional controls both sides of the "deal".

Outside employment, in which the interests of one job conflict with the other.

Nepotism is when a person uses his/her authority to facilitate employment of the spouse, child, or close relatives. Also, nepotism is present when goods and/or services are sought only from a relative's firm.

When *small gifts and kinds* are received from friends or a company controlled by his/her friends.

Intellectual bias while peer-reviewing a research paper. The reviewer rejects the paper when it competes one of his own research interest or accepts a research manuscript when one of his own stands to benefit from it.

In functional terms, COI can be divided as per the source (individual, group), authority position, and the secondary interest factor it involves (money, time, commitment).

COI in anesthesiology may refer to any real or perceived conflicts of interest relating to any form including, any direct or indirect funding source(s) that supports investigators (e.g. local research foundation, departmental/hospital/institutional funds). COI occurring due to undue influence arising out of commercial association may involve consultation, equity interests, or patent-licensing arrangement also calls for due consideration and monitoring.[24,25]

CONFLICT-OF-INTEREST SITUATIONS IN ANESTHESIOLOGY

Clinical Anesthesiology Practice

Typically, anesthesia practice involves use of drugs, devices, and techniques.[20] Each one of them requires close decision-making to cohere the best possible combination to facilitate anesthesia for a particular surgical situation. It is the prerogative of the anesthesiologist to decide on anesthetic agents, airway/monitoring devices, and the anesthesia technique for the perioperative course of a surgical patient. In anesthesiology, due to a relative lack of a patient-anesthesiologist relationship,[26] there is a potential for bias because neither the patient

---

Box 3: Personal conflict-of-interest of anesthesiologists

- The anesthesiologist-in-charge can be charged with personal conflict-of-interest if the patient suffers physically, mentally, vocationally, financially or spiritually in the process of going through perioperative anesthesia care due to:
- Moves away from set standards and practice guidelines citing his/her experience and/or philosophical premise. Further he/she is not able to generate representative objective evidence to back the claims.
- Administers anesthesia to same set of patients differently.
- Undertakes clinical decision-making/actions are far removed from peer physicians.
- Indulge in frequent follow-ups, which by definition of care are deemed unnecessary.
- Interacts overly with patients on social front.
- Makes subtle/explicit sexual advances towards female patients.
- Involves in activity that can be billed under the term 'nepotism'.

desires nor he/she questions the integrity of anesthesiologists' choices. Further, more often than not, the anesthesiologist does not possess the necessary motivation and time to explain intricacies and issues to the patient. The anesthesiologist being largely dry to patients' subtle needs, rides on essential nature of anesthesia care delivery (one requires anesthesia for surgery anyway) to do whatever they want to do and not care about the specific implications, cost or possible fallout of their decisions. Over the years, because the rapidly evolving field of anesthesiology has given more impetus to development of mechanisms and machines, the culture of brewing patient-physician relationship has taken a back-seat. Therefore, the anesthesiologists who usually have short and transitory subjective exchanges with their patients, the real-time interaction with machines and drugs becomes a primary interest, and relatively, the anesthetized and still patient become secondary object of interest. This relative lack of a patient-physician bond in conjunction with general human tendency towards other interests gives rise to ground for complex secondary COI, which are difficult to perceive and identify, and the most difficult to investigate and manage. Moreover, in order to ensure a safe anesthesia sojourn and return to consciousness, even when resorting to a shared decision approach,[27] a fairly informed patient entrusts the anesthesiologist to go ahead with his/her plan on-the-go. The anesthesiologist, who is otherwise supposed to function within the ambit of clinical guidelines and standard of conduct, still gets enough leeway to activate conflicted decisions without getting marked as such (Box 4).

Anesthesiology Research

In anesthesiology, the major quantum of research involves drug, devices, and the use of different techniques. Since research in anesthesiology toes patient's need, investigator will, and finances, there is always a possibility that COI situations would arise. Therefore, handling clinical practice of anesthesiology and related research would always have a real-and-present chance that COI would situate itself and influence the research proceeds (hypothesis, objectives, conduct, evidence generation, publication) accordingly. Moreover, over-and-above the personal interests that the anesthesiologist may have, there may be other interests which may trigger a COI scenario. The acute conflation of healthy professional

---

Box 4: Plausible COI situations in clinical anesthesiology

- **Establishing upper airway with supraglottic airways (SGAs) as a first choice device:** For prolonged abdomino-pelvic surgery with contentious intraoperative position changes when and endotracheal airway is deemed to be safe upfront; in unusual positions (lateral, prone), etc. Clearly, going for SGAs as a first choice is fraught with risk of pulmonary aspiration of gastric contents, loss of airway, and hypoxemia. Routine employment of SGAs in elective surgical setting hints COI of the professional.
- **The use of newer and costly inhalation anesthetics (sevoflurane, desflurane, xenon) and intravenous induction agents (propofol, etomidate):** When equally efficient low-cost alternatives are available may reflect a potential COI scenario, especially when the anesthesiologist is soliciting the company with extraordinary academics (giving lecture, being on advisory board) and research (doing study on particular inhalation agent, serial publishing on same agents, giving thesis/research scholars the topics relating to inhalation agents).
- **Employing unnecessary invasive monitoring:** For short-duration surgery when standard monitoring would suffice for clinical need and as measurable variables of research.

interests (subspecialty inclinations, a preference for a particular drugs/devices/technique) with specific targeted interests like, promotion, recognition and awards, and financial returns, invariably results in a significant COI platform.

Anesthesiology Training and Education

Like clinical medicine practice and research, anesthesiology training and education is not free from COI situations. An investigator is likely to give the thesis scholar a topic that involves his/her area of interest irrespective of the difficulties therein; he/she may not be forthcoming on feasibility issues and the scope of the study area. Many a times, the anesthesiology trainees are allowed to learn a general technique first-up on actual patients without the mandatory pre-training on simulators.[28] Sometimes, the postgraduate residents are instructed to attend lectures with free luncheon on topics content beyond the scope of their curriculum. There are also instances where the trainees are allowed to use patients as training models, especially when they belong to free-category, thus exposing them to risk of complications owing to wrong techniques (no-effect, LA/neurolytic agent toxicity), over-exposure to radiation (during fluoroscopy guided pain blocks), and from failure to establish invasive monitoring (failed arterial puncture, catching carotid artery during internal jugular vein cannulation).

EVALUATION AND MANAGEMENT OF CONFLICT-OF-INTEREST

A typical COI situation where financial and/or non-financial secondary interests runs over the primary interest, needs to be analyzed first for its existence, then for its quantum, the harm it entails, and how it can be limited, managed or eliminated. *Financial* COI, for its objective presence, is fairly amenable to interpretation and enforcement by policy instruments. The *non-financial* COI are not only difficult to identify and analyze; for management, they are too complex to be contained within a structural realm. However, they are no less important and may have consequences that are far-reaching and more damaging with a long-term reverberating impact. In *Anesthesiology*, whereas a financial COI which actualizes harm is considered significant, at present, the comprehensive assessment of non-financial interest seems to be out of bounds. The clinical and academic Anesthesiology institutions, fraternity, and professional stakeholders who are entrusted with primary interest servitude, apparently, have only a general know-how of COI and usually follow the policies derived from other branches of medicine. Therefore, dedicated COI policy(s) governing anesthesiology sciences (practice, academic, research) is the need-of-the-hour. For Anesthesiology, the following strategies to evaluate and manage COI may be considered.

Evaluation of Conflict-of-Interest

The current scenario of practice of Anesthesiology is far from being non-controversial. Every-now-and-then the anesthesiologists are tapped on the wrist by surgeons' accusations, litigating patients, and competitive fraternal peers citing inconsistency and conduct. Ethical analysis and legal recourse notwithstanding, whenever an awkward situation puts professionals' and/or institutions' decision-making into a spot, the investigation into a possible COI trigger lurks around. Therefore, the individual professional anesthesiologists and the specialty office bearers should possess comprehensive clarity on the nuances of COI evaluation to be able to withstand deliberations on the content and the line of scrutiny. In principle, evaluation of a COI circumstance is based on the following:

Proportionality

Whenever a COI situation is considered, first the expected benefit from secondary interest is valuated and then whether it outweighs the bias it entails. Sometimes, secondary COI could be allowed to an extent if it benefits the primary cause (*valid-COI*). Therefore, for every COI situation, it is important to evaluate and balance the risk: benefit ratio arising out of the secondary interest.

Assessment of Undue Influence

The size and value of secondary interest should always be analyzed for its influence over the primary interest. Even small gifts, when given frequently in order to create and sustain physician-industry relationship, may bring about insidious subconscious changes in individual behavior. On most occasions, the professionals are either oblivious or are unaware of the changes in their behavior. Further, *undue influence* should be considered in the light of duration and extent of relationship.[29] The duration and closeness of professional's relation with industry sponsor heightens the risk of COI. The negative effects of COI are more pronounced if the latitude and traction of the professional (because of high institutional position and reputation) influence practice or research proceeds.

Assessment of Seriousness of Harm due to COI

The COI which has an amplification impact on a large number of patients are considered more serious. When compared to investigator-initiated studies, the scope of harm due COI in research is greatest with clinical trials.[30] Therefore, the evidence generated during different phases of clinical trials which ultimately are applied to population at large, require greater diligence and monitoring.

Accountability and Transparency

If the research investigator is allowed to be less accountable for his/her actions and decisions to patients, participants, peers, institution, and health mechanisms of the state, the probability of harm due to COI increases. Institutions should take initiatives for accountability of healthcare delivery and research by promoting the disclosure clause, investigating the disclosed content routinely, managing the disclosure, and if required, prohibiting the investigator to participate in research.[9] Importantly, institution COI policy should reflect their responsibility towards public in responding to query and grievances; justify remedial actions; and adjudicate penalty or compensation in case 'harm' has occurred due to issues with observance and handling of COI policies.

Principles of COI Management

The evaluation and management of COI in *Anesthesiology* is a labor-intensive, contentious, and sometimes, an investigative process. It involves three major aspects; *First*, to identify and situate COI in a particular context/circumstance; *second*, disclosure of the COI; and *third*, the management of COI. Any research, clinical procedure, or related activity in Anesthesiology that is funded by a private organization (pharmaceutical industry, device firms) should be looked into from the outset for the presence of financial secondary interest. Even if it seems to be clean, the designated process needs to be monitored through its course. *Finally,* the research outcome warrants diligent scrutiny to ensure that the substantiated evidence is free from the influence of secondary interests. While cornerstone of managing financial COI in Anesthesiology is 'Disclosure',[30] ethical evaluation of the research proposal, monitoring of conduct of ongoing research, participation of stakeholders in establishing validity (internal, external) of research, and analyzing results for framing evidence for publication, are key to prevention. A general framework of controlling governance and policy of handling COI within a research institution is presented (Fig. 1).

Tools for Managing COI

Disclosure (for financial COI): Disclosure is considered the best way to manage a financial COI.[31] Since a research can be affected by COI at every stage of development (hypothesis, methods, result interpretation, evidence creation), a proactive approach to disclosure of COI is desirable. However, there are a few concerns to settle. *First,* there remains a sensitive ethical issue of confidentiality and that any disclosure as a part of self-report or by institutional arrangement, should get limited dissemination within the institution;[32] *second* an adequate 'disclosure' should be presented in simple and understandable language, and open to critical interpretation; and *third,* the disclosure which usually depends on self-declaration and self-reports, is vulnerable to subjective manipulations. Further, disclosure only offers to limit financial COI and does not eliminate it completely. Marcia Angell's school of thought, though radical, aims at a 'zero tolerance' dictum, i.e. there should not be any financial COI whatsoever such that manipulations

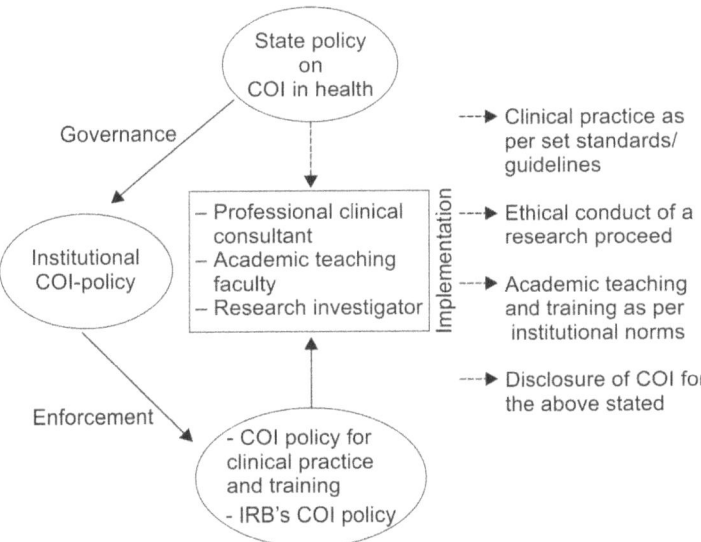

Fig. 1: COI policy conglomerate for individual professional and researcher anesthesiologist.

around controlling and/or filtering disclosure cease to exist.[33] Many research societies have now adopted the zero-tolerance policy (e.g. American Society of Gene Therapy [ASGT]).[34] Similarly, many Journals have now stopped manuscript submissions of research funded by tobacco industry.[35] Recently, the noted writer Arundhati Roy employed zero-tolerance policy to recuse herself from a literary fest because it was sponsored by mining industry.

Reflexivity (for non-financial COI): Non-financial COI is extremely difficult to pin-point. Recently, Bero and Grundy presented a multidisciplinary perspective drawn from social sciences to facilitate management of non-financial COI.[36] They suggested that inability to separate one's general interests from non-financial COI is the main reason for difficulty. They proposed 'reflexivity' as an extraordinary tool to manage non-financial COI. Analysis of non-financial interest based on 'reflexivity' essentially includes the following tenets:

Differentiating Conflict-of-Interest from General Interests

There is a possibility that influence of an individual's position or institutions' stance which the people rely on, affects decision-making. Generally, COI stands separated from general "interest" if:

- It is possible to eliminate COI altogether from a set of circumstances
- Recusal is the only way an interest can be eliminated then it is possibly an interest and not a COI.
- Unlike general "interest", the direction of bias created due to a COI is stable within a particular set of circumstances
- The effect of COI can be widespread and its scope unlimited. A general "interest" has a limited impact. For example, a sponsor may be interested in amplifying a particular view point, strive to ensure representation in decision-making, and invest in widespread dissemination of the intended evidence.
- One of the interests in conflict has a clear ethical claim to priority.

Heightened 'Disclosure'

'Reflexivity' as a tool for managing non-financial interest attempts to seek heightened 'disclosure' in addition to routine disclosure required for a financial COI.[37] 'Reflexivity' account for the possible influence of personal and professional *identity* and *interest* on decision-making process, direction of research, and the dissemination of evidence. The 'heightened disclosure' advocates greater information sharing on investigator's/clinicians' personal and professional identity, researcher's position statement, favored area of interest, and views on particular concepts and the research question.

Analyzing Influence of Interest and Identities on Research

The final aspect of 'reflexivity' enables one to look into possible influence of the identity of the investigator and/or institutional position and policy on research. COI policy primarily targets to minimize influence of secondary interest by:
- Enforcing implementation of standards of research conduct
- Reducing natural and inventive bias
- Publishing research in timely manner
- Development of practice guidelines based on research evidence
- Placing efforts to sustain public confidence in professional judgment.

Applied Management of Conflict-of-Interest

Individual clinical anesthesiologists and researchers should always exercise due care to identify potential COI and manage accordingly. Apart from the common approaches to managing COI, such as, disclosure, recusal, substitution or the termination of relationship, the following mechanisms should also be considered wherever applicable:

COI-Resolution: The Proactive Approach[38]

- Anesthesiology professional should follow the dictum *"I will practice my profession with conscience and dignity; and the health of my patient will be my first priority"* (WMA, Declaration of Geneva, 1948)
- Anesthesiologists must get into a reasonable interaction with the patients to help them make informed choices (*Principle of Autonomy*)
- Patient's benefit must always get first priority (*Principle of Beneficence*)
- Always consider that one's action or decision do not result in harm to the patient (Primum Nocere, *Principle of Non-maleficence*)
- Anesthesiologists should be fair to every patient and give them equal entitlement (Equity, Equality; *Principle of Justice*).

COI-Resolution: The Considered Approach

Every anesthesiologist should strive to nullify COI by:
- Retaining primary responsibility and duty to the patient
- Undertake independent judgement to justify his/her actions that has a potential to harm the patients (continuous risk-benefit analysis)
- Ensure not to accede to any unreasonable request for the third party services (travel allowance, hotel stays, paid lectures, conference registrations, patent facilitation)
- Always disclose financial COI at every stage of research as appropriate.

COI-Resolution: The Post hoc Approach

- Report COI if it is identified after the research
- Give solutions to conflict-prone clinical situations
- Suggest changes in clinical practice and research
- Work towards enhancement of awareness and accountability of COI
- Suggest modifications in the institutional COI policy.

CONCLUSION

Conflict-of-Interest is a clear and present nuance that can hamper practice and research in Anesthesiology. COI in Anesthesiology may result in harm to the anesthesia care service 'recipient' (the patients); the public at large (loss of confidence/trust); the science (conflicted evidence); and the 'provider' clinical anesthesiologist, investigators, institution (legal implications). A comprehensive basic and applied knowledge of COI will help anesthesiology healthcare institutions and individuals to ward off unknown challenges outside the area and scope of their domain. Moreover, getting aware and oriented about COI presence and implications would place them on a solid foundation of moral high ground in regard to patient care, clinical research, and advancement of science.

REFERENCES

1. Lo B, Field MJ. Conflict of Interest in Medical Research, Education and Practice. Institute of Medicine (US) Committee on Conflict of Interest in Medical Research, Education and Practice. National Academic Press (US). 2009.
2. Hemachuda T. Conflict of Interest and medical sciences. J Med Assoc Thai. 1999;82: 844-7.
3. Waisel DB. Ethics and conflicts of interest in anesthesia practice. In: Longnecker DE, Brown DL, Newman MF, Zappol WM, (Ed). Anesthesiology, 2nd edn, 2012. McGraw Hill.
4. Hoffman R, Martin D. Anesthesiologist. The History of Modern Anesthesia. Pennsylvania Society of Anesthesiologists. http://www.psanes.org/home/tabid/37/anid/43/default.aspx#20th_Century; (Accessed on July 10, 2017).
5. Thompson DF. Understanding conflicts of interest. N Engl J Med. 1993;329:573-6.
6. Lockhart A, Brose M, Kim E, et al. Physician and stakeholder perceptions of conflict of interest policies in oncology. J Clin Oncol. 2013;31:1677-82.
7. Braun AR, Leslie K, Morgan C, et al. Patients' knowledge of the qualifications and the roles of anaesthetist. Anaesth Intensive Care. 2007;35:570-4.
8. Bradley SG. Managing Conflicting Interests. In: Magrina FL, (Ed). Scientific Integrity: An Introductory Text with Cases. Washington, DC: American Society for Microbiology. 2000: p.131-57.
9. Bekelman JE, Li Y. Scope and impact of financial conflicts of interest in biomedical research. JAMA. 2003;289:454-65.
10. Fugh-Berman A, Ahari S. Following the script: how drug reps make friends and influence doctors. PLoS Medicine. 2007;4:e150.
11. Sah S. Conflicts of Interest and your physician: psychological processes that cause unexpected changes in behavior. J Law Med Ethics. 2012;40:482-7.
12. Hemingway E. For whom the bell tolls. Simon and Schuster USA 1996.
13. Waltz P, Zuckerbraun BS. Inferior vena cava filters in trauma patients—for whom the benefit tolls? JAMA Surgery. 2017;152:81.
14. Brandt A M. Inventing conflicts of interest: a history of tobacco industry tactics. Am J Public Health. 2012;102:63-71.
15. Oreskes N, Conway E. Merchants of Doubt: How a handful of Scientists Obscured the Truth on Issues from Tobacco Smoke to Global Warming. New York NY: Bloomsbury Press; 2010.
16. Brandt AM. The cigarette century: the rise, fall, and deadly persistence of the product that defined America. New York, NY: Basic Books 2007.
17. Markel H. Patents, Profits, and the American People—The Bayh–Dole Act of 1980. N Engl J Med. 2013;369:794-6.
18. Objectivity in research; final rule. US Public Health Service. Fed Regist 1995;60: 35810-9.
19. Department of Human and Health Services. Responsibility of applicants for promoting objectivity in research for which public health service funding is sought and responsible prospective contractors. Final rule. Fed Regist 2011;76:53256-93.
20. Todd MM, Saidman LJ: Academic-industrial relationships: The good, the bad, and the ugly. Anesthesiology. 1997;87:197-200.
21. Tetzlaff JE. Professionalism in Anesthesiology: What is it? or "I know when I see it". Anesthesiology 2009;110:700-2.
22. Katz JD. Conflict and its resolution in the operating room. J Clin Anesth. 2007;19:152-8.
23. Bion J. Financial and intellectual conflicts of interest: confusion and clarity. Curr Opin Crit Care. 2009;15:583-90.

24. Bero LA. Managing financial conflicts of interest in research. Am Coll Dent. 2005;72:4-9.
25. Policy statement regarding application of Harvard University conflict of interest policies to the granting of licenses. Policies and Procedures. Harvard Office of Techno-logy Department. http://otd.harvard.edu/facultyinventors/resources/policies-and-procedures/policy-statement-for-conflict-of-interest-in-licensing/ (Accessed on July 11, 2017).
26. Egbert LD, Jackson SH. Therapeutic benefit of anesthesiologist-patient relationship. Anesthesiology. 2013;119:1465-8.
27. Flierler WJ, Numbling M, Kasper J, et al. Implementation of shared decision making in anaesthesia and its influence on patient satisfaction. Anaesthesia. 2013;68:713-22.
28. Zhang M-Y, Cheng X, Luo L-P, et al. Clinical simulation training improves the clinical performance of Chinese medical students. Med Edu Online. 2015;20:10.3402/meo.v20.28796.
29. Bodenheimer T. Uneasy Alliance — Clinical Investigators and the Pharmaceutical Industry. N Engl J Med. 2000;342:1539-44.
30. Recognizing and Managing Personal Conflicts of Interest. Council on Government Relations (COGR), Winter 2002. From http://www.cogr.edu
31. Reider B, Poehling GG, Lubowitz JH, et al. Disclosure of conflict of interest. Arthroscopy. 2011;27:1167.
32. Grady C, Horstmann E, Sussman JS, et al. The limits of disclosure: What research subjects want to know about investigator financial interests? J Law Med Ethics. 2006; 34:592-9.
33. Angel M. Is Academic Medicine for Sale? N Engl J Med. 2000;342:1516-18.
34. Policy of The American Society of Gene Therapy financial conflict of interest in clinical research. Adopted April 5, 2000. (http://www.asgct.org/position_statements/conflict_of_interest.php, Accessed on July 11, 2017)
35. Ruff K. Scientific journals and conflict of interest disclosure: What progress has been made? Environmental Health 2015;14:45. doi: 10.1186/s12940-015-0035-6.
36. Bero LA, Grundy Q. Why having a (nonfinancial) interest is not a conflict of interest. PLoS Biol 2016;14:e2001221.
37. Siemensma F, Masel GR, Cameron W. Conflicts of interest: the universal blind spot. Melbourne: Leo Cussen Institute, 2000.
38. Beauchamp TL, Childress JF. Principles of biomedical ethics, 5th edn. Oxford University Press, New York, NY 2001.

CHAPTER 2

Understanding Hemostasis: The Knowns and the Unknowns

Anil Karlekar

KEY POINTS

- Physiological preparedness of blood to readily form clots when required, is continually balanced by ongoing processes that prevent unnecessary coagulation, with a tilt in favor of the latter.
- No amount of clot formation by itself can prevent blood loss if the breached vessels size is bigger than 50 μm.
- Platelets play an important role in clot formation and justifiably are target of various anticoagulation strategies. They also have a role to play in immunothrombosis and netosis.
- Controversy around cardiovascular safety of NSAIDs is gradually being resolved. Naproxen appears to be a safe choice for pain relief in patients with cardiovascular disease.
- Deranged coagulation and pathological thrombosis is equally challenging for perioperative physician, the risk of VTE and PE is very real and yet prophylaxis on the ground has discernible gaps.
- Surgical patients on antithrombotics require careful planning of interval between the last dose of the antithrombotic agent and the elective surgery or the placement/removal of catheters for neuraxial anesthesia.

INTRODUCTION

Hemostasis is the physiological process of maintaining blood circulation in the event of a breach in integrity of vessel wall (like in trauma) by initially forming a localized clot to contain blood loss, restricting the clot to the site of breach only and later actively dissolving the clot as a part of repair to restore normal circulation through the affected vessels. Hemostasis, thus, is one of the most finely balanced physiological process involving coagulation when required followed by appropriately timed lysis of the clot formed. The steps of coagulation and clot dissolution are interlinked and regulated in such a precise manner that forward steps in many instances, would simultaneously set in motion their own inhibition to contain an overwhelming wave that could engulf the whole being.

Anesthesiologists, as perioperative physicians, are increasingly involved in crucial decision making related to hemostasis. The common situations related to altered physiology routinely confronted are given further

Glossary of Terms often used in the Context of Hemostasis

- **Platelet adhesion:** Platelets adhering with exposed tissues like collagen
- **Platelet aggregation:** Clumping of platelets with other platelets
- **Cell adhesion molecules (CAM)** are proteins located on the cell surfaces involved in binding with other cells or with other extracellular matrix. *Integrins and Selectins* are Glycoprotein (GP) CAMS located on platelets. *Integrins* are calcium independent and involved with cell to extracellular matrix interactions. Integrins GPs form diverse platelet receptors from a combination of 20 α and 8 β subunits. *Selectins* are calcium dependent, platelet-selectin is released from alpha granules of platelets, promote adhesion with leucocytes and expression of tissue factor on monocytes that further amplifies coagulation.
- **Zymogens** are inactive circulating coagulation factors, and are termed serine proteases once activated.
- **Serine** is a nonessential amino acid and serine protease are enzymes that cleave proteins.
- **Serpins** are the inhibitor serine proteases; antithrombin is the most important serpin.
- **Ligand** is a molecule like hormone or transmitter that binds to a receptor.
- **UFH:** Unfractionated Heparin
- **Heparan sulfate** (and heparin) are complex, acidic polysaccharides belonging to the glycosaminoglycan (GAG) family, found in higher organisms on the cell surface or in the extracellular matrix and responsible for inhibiting thrombin by activating/enhancing antithrombin.
- **LMWH:** Low Molecular Weight Heparin
- **PCC:** Prothrombin Complex Concentrates, prepared from pooled plasma and has vitamin K dependent coagulation factors II, VII, IX and X and inhibitors protein C, S, antithrombin and heparin.

- Surgical patients receiving anticoagulants preoperatively may not only be confronted with excessive intraoperative blood loss, they may have limited options to choose from the anesthetic techniques available to them.
- Surgery itself involves *intentional* breach of vascular integrity of varying scale resulting in blood loss on one hand and triggering a state of inflammation in response to what body perceives as *an assault*. Surgery thus triggers the process of coagulation to arrest the *iatrogenic* blood loss, resulting in a *hypercoagulable* state perioperatively.
- Intravenous fluids, blood/blood products and anticoagulants/procoagulants are ordered perioperatively, each affecting hemostasis, directly or indirectly. In addition to managing surgery related blood loss on one hand, anesthesiologists are expected to prescribe appropriately timed anticoagulants postoperatively either for prophylaxis of dreaded venous thromboembolism (VTE) or for therapeutic use in conditions like implanted devices.

Therefore, anesthesiologists ought to have a comprehensive understanding of hemostasis to help them manage perioperative disturbances of coagulation, whether due to disease states or as a result of pharmacological interventions.

PHYSIOLOGY OF HEMOSTATSIS

Hemostasis comprises of two distinct opposing yet interrelated processes, *'coagulation'* and *'prevention of undesirable coagulation and clot lysis'* and can be described as a 4-component process:[1]
- Initiation (trigger),
- Acceleration (akin to explosion of biologic activity),
- Control (limiting coagulation locally) and
- Lysis (recanalization)

Elements of Coagulation

Coagulation involves three biologic elements: *the vascular (endothelium), platelets* and *plasma factors* to form an effective clot at the site of injury (*see* Fig. 1A for basic coagulation schema and Table 1 for plasma factors). It is noteworthy that all the required 'ingredients' to form a clot are either circulating in blood itself or are available in subendothelial layers across body, albeit in inactive forms. Counter-regulatory set of events too are initiated simultaneously to ensure clot is restricted to site of injury and help restore normalcy once bleeding is controlled.

Vascular Endothelium

Vascular response to injury, in order to minimize blood loss, is not restricted to vasoconstriction only. While non-thrombogenic surfaces of endothelium and other mediators ensure uninterrupted circulation in health, it goes through changes to arrest bleeding when challenged. Undisturbed vascular endothelium in health keeps the coagulation under control by:
a. Maintaining its inherent antifibrinolytic and antiplatelet character (prevents adhesion, activation, secretion and aggregation of platelets) by producing and releasing nitric oxide, prostacyclin and CD39.
b. Inhibiting thrombin through Tissue Factor Pathway Inhibitor (TFPI), Antithrombin (AT), Protein S, Heparin factor II, Heparan Sulfate, Thrombomodulin (TM) and Dermatan Sulfate.

When challenged, vascular endothelium supports coagulation by:
- Suspending a and b above (Fig. 1A).
- Promoting platelet adhesion (with tissue) and aggregation (amongst themselves).
- Accelerating thrombin formation by providing the essential phospholipid surface, exposing tissue vWF and P-selectin for platelet attachment.
- Secreting Tissue Factor and Factor V and modulating fibrinolytic response by releasing PAI-1(inhibits tPA/urokinase) (Fig. 1A).

While the finely calibrated response is initiated in the event of a disrupted vessel, vasoconstriction and eventual stable clot can arrest bleeding only in vessels smaller than 50 µm, a fact worth remembering during surgery to emphasize the importance of meticulous surgical hemostasis.[1] In the event of pathological atherosclerotic plaque formation and thrombotic diseases, deranged vascular endothelial goes through similar processes.

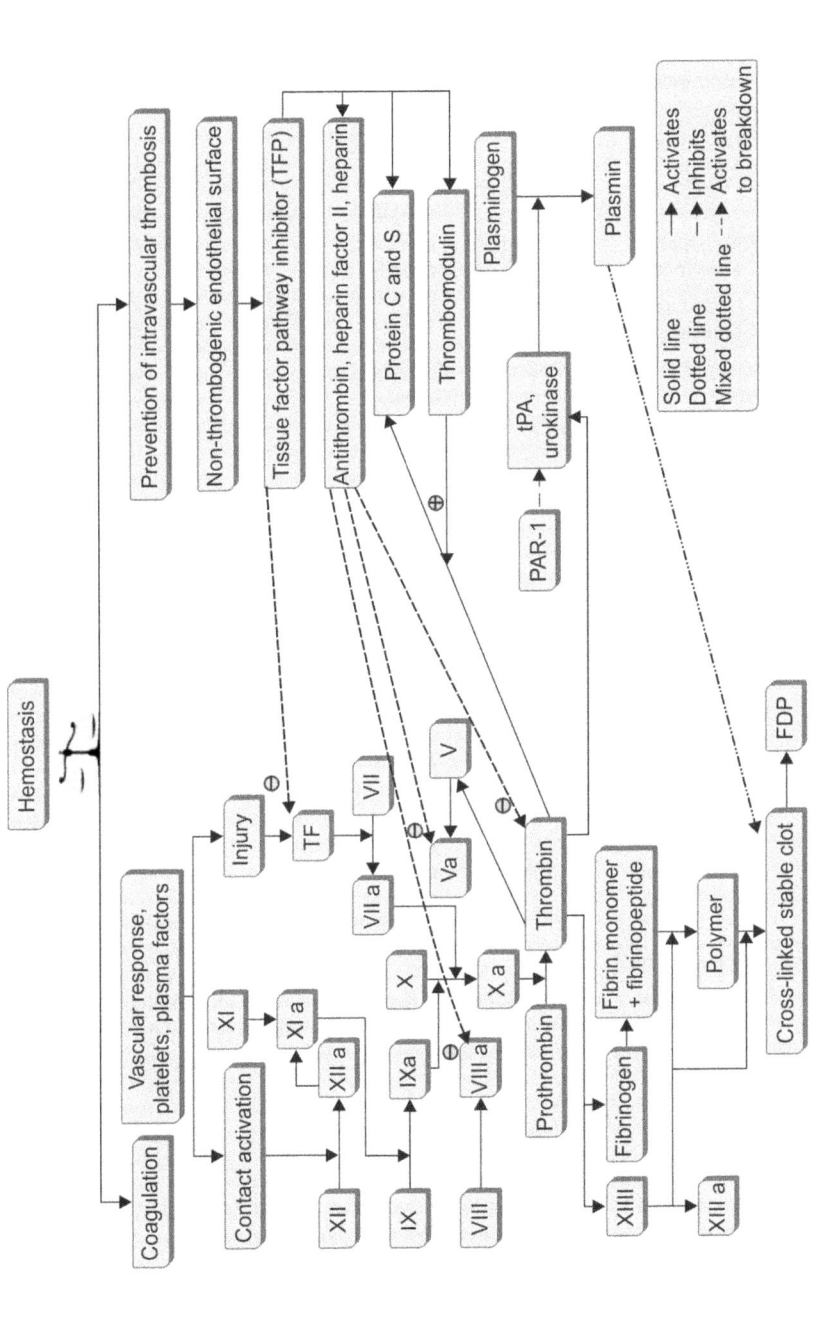

Fig. 1A: Basic hemostasis schema depicting coagulation and its counter-regulation that ensures fluidity of blood and its circulation. Thrombin is central to coagulation like plasmin is central to clot lysis.

Table 1: Plasma coagulation factors

Factor	Name	Type	Source	Dependent on	Available in
I	Fibrinogen	Zymogen	Liver		Cryo, FFP
II	Prothrombin	Zymogen	Liver	Vit K	FFP, PCC
III	Tissue factor (Thromboplastin)	Cofactor	Platelets, endothelium		
IV	Calcium	Cofactor	Bone and from GI		IV preparations
V	Proaccelarin (Labile factor)	Cofactor	Liver and platelets		FFP
VII	Proconvertin (Stabilizing factor)	Zymogen	Liver	Vit K	Factor VII, PCC
VIII	Antihemophilic factor A, Antihemophilic globulin	Cofactor	Endothelium (blood vessels), platelets		Cryo, FFP
IX	Antihemophilic factor B, Plasma thromboplastin component, Christmas factor	Zymogen	Liver	Vit K	FFP, PCC
X	Stuart-Prower factor	Zymogen	Liver	Vit K	FFP, PCC
XI	Plasma thromboplastin antecedent	Zymogen	Liver		FFP
XII	Hageman factor	Zymogen	Liver		----
XIII	Fibrin stabilizing factor	Zymogen	Liver		FFP, Cryo
vWF	von Willebrand Factor	Cofactor	Injured tissue, Endothelium		Cryo, FFP
Serpins	Protein C and S		Liver	Vit K	
	Antithrombin		Traditionally FFP was administered to substitute deficient antithrombin. Now, concentrates from human plasma and goat milk are also available		

Platelets

Platelets the anucleated smallest blood particles (diameter 2-3 mm, normal blood count 150–400 × 10^3 per mL, average lifespan 5-9 days) play a key role in coagulation and are vital to hemostasis. The role of platelets in hemostasis could be summed up as under:

- ❑ As the first responders earning them the title of 'circulating band-aids', platelet reach the damaged intima, adhere to the tissues and try to plug the gap physically, though such a platelet-only clot is inherently unstable.

- As the coagulation process continues, the platelets get *activated* through several mechanisms and undergo conformational changes that expose platelet receptors and binding sites including essential phospholipid surfaces. They release several chemicals which are stored in granules and lysosomes as follows:
    - Dense granules — ADP, ATP, serotonin (further platelet activation)
    - Alpha granules — Fibrinogen, fibronectin, vitronectin, vWF (promote adhesion)
    - Lysosomal granules — Glycosidases and proteases (so far unclear function).

The activation of platelets along with sequential activation of plasma coagulation factors lead to a chain of events resulting in tissue, platelets and fibrin coming together to convert the unstable soft clot into insoluble clot.

Platelets, though mainly known for their important role in hemostasis, have also been implicated in diabetes, renal diseases, tumor genesis, cardiovascular and Alzheimer's disease. The change in the face of innocent looking inactive platelets can be credited to the plethora of receptors that open up in response to diverse stimuli. Platelet receptors[2-5] play a crucial role in platelet functioning, and in the context of hemostasis, receptor specific agonists and antagonists make the basis of many therapeutic interventions (Tables 2A and 2B).

Platelet and endothelium interact in multiple ways, platelets are said to *adhere* to tissues and *aggregate* amongst themselves. Endothelial cells convert arachidonic acid to prostacyclin with the help of cyclooxygenase and prostacyclin synthase. Prostacyclin inhibits platelet aggregation and dilates vessels. Platelet through their own cyclooxygenase forms thromboxane A2 which promotes aggregation and is a vasoconstrictor. Low dose aspirin inhibits platelet COX but not endothelial COX, thus while thromboxane synthesis ceases, endothelial production of prostacyclin continues. The selective platelet inhibition with low dose aspirin produces desired reduced platelet activation and aggregation without affecting prostacyclin induced vasodilation. High dose aspirin blocks both platelets as well as endothelial COX, negating the intended effect of platelet inhibition as accompanying vasoconstriction favors stasis and possible thrombosis.[6]

Platelet microvesicles[7] were discovered when clotting of blood was found prolonged following centrifugation, further confirmed by electron microscopy. Microvesicles are released by cell membranes of various cells including platelets during activation or apoptosis. Platelet microvesicles are most abundant in plasma and are procoagulant. They are produced by multiple pathways as a part of platelet activation and are accompanied by movement of phosphatidylserine that acts on Factor X and prothrombin, propagating coagulation.

Circulating platelet microvesicles are higher in females until menopause. Other conditions that are associated with higher levels are systemic lupus erythematosus, acute coronary syndrome, venous thromboembolism, myeloproliferative diseases, diabetes and chronic renal failure. Though not yet available for routine testing, their estimation could possibly predict bleeding in surgical patients particularly cardiac surgery. Future developments may place platelet microvesicles count as part of platelet function assessment and their transfusion to control bleeding.

Table 2A: Know your drugs: antiplatelet agents

Receptors	Agonist	Antagonist	Route	Rveversibility	Caution	Comments	Recommended interval before intervention
P2Y1 and P2Y$_{12}$	ADP	Ticlopidine	Oral	Irreversible	Low blood counts	Has generally been replaced by newer drugs	
		Clopidogrel	Oral	Irreversible	Incidence of resistance is high, almost 30% are non-responders. Risk of bleeding+	Delayed prodrug activation in liver, needs loading dose	D/C 5 to 7 days prior to elective surgery or catheter placement
		Prasugrel	Oral	Irreversible	Higher risk of bleeding: avoid in >75 years, wt <60kg, in h/o stroke, TIA	More predictable platelet blockage.	D/C 7–10 days prior to catheter placement
		Ticagrelor	Oral	Reversible	May cause dyspnea, ventricular pauses. Increases uric acid and creatinine. Dose of aspirin should be kept < 100 mg	Potent blocker. Better outcomes in ACS, MI without increasing risk of bleeding.	D/C 5 days prior to catheter placement.
		Cangrelor	IV	Reversible	May cause dyspnea	Has been suggested for 'platelet anesthesia' during CPB to protect platelets from activation and consumption, to eventually reduce bleeding. May have a role in HIT.	Has rapid onset and offset, complete recovery of platelet function within 1–2 hours. Delay intervention 1–6 hours.
		Elenogrel	IV as well as oral	Reversible	Dyspnea	Rapid and profound platelet blockade without increased bleeding risk.	Needs further evaluation
Thromboxane A2 receptor	Thromboxane	Aspirin	Oral/IV	Irreversible	GI bleed	Part of Dual Antiplatelet therapy and between the two, aspirin is mostly continued perioperatively. May be discontinued for 0–5 days	

(ACS: Acute coronary syndrome; CPB: Cardiopulmonary bypass; HIT: Heparin induced thrombocytopenia)

Table 2B: Know your drugs: antiplatelet agents used during percutaneous coronary intervention (PCI)

Receptors	Agonists	Antagonists	Route	Reversibility	Comments	Recommended interval before intervention
GPIIb/IIIa	Act at the final common pathway of platelet aggregation involving fibrinogen, forming interplatelet bridges.	Abciximab	IV	Reversible	Has onset of action, long biological activity	Advisable to delay catheter placement for at least 24–48 hours
		Tirofiban	IV	Reversible	Effect on platelets disappears soon after discontinuation of infusion	Advisable to delay catheter placement for at least 4–8 hours
		Eptifitide	IV	Reversible		

Platelets also play a role in infections.[8] Coordinated intravascular coagulation in response to pathogens in blood has been termed *Immunothrombosis*.[9] In order to confine the pathogens, platelets along with other immune cells tend to form a physical barrier around them in the form of a thrombus, thus leading to a prothrombotic state.

Plasma Factors

Circulating inactive precursors (zymogens) and cofactors together make the plasma components for hemostasis. Following an initial activation trigger, like an injury, the zymogens and cofactors get activated sequentially, the product of one reaction, a serine protease, causing activation of the next. Many of these reactions require Ca^{++} and a phospholipid surface that is provided by activated platelets and endothelium and occasionally even white cell.

It may be worthwhile recalling that plasma factors and cofactors (like Tissue Factor and Factor V), mostly synthesized in liver, have been identified as Roman numerals and/or names (Table 1) as they were discovered and not in the sequence that they participate in the process of coagulation. Traditionally coagulation has been taught as comprising of intrinsic and extrinsic pathways, both merging finally into a common pathway. However, it is now known that the in-vivo coagulation does not happen compartmentalized into intrinsic or extrinsic pathways. These pathways crisscross, are highly interactive, work on feedback loops and the two probably complement each other. Thus, *initiation* of coagulation happens through contact activation while *amplification* and *propagation* involves intrinsic and extrinsic pathways leading to a common pathway of activated factor X and thrombin. Thrombin converts fibrinogen to fibrin which enmeshes activated platelets and finally forms a stable clot (Figs. 1A and 1B).

The complexity of nomenclature of plasma coagulation factors will remain incomplete without mentioning *von Willebrand Factor* (*vWF*).[10] It circulates in plasma but is not a coagulation factor. vWF in its normal inactive coiled form

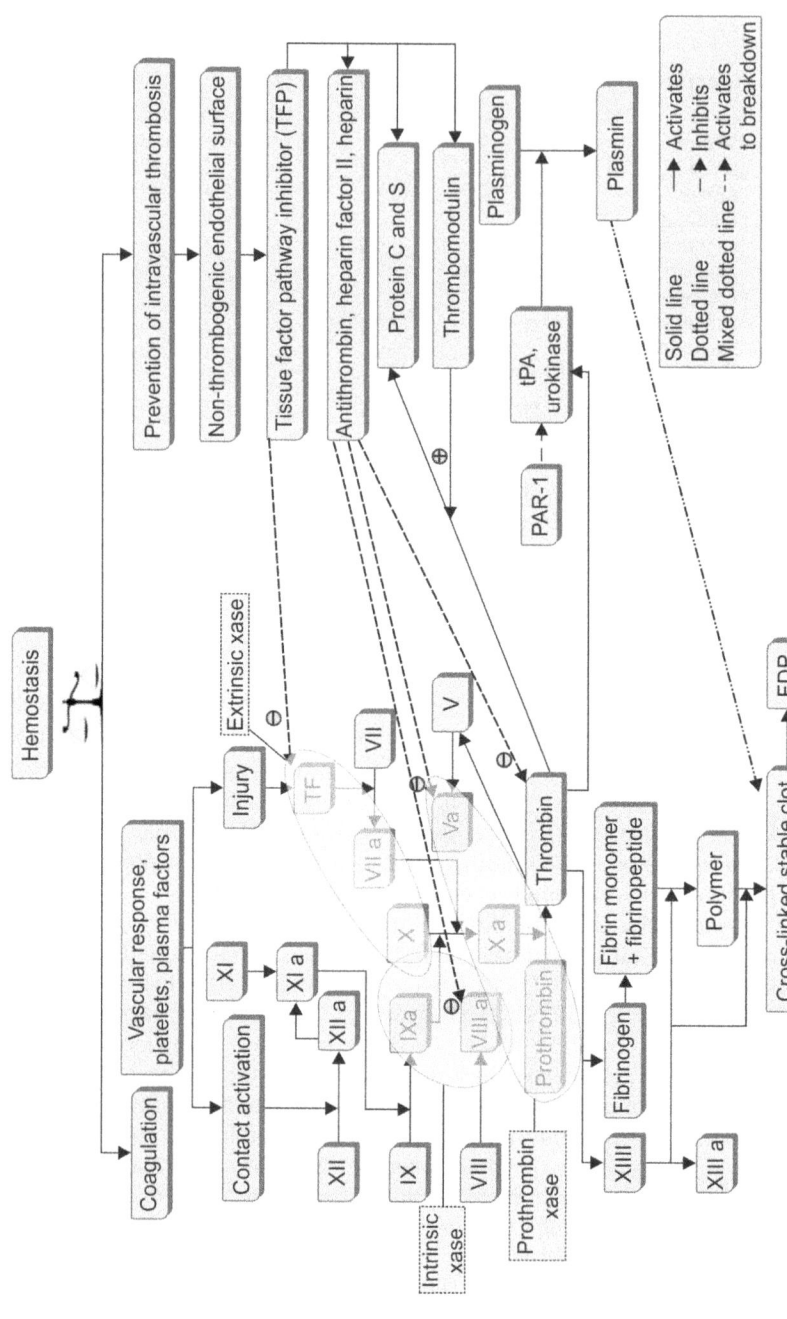

Fig. 1B: Basic hemostasis schema with superimposed three procoagulant complexes, Prothrombin Xase, Extrinsic Xase and Intrinsic Xases, composition of each depicted within the respective shaded area. Each complex comprises of one serine protease (VIIa, IXa and Xa), cofactor (VIIIa, Va, TF) and a negatively charged cell surface that is provided by cells (platelets, monocytes). These membrane-bound complexes localize enzymatic activity.

functions as a protector carrier of Factor VIII, saving it from proteolytic enzymes. It can also be expressed from injured tissue and endothelium. Injury induced endothelial disruption binds vWF, it uncoils as part of activation, facilitating platelet trapping beginning the hemostasis with the soft clot. vWF released by endothelium, facilitates factor IX to reach activated platelet (GP1b, IX), a crucial step in keeping platelets and fibrinogen together to form clot, thus earning it term of 'glue'.

Hemophilia, a bleeding disorder, is distinct from vWF-deficiency induced bleeding disorder, von Willebrand Disease (vWD). Deficiency of F VIII causes Hemophilia A and that of F IX is called Hemophilia B. Hemophilia leads to bleeding due to lack of fibrin as F VIII or F IX are deficient; vWD causes bleeding as platelets fail to stick together to form the plug in absence of vWF. vWD is underdiagnosed, and a deficient vWF would lead to lower levels of unprotected F VIII too, and is often misdiagnosed as hemophilia.

Desmopressin (DDAVP), a synthetic analogue of vasopressin (ADH) promotes release of vWF and F VIII from endothelial cells as well as platelets and has been used to control bleeding in Hemophilia A.[11] Novel approaches to manage bleeding in hemophiliacs like emicizumab (a recombinant antibody that binds F IX and F X together obviating the need of F VIII in the coagulation cascade), concizumab (an antibody against TFPI), antithrombin gene silencing and gene therapy are under various stages of development, and may become available in near future.

Coagulation Cascade (Fig. 1A)

Contact activation, the initial step, triggered by *contact*, involves factor XII, high molecular weight kininogen (HMWK), prekallikrein (PK) and factor IX. HMWK anchors PK and F XI to exposed tissue or activated platelets. F XII is said to be activated by exposed sub-endothelial collagen, activated platelets or autoactivation. Activated F XII cleaves F XI and PK, triggering production of bradykinin, thought to be responsible for complement activation and fibrinolysis, hitherto associated with consumption coagulopathy and bleeding following cardiopulmonary bypass. Deficiency of F XII though has not been found to cause coagulation disorders in humans.

Intrinsic and Extrinsic Coagulation Pathways

Intrinsic pathway can be said to start with contact activation forming F IXa from F IX. F IXa then acts on F X to form F Xa in the presence of cofactor-VIII and Ca^{++} on the phospholipid surface of platelet that gets exposed subsequent to activation.

Extrinsic pathway, as the name suggests was thought to be triggered by extravascular substances (tissue factor) independent of F XII of the contact activation. The line of distinction between intrinsic and extrinsic pathways gets blurred as one realizes that tissue factor can actually be produced by endothelial cells under varied pathological conditions like sepsis, ischemia and reperfusion. Tissue factor converts F VII to F VIIa which converts F X to F Xa as a part of common pathway and also acts as a cofactor for F VIIa mediated F X activation. Interestingly, F VII and F X then activate each other facilitated by platelet phospholipid surface and Ca^+.

Common Pathway

The common pathway depends on Vit K dependent complexes for hemostatic balance, each one has a factor, a cofactor, a negatively charged cell surface along with either F X/Xa or prothrombin/thrombin[12] (Fig. 1B). These vitamin K dependent complexes are:

- Extrinsic X'ase' (VIIa, IX, TF, X)
- Intrinsic X'ase' (VIIIa, IXa, X)
- Prothrombin'ase' (Xa,Va, Prothrombin) and
- Protein C'ase' (Thrombin, Thrombomodulin, Protein C)

These complexes are bound to membranes and serve to localize the enzymatic activity to specific sites. Prothrombinase complex converts prothrombin to active thrombin. Functionally, thrombin, the active form of inactive plasma factor prothrombin, is central to coagulation process. It is the key regulator for final step of fibrin generation from fibrinogen, as well as for initiating downregulation of hemostasis to limit its spread. Thrombin is unique in its role of sustaining the cascade by a feedback mechanism wherein it promotes its own production. Understandably, being two common final steps of the cascade, thrombin and Factor X are the target of many therapeutic anticoagulation strategies (Fig. 1C).

Thrombin initiates several processes (Fig. 1A). It breaks fibrinogen to soluble fibrin monomer + polypeptide fragments called fibrinopeptides A and B. Monomers come together to form polymer. It activates factor VIII and factor XI as well as activates F XIII to F XIIIa which strenghthens bonds between adjacent fibrin polymers and forms the insoluble clot enmeshing critical mass of active and aggregated platelets and other cells. Thrombin also activates more platelets and other mediators that results in more thrombin generation thus resulting in 'thrombin burst', a multiplier of action. It modulates coagulation by simultaneous release of tPA, prostacyclin and nitric oxide. With thrombomodulin, thrombin activates protein C, that inactivates FVa and FVIIIa, helped by protein S. It also has a role to play in inflammation and mitogenesis involving leucocytes and macrophages.

PLASMA FACTORS REGULATING COAGULATION

Coagulation is counterbalanced by serine protease inhibitors, the serpines. Antithrombin (previously known as antithrombin III) is the most potent inhibitor. It mainly inhibits thrombin by binding to its active site and to some extent inhibits XIIa, XIa, IXa, Xa, kallikrein and fibrinolytic molecule plasmin as well. Antithrombin can not reach thrombin bound to fibrin, protected by platelets. Antithrombin is inactive while circulating, it is the heparan of endothelial layer that unfolds its activity. Heparin has the same pentasaccharide sequence as that of heparan, and its acts by accelerating antithrombin action. Cardiopulmonary bypass (CPB) causes low levels of antithrombin by dilution as well as by consumption. Patients with low levels of antithrombin also have higher risk of deep vein thrombosis, its addition may help reduce the risk of thrombosis.[13] The so called 'resistance' to heparin is likely due to deficiency of antithrombin and has been mostly managed by transfusion of fresh frozen plasma, providing antithrombin from an extraneous source. Concentrates of antithrombin from human plasma and the one produced from goat milk are also available now and are preferred over fresh frozen plasma.[9]

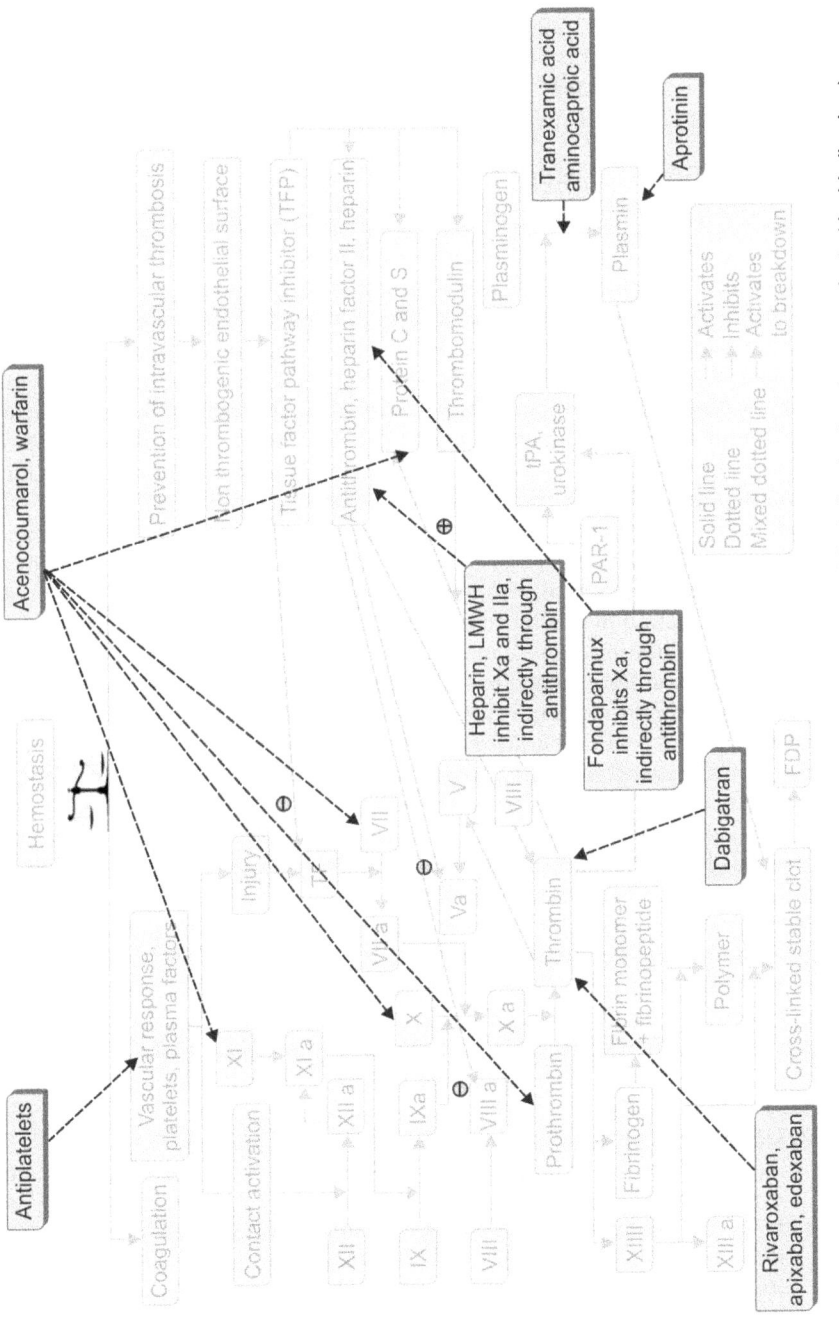

Fig. 1C: Hemostasis schema depicting site of action of antithrombotics (single line box) and procoagulants (double line box).

α1-antitrypsin, α2-macroglobulin, heparin factor II, and α2 antiplasmin at different levels inhibit coagulation. Activated by thrombin, protein C inactivates factor Va and VIIIa and requires Ca^{++}, phospholipid surface and protein S as cofactor. Both proteins C and S are vitamn K dependent. Thrombomodulin released by endothelium accelerates thrombin activation of protein C by several times. Tissue factor pathway inhibitor (TFPI) produced by endothelium and platelets, blocks TF + F VIIa induced F X activation in the extrinsic pathway.

CYCLOOXYGENASE, NSAIDS, CARDIOVASCULAR SAFETY AND PLATELET INHIBITION

Cooxygenase (COX) catalyzes the conversion of arachidonic acid into prostaglandin H_2 and further into prostanoids by actions of isomerase. Cyclooxygenase has two isomers, COX-1 and COX-2. COX-1 is a constitutive enzyme, stimulated by hormones or growth factors, has mostly a protective role and is active in most tissues like heart, kidney and platelets while COX-2 is an inducible enzyme released in response to cytokines and mitogens in conditions like atherosclerosis, ischemia and malignancy; while normal endothelium expresses COX-2 in response to shear stress, COX-1, is involved in regulation of processes like platelet aggregation, thrombosis, gastric cytoprotection and kidney function.

Platelets contain only COX-1, and its inhibition would block thromboxane A_2 (Tx_2) production and result in suppressing platelets aggregation and local vasoconstriction. Endothelial cells express COX-2 in response to shear stress promoting production of prostacyclin that extends protection by way of causing vasodilatation, inhibiting smooth muscle proliferation and antagonizing platelet aggregation. Interestingly, small dose of aspirin only blocks COX-1 at the platelets thus preventing clot formation, while higher dose of aspirin, additionally blocks cyclooxygenase at endothelium as well, limiting prostacyclin production leading to local vasoconstriction and allowing smooth muscle proliferation, thus negating the advantages if platelets were to be blocked alone. Additionally, COX-1 blockers, besides thromboxane A_2 production by platelets, would also limit release of protective prostaglandins by gastric mucosa increasing the risk of gastrointestinal toxicity including bleeding.

NSAIDs primarily used for treatment of fever, inflammation and pain, could thus be safe if they selectively blocked COX-2 only, the rationale for developing coxibs, introduced in 1998. Coxibs and traditional NSAIDs have been studied for their selectivity for COX-1 and COX-2 inhibition, and for their cardiovascular safety when used for pain relief. A summary of the effects that COX isomers block in the context of cardiovascular system and kidney is presented for easier understanding:

- ❑ COX-1 catalyses production of
  - ➢ TxA_2 in *platelets* (platelet activation, vasoconstriction, necessary in the event of bleeding) and *mesangial cells in kidney* (vasoconstriction);
  - ➢ PGE_2 in *vascular endothelium* (platelet inhibition, antiadhesion, antithrombotic, protection against oxidative injury) and in *collecting ducts of kidneys* (natriuresis, diuresis) and
  - ➢ PGI_2 in *endothelium* and *smooth muscles* (similar effects as by PGE_2: platelet inhibition, antiadhesion, antithrombotic, protection against oxidative injury).

Inhibition is desirable to prevent atherogenesis and thrombosis (by blocking platelet activation).
- COX-2 catalyzes production of
  - PGE_2 and PGI_2 in *endothelium* and *smooth muscles* (platelet inhibition, antiadhesion, antithrombotic, protection against oxidative injury), *cardiomyocytes* (ischemic preconditioning, antiarrhythmic, protection against ischemic injury) and *macula densa* (renin release, ? undesirable) and *medullary interstitium* (maintains medullary flow and diuresis) of kidneys.
  - TxA_2 and PGE_2 in *macrophages* (inflammation)
  - PGF_{2a} in *fibroblasts of heart* (fibrosis, arrhythmia)

Inhibition is desirable mainly for an anti-inflammatory effect and antiarrhythmic/antifibrotic effect/renin release.

Apart from aspirin which is specifically prescribed in low doses for platelet inhibition, other traditional NSAIDs and coxibs are used for their analgesic, antipyretic and anti-inflammatory effects through COX-2 inhibition. Since most of the NSAIDs are nonselective, the concern is related to their simultaneous inhibition of PGE_2 and PGI_2, that can precipitate myocardial infarction, stroke, heart failure, hypertension, venous thrombosis and kidney failure. In addition, it is known that some relatively selective COX-2 inhibitor NSAIDs may lose their selectivity in higher doses.

Use of NSAIDs in Patients with Higher Risk of Cardiovascular Disease

Following are conclusions drawn from the position paper by European Society of Cardiology on cardiovascular safety of non-aspirin NSAIDs (based on largest metanalysis of RCTs, 2013):[14,15]
- Commonly used diclofenac, high dose ibuprofen, and coxibs, all have similar risk profile for likelihood of causing cardiovascular events, independent of baseline characteristics.
- Naproxen did not increase the risk of major vascular events.
- All non-aspirin NSAIDs roughly doubled the risk of heart failure.

In addition, it appears on the basis of other observational studies that the neither the shorter duration of treatment nor lower doses make diclofenac any safer.

Use of Coxibs/Traditional NSAIDs for Postoperative Pain Relief

- Cardiac surgery: Small volume RCTs[14] suggest that
  - Coxibs increase the risk of cardiovascular events in CABG patients
  - Higher incidence of sternal wound infection was found with coxibs after cardiac surgery.
  - The incidence of myocardial infarction was *not* found to be higher in patients undergoing cardiothoracic surgery when traditional NSAIDs were added.
  - Naproxen appeared to be a safe analgesic for postoperative pain relief.
- Noncardiac surgery:
  - No evidence of higher incidence of thromboembolic or other cardiovascular events was found either with coxibs or traditional NSAIDs, though caution is warranted.

> However, the use of coxibs or NSAIDs is best avoided in patients with ischemic heart disease or history of stroke.

Concomitant Use of Coxibs/Traditional NSAIDs and Antithrombotic Treatment

- Risk of bleeding is higher
- Patients with atrial fibrillation using NSAIDs had higher risk of thromboembolism.

NSAIDs and Atrial Fibrillation (AF)

- The risk of developing AF appears higher with use of NSAIDs, particularly diclofenac.

THROMBOSIS[8]

Normal hemostasis when overtaken by pathological factors may lead to uncontrolled clot formation causing occlusion of the vessel, artery or a vein. Arterial thrombi are rich in platelets and form in and around a ruptured plaque. Venous clots are rich in fibrin with activated platelets and RBCs and may occur despite an intact endothelium.

Arterial thrombosis is seen mostly in the setting of atherosclerotic plaque rupture, leading to platelet aggregation and clot formation, like in MI or ischemic stroke. Arterial thrombi are treated with therapies that aim to inhibit platelet activation and aggregation, forming the basis of usage of antiplatelet drugs in coronary artery disease. For the same reason, the role of antiplatelet drugs in 'Angina and No Obstructive Coronary Artery' disease (ANOCA) and 'MI and Non-obstructed Coronary Artery' disease (MINOCA) is unclear. The risk factors for developing arterial thrombosis include hypertension, high levels of LDL cholesterol, smoking, diabetes, pregnancy, age, chemotherapy, infections and high levels of vWF. Some of the mechanism that lead to pathological arterial thrombosis include extraneous sources of procoagulants or compromised antithrombotic character of normal endothelium. Tissue Factor (TF), which is normally released by subendothelial adventitia and smooth muscle, is also expressed by *monocytes and tumor-secreted microparticles*, and can initiate thrombin generation leading to coagulation. *High shear stress and epinephrine* can secrete large amount of vWF that entrap platelets to intact endothelium causing arterial thrombosis. *Pathogens* can bring platelets and neutrophils to form what is called Neutrophil Extracellular Trap (NET) which is highly thrombotic and resistant to tPA.

Venous thrombi mainly comprise of fibrin, RBCs and the mandatory platelets, and the treatment is targeted at coagulation factors that finally convert fibrinogen to fibrin. Venous thrombosis is favored by low shear flow even with intact endothelium, leaving thrombi loosely adherent and easy to dislodge. A state of inflammation is said to activate endothelium, leading to vWF secretion and attaching platelets and leucocytes. Activated leucocytes are the source of TF, triggering the coagulation cascade. Sluggish venous flow, hypoxemia and altered shape of the RBCs favor venous thrombosis.

Venous thromboembolism (VTE) includes pulmonary embolism (PE) and deep venous thrombosis (DVT). VTE occurs more often than it is diagnosed, is a common clinical problem and is associated with substantial morbidity and mortality.[16] In United States alone, 150,000 to 200,000 deaths are attributed to pulmonary embolism, considered the most common preventable cause of hospital deaths. Though all hospitalized patients are at risk and have at least one risk factor for VTE, certain group of patients like those suffering from malignancy, patients immobilized for any reason and postoperative patients are more at risk. Anesthesiologists as perioperative physicians should not only be aware of the risk of VTE but are also expected to initiate prophylactic measures against what is potentially a fatal complication. It is estimated that between 5% and 10% of all in-hospital deaths are a direct result of PE.[17-19]

Following are the risk factors for VTE:
- Age > 40 years irrespective of sex, race.
- Obesity, particularly for cerebral venous thrombosis in women taking oral contraceptives.
- Cerebral venous thrombosis occurs more frequently in anemics, particularly among men. Endothelial hypoxia has been suggested as a probable cause.
- Prior episodes of VTE, atherothrombosis including MI; higher levels of D-dimers.
- Higher levels of estrogens like in pregnancy, obesity, taking oral contraceptives. Higher levels of estrogens associated with pregnancy and childbirth cause a rise in coagulation factors to meet the challenge of blood loss, thus increasing the risk of VTE.
- Multiple pregnancies and older maternal age.
- Immobility related to bed rest, long distance travel.
- Surgical patients are particularly at risk. Patients of advanced age, increasing degree of invasiveness of surgery, type and duration of anesthesia, requirement for immobilization, sepsis and some other comorbidities like heart diseases and recent stroke are known to add to the risk.
- Advanced malignancy as well as chemotherapy are associated with VTE. TF released by micro-vesicles produced by tumor cells has been held responsible for initiating thrombosis.
- And finally, genetic mutations too may be the cause of increased risk of thrombosis. Factor V Leiden, said to be due to mutation, results in a form of protein C that fails to inactivate Factor V. Mutations of prothrombin, fibrinogen, antithrombin, protein C and S also have been implicated for increased risk of thrombosis. For reasons that remain unexplained, non-O blood groups are said be associated with higher risk.

Caprini Score, modified and recommended by ACCP (Guidelines 2012) is the most widely accepted risk assessment tool.[20]

Immunothrombosis[8]

Infection as a risk factor for thrombosis, arterial as well as venous, and atherosclerosis is getting established, as convincing evidence is accumulating.[21] Coordinated intravascular coagulation in response to pathogens in blood has been termed *Immunothrombosis*. In order to confine the pathogens, platelets along with other immune cells tend to form a physical barrier around them in the form of a thrombus, thus leading to a prothrombotic state. Platelets are believed to secrete chemokines in response to infections, leading to sequestration and destruction of bacteria. HIV, HCV and Dengue viruses are also known to lead to prothrombotic state. Other immune cells like monocytes are known to release TF, while neutrophils go through a process called *netosis*. Netosis is the formation of neutrophils extracellular traps (NET) from the DNA released by neutrophils. While NET form part of immune response to contain infections, simultaneous activation of platelets and increased thrombin level create a prothrombotic state. Levels of NET have been associated with myocardial infarction.[22]

Anticoagulants and Antiplatelet Drugs, Risk of Bleeding and Choice of Anesthetic Technique

Anesthesiologists are often faced with patients who are on anticoagulants; such patients are not only likely to have excessive perioperative surgical bleeding; these drugs may also influence the choice of anesthetic technique specifically regional blocks. The risk of bleeding in the closed space of spinal canal leading to hematomas and serious neurological complications, mandates careful evaluation and weighing of the risk against possible benefits. The risk of bleeding is maximum at the time of needle puncture and placement of catheter or when it is being withdrawn[23,24] Tables 2A to 2D).

Anesthesiologists should be familiar with specific reversal agents[25] for anticoagulants. While antidotes for many anticoagulants like heparin (protamine) and vitamin K antagonists (FFP, PCC) are common knowledge, recent developments for direct oral anticoagulants (DOAC) are worth mentioning. Idarucizumab has recently been approved for reversal of dabigatran. Ciraparantag holds promise to be a universal antidote once investigations are complete.[23]

For details, readers are advised to refer to two excellent articles on the subject.[23,24]

CONCLUSION

Hemostasis is complex and its understanding is essential for judicious use of the large number of existing procoagulant and anticoagulant agents as well as the new ones that are continuously being added. In addition to drugs, variety of fluids that are invariably being used by perioperative physicians, also affect coagulation process. Shorter duration and reversibility of action of drugs, in addition to point of care tests, like those for platelet function, will help physicians take decisions that will ensure safer perioperative passage to many vulnerable patients.

Declaration

The author does not claim any original research work forming the basis of the chapter. The contents are based on available literature on the subject including published guidelines and position papers. The author has on occassions, in attempt to make a complex subject easy to understand, has used his interpretation.

Table 2C: Know your drugs: direct oral anticoagulants (DOAC), used in nonvalvular atrial fibrillation, DVT and PE (prevention and treatment)

Site/Mechanism of action	Antagonist	Route	Caution	Notes	Recommended interval before intervention
	Rivaroxaban	Oral	Prolonged action in renal failure	35% renal excretion	Effect lasts for 24 hours. Increased interval recommended in renal failure
Direct factor Xa inhibitor	Apixaban	Oral	Action prolonged in renal failure	25% renal excretion	Effect lasts for 24 hours. Increased interval recommended in renal failure
	Edoxaban	Oral	Action prolonged in renal failure	50% renal excretion	Effect lasts for 24 hours. Increased interval recommended in renal failure
Direct thrombin (IIa) inhibition	Dabigatran	Oral	Action prolonged in renal failure	80% renal excretion. Main advantage is reduced occurrence of intracranial bleeding compared to vit K antagonists	Effect lasts for 48 hours. Increased interval recommended in renal failure

Table 2D: Know your drugs: anticoagulants

Site/Mechanism of action	Antagonist	Route	Comments	Recommended interval for intervention
Vit K antagonists (Inhibit Vit K dependent plasma factors)	Acenocoumarol	Oral	Effect can be monitored with INR. Ideally should be < 1.5	Effect lasts 48–120 hours	Though FFP has been traditionally used to reverse its effect, Prothrombin Complex Concentrate (PCC) is now available: avoids both blood-product related complications and volume overload
	Warfarin	Oral	Effect can be monitored with INR. Ideally should be < 1.5	Effect lasts 48–96 hours	
Indirect inhibition of Xa and IIa (equal) through antithrombin	Unfractionated heparin (UFH)	IV/SC	Effect can be monitored by PTTK and ACT	Effect may last 1–3 hours. Intervention timing 2–4 hours
Indirect inhibition of Xa and IIa (Xa > IIa)	LMWH (enoxaparin, dalteparin)	SC	Caution in renal failure as elimination is dose dependent	Dose dependent deferment of catheter placement, >24 hours in case of therapeutic doses, 12 hours in case of prophylactic doses
Indirect inhibition of Xa	Fondaparinux	SC	100% elimination through kidneys	Interval for placement 36–42 hours. Effect may last up to 96 hours

(FFP: Fresh frozen plasma; LMWH: Low molecular weight heparin; INR: International normalized ratio; SC: Subcutaneous)

ACKNOWLEDGMENTS

The author is indebted to Dr V P Kumra and Dr Raminder Sehgal for their constant support and wise counsel.

The author is also thankful to Dr Devesh Dutta and Dr Neha Arora (Quality, FEHI) for help in drawing up coagulation schema.

REFERENCES

1. Spiess BD. Transfusion Medicine and Coagulation Disorders. In: Kaplan's Cardiac Anesthesia fo Cardiac and Noncardiac surgery Elsevier: 7th edition; 2017. pp 1249.
2. Abrams CA. Platelet biology. In: UpToDate, Post TW (Ed), UpToDate, Waltham, MA. (Accessed on January 04, 2016).
3. Ghoshal K, Bhattacharyya M. Overview of Platelet Physiology: Its Hemostatic and Nonhemostatic Role in Disease Pathogenesis. The Scientific World Journal (2014). 2014:781857.10.1155/2014/781857 (PMC Free article).
4. Kauskot A, Hoylaerts MF. "Platelet receptors" Handbook of Experimental Pharmacology. 2012;(210):23-57.
5. Saboor M, Ayub Q, Samina Ilyas, et al. Platelet receptors: An instrumental of platelet physiology. Pak J Med Sci. 2013;29(3):891-6. doi: http://dx.doi.org/10.12669/pjms. 293.3497.
6. Spiess BD. Transfusion Medicine and Coagulation Disorders. In: Kaplan's Cardiac Anesthesia for Cardiac and Noncardiac surgery Elsevier: 7th edition; 2017; pp 1256.
7. Tempo JA, Englyst NA, Holloway JA, et al. Platelet Microvesicles (Microparticles) in Cardiac Surgery. Journal of Cardiothoracic and Vascular Anesthesia. 2016;30:222-8.
8. Koupenova M, Kehrel BE, Corkrey HA, et al. Thrombosis and Platelets: An Update. Eur Heart. J. 2017;38:785-91.
9. Engelmann B, Massberg S. Thrombosis as an intravascular effector of innate immunity. Nat Rev Immunol. 2013;13:34-45.
10. Spiess BD. Transfusion Medicine and Coagulation Disorders. In: Kaplan's Cardiac Anesthesia for Cardiac and Noncardiac Surgery. Elsevier: 7th edition; 2017; pp 1253.
11. W Keith Hoots, Amy D Shapiro. Hemophilia A and B: Routine management including prophylaxis. In: UpToDate, Post TW (Ed), UpToDate, Waltham, MA. Accessed on April 22, 2017.
12. Mann KG, Brummel-Ziedins K. Normal Coagulation. In Rutherford's Vascular Surgery E-book. Elseviers:8th Edition 2014: pp 528-47.
13. Ranucci M, Baryshnikova E, Crapelli GB, et al.: Pre-operative antithrombin supplementation in cardiac surgery: a randomized controlled trial. J Thorac Cardiovasc Surg. 2013;145:1393-9 PMID 23102903.
14. Schmidt M, Lamberts M, Olsen AMS, et al. Cardiovascular safety of nonaspirin nonsteroidal anti-inflammatory drugs: review and position paper by the working group for Cardiovascular Pharmacotherapy of European Society of Cardiology. European Heart Journal 2016;37:1015-23.
15. Coxib and traditional NSAID Trialists' (CNT) Collaboration, Bhala N, Emberson J, Merhi A, Abramson S, et al. Vascular and upper gastrointestinal effects of non-steroidal anti-inflammatory drugs: meta analyses of individual participant data from randomised trials. Lancet. 2013;382:769-79.
16. Geerts WH, Pineo GF, Heit JA, et al. Prevention of venous thromboembolism: The Seventh ACCP Conference on Antithrombotic and Thrombolytic Therapy. Chest. 2004;126:338S-400S. [PMID: 15383478]
17. Lindblad B, Sternby NH, Bergqvist D. Incidence of venous thromboembolism verified by necropsy over 30 years. BMJ. 1991;302:709-11. [PMID: 2021744]

18. Sandler DA, Martin JF. Autopsy proven pulmonary embolism in hospital patients: are we detecting enough deep vein thrombosis? J R Soc Med. 1989;82:203-5. [PMID: 2716016].
19. Alikhan R, Peters F, Wilmott R, et al. Fatal pulmonary embolism in hospitalised patients: a necropsy review. J Clin Pathol. 2004;57:1254-7. [PMID: 15563663]
20. Gould MK, Garcia DA, Wren SM, et al. Prevention of VTE in nonorthopedic surgical patients: antithrombotic therapy and prevention of thrombosis, 9th ed: American College of Chest Physicians evidence-based clinical practical guidelines. Chest. 2012; 141:e227S.
21. Campbell LA, Rosenfeld ME. Infection and atherosclerosis development. Arch Med Res. 2015;46:339-50.
22. Mangold A, Alias S, Scherz T, et al. Coronary neutrophil extracellular trap burden and deoxyribonuclease activity in ST-elevation acute coronary syndrome are predictors of ST-segment resolution and infarct size. Circ Res. 2015;116:1182-92.
23. Yurttas T. Perioperative management of antithrombotic therapies. Curr Opin Anesthesiol 2017, 30:000–000. DOI:10.1097/ACO.0000000000000481. Ahead of print. Accessed May 25, 2017.
24. Rosenquist R. Neuraxial (spinal, epidural) anesthesia/analgesia techniques in patients receiving anticoagulant or antiplatelet medication. In: UpToDate, Post TW (Ed), UpToDate, Waltham MA. (Accessed on May 15, 2017.)
25. Raval AN, Cigarroa JE, Chung MK, et al. American Heart Association Clinical Pharmacology Subcommittee of the Acute Cardiac Care and General Cardiology Committee of the Council on Clinical Cardiology; Council on Cardiovascular Disease in the Young; and Council on Quality of Care and Outcomes Research. Management of patients on non-vitamin K antagonist oral anticoagulants in the acute care and periprocedural setting. A scientific statement from American Heart Association. Circulation 2017;135:e604-e633.

CHAPTER 3

Moving away from Null Hypothesis Significance Testing

LN Yaddanapudi

KEY POINTS

- Null hypothesis significance testing (NHST) framework with the associated p-values does not serve to produce firm evidence for or against the research hypothesis.
- There are a number of intrinsic problems with NHST and p-values.
- There are other extrinsic problems such as p-hacking, flexible and undocumented analytic decisions and publication bias with this framework.
- More attention to framing of the hypothesis, data collection, validation and analysis, full disclosure of all data and results along with effect sizes is recommended.
- Predictive model building should be promoted.

INTRODUCTION

Most research in anesthesiology, in India as well as internationally, seems to be focused on null hypothesis significance testing (NHST). This reliance on NHST devalues our science, while promoting unjustifiable trust in so-called "statistical significance" leading to irrational practices.

What We are Looking for?

We want to find out if the treatment we administer to the patient produces a greater degree of desirable change compared to a standard treatment or no treatment. We are looking for the probability that the change that we see is because of the treatment and not because of intrinsic variability of the patient population or because of random chance. That is, if we administer a drug, we want to know if the change we see is because of the drug.

Procedure of NHST

A treatment (a new drug, a new procedure) is administered to one group of patients (called Test group), while a traditional/standard/old treatment is administered to a second group (called Control group). Some measurement of an outcome of interest is made in both groups. The difference between the two groups is calculated. Using a statistical procedure of estimating a test statistic (e.g. t value in t-test, F in ANOVA, etc.), the investigator estimates the probability of the observed data occurring, when in fact there is no difference between the drugs. We make an arbitrary cut-off of this probability below which we say that there is a significant difference at a value of 0.05. However, there is nothing sacrosanct about this conventional cut-off value. It was originally suggested as a convenient value by Sir Ronald Fisher[1] who wrote "... it is convenient to draw the line at about a level at which we can say: 'Either there is something in the treatment, or a coincidence has occurred such as does not occur more than once in twenty trials.'"

Assumptions of NHST

In NHST the investigator assumes a null hypothesis, i.e. the treatment administered has made no difference to the outcome. NHST assumes that there was no baseline difference between the two groups. It also assumes that the patients had been allocated to the two groups completely randomly and that there was no bias in measurement of the outcome. When any of these assumptions are violated, as they often are, NHST loses its validity.

Even when the null hypothesis is true, there would be a variation in the outcome in the two groups because of one or more of the following reasons: biological variation in the patients, inefficient design of the study, small sample size, imprecise measurements due to the instruments/scales used, lack of training of observers, errors by the measuring personnel, etc.

What about the Alternate Hypothesis?

A p-value of 0.05 means that the degree of difference in the outcome found between the two groups could have arisen in 5% of the cases where there is no real difference between the treatments. This says nothing about the situation where the effects of the drugs are actually different. In this case the chances of detecting the difference that has been seen will be entirely different and not 5% or the complement of it, i.e. 95%. In addition, for any given null hypothesis there are theoretically infinite number of alternate hypotheses, i.e. there are many ways in which the new treatment differs from the control. In most cases the researchers do not even specify a single alternate hypothesis. And we do not know the probability distribution of any of these alternate hypotheses.

Let me give an example: The baseline rate of postoperative nausea (PN) is 80% in a given patient population. A new prophylactic anti-emetic, Nospew, is claimed to reduce this by half. We find the control group has an 80% incidence of PN while the test group has 40%. Let us say this difference is statistically significant at the 0.05 level, i.e. $p < 0.05$. This gives us two possible explanations:
1. The null is true, and we have found a rare event, or
2. The null is not true.

The p-value does not distinguish between the two cases.

In other words, there is a 5% probability of finding a 40% difference in the incidence of PN when Nospew does **not** work. Even when there is no difference between Nospew and placebo, there is a difference in the outcome between the two groups, due to the reasons listed above. Figure 1 shows what the probability distribution of this effect would be. For simplicity I have assumed this is a unimodal normal distribution. As you can see, in a small number of cases, the difference between the groups would be as large as 40% in our example.

We do not know, and the data do not say, anything about the case where Nospew actually works and reduces the incidence of PN by half. In addition,

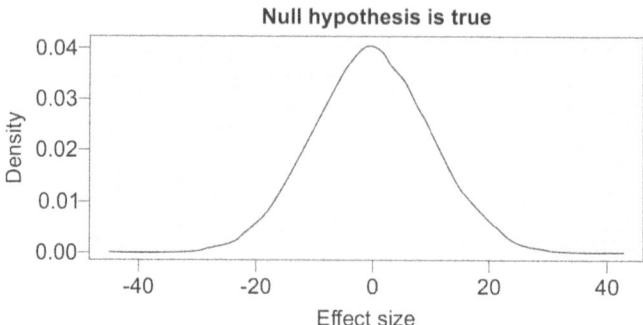

Fig. 1: The probability distribution of the effect size when the null hypothesis is true, i.e. the treatment being investigated has no effect.

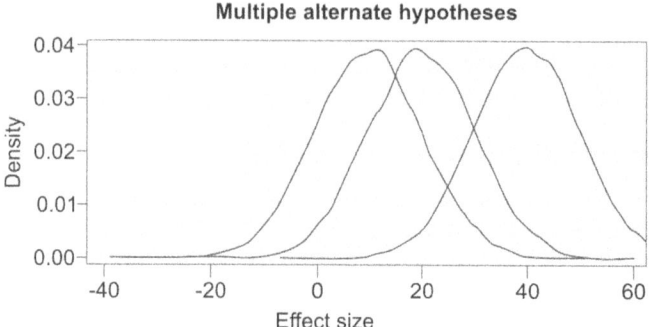

Fig. 2: The probability distribution of the effect size when three alternate hypotheses (with small, medium and large effect sizes) are true.

Nospew may be effective, but may only decrease PN by a third, or a quarter or any other fraction. It may even increase the incidence of PN. The probability of a decrease by 50% (that we actually found) occurring by chance in any of these settings would be different than in the first case. In Figure 2, I show the possible probability distribution of the effect in three different cases, where Nospew has a small, medium and large effect. Again, for simplicity I assume unimodal normal distribution for all these effect sizes, with the same standard deviation. As you can see, the probability of finding a decrease in PN to 40% is different under each of these scenarios. Realistically, the distributions will probably not be normal and will have varying standard deviations, giving a much larger variation in the probability of detecting the 40% difference.

However, you would expect the probability to be higher than with the null hypothesis true. But would this be 100–5 = 95%? This is not true, as explained by Colquhoun[2] in simple mathematical terms. Sellke et al.[3] have shown that even in the most optimistic scenarios, the probability of finding the actual difference is not more than about 70%.

This sort of optimistic approach does not take into account the real world scenarios detailed below.

In the Real World there is no Null

In the real world, the null hypothesis is almost never true. No two groups of people are identical. No two drugs are exactly equal in all their effects. In addition, no drug or treatment arrives at the stage where it is subjected to a randomised controlled trial without evidence that it has some desired effect in the form of tissue/animal/Phase I and II trials. Therefore the, null hypothesis should always be rejected in every trial, which makes the whole process of significance testing infructuous.

The p-value Depends on the Sample Size

It is a commonplace among statisticians that the p-value is a measure of sample size. Any degree of difference between two groups becomes statistically significant, i.e. produces a small enough p-value, if one takes a large enough sample. As long ago as 1966, Bahadur[4] showed that the null hypothesis becomes "more and more incredible as the sample size increases, when a non-null distribution obtains".

Let us take an example. All calculations in this example are done using the on-line statistical software OpenEpi (version 3.03).[5] Consider a drug Lospew, which reduces the incidence of PN marginally. About 80% of the Control group and 70% of the Test group suffer PN. The absolute reduction of PN is 10%. If we have 10 patients in each group, the p-value of the chi-square test is 0.5. By increasing the sample size to 100 patients per group, the p-value becomes 0.07. This can further be reduced to a "statistically significant" value of 0.0000002 by taking 1000 patients in each group. For the same absolute difference of 10%, naive researchers would conclude that in the first case there was no difference between the groups, while in the third case there is powerful evidence of difference.

One of the examples of misplaced reliance on p-values to decide standards of practice is the Physicians Health Study of oral aspirin to prevent myocardial infarction (MI).[6] In a sample of 22,000 patients, a statistically significant ($p < 0.00001$) reduction in incidence of MI was found on interim analysis. The study was terminated early and aspirin was recommended for general prevention. However, the actual effect size was very small with a risk difference of 0.77%. An R of 0.001 meant that intake of aspirin explained only about 0.1% of the decrease in the incidence of MI. A large number of patients were treated with prophylactic aspirin due to this study. Later studies showed an even smaller effect, and the recommendation has now been modified.

Conversely, a high p-value is also uninformative. It indicates that either (a) the null hypothesis is true and there is no effect, or (b) there is an actual difference, but you have failed to find it because of using a sample size calculated to detect a larger effect, bad design or bad execution of the study etc. In other words, a large Type II error (false negative) in conventional terms.

Another facet of the same problem is the manipulation of the sample size calculation that most researchers practice. If I want to detect a possible decrease of 10% in PN, I will need 327 patients in each group. To detect a difference of 20%, the sample size decreases to 94 per group. If there are logistical difficulties in recruiting nearly 200 patients, I reduce the number required to 28 per group by looking for a difference of 40%. In the real world, almost all drugs improve outcomes only marginally. A new drug which decreases the incidence of a harmful outcome by half is very rare indeed. The chances are, the new drug Lospew actually reduces the incidence of PN somewhere on the order of 10–20%, which can be estimated from earlier studies of the drug in animal or early phase human studies as well as the effect found with related drugs in practice. By ignoring the actually probable effect size based on biological plausibility, and unethically inflating the effect size to be detected, we have managed to decrease the number of patients to be recruited, but have greatly increased the chances of not finding any effect at all. In other words, we have decreased the power of the test.

Regression to the Mean

In Ioannidis' 2005 study[7] 45 out of 49 highly cited clinical research studies claimed the intervention was effective. In later literature no attempts at replication have been made of 11 of these studies. Of the remaining 34, seven (16%) have subsequently been contradicted and another 7 (16%) have been found to have smaller effect sizes. Part of the explanation for this phenomenon is as follows: Only "significant" results are published. Historically most scientific hypotheses are false. Therefore in most trials the null hypothesis is true and the "significant" results are actually rare events. Consequently most attempts at confirming the findings in another trial fail, or at least the effect size is smaller. Hence, the regression to the mean. Other reasons include the inflated effect size when a true discovery is claimed based on a significance test in an underpowered study, flexible analyses and selective reporting, and conflicts of interest of the authors.[8]

Attempts to Reduce the Problem

In a bid to reduce the problems of finding statistically significant but clinically irrelevant findings, some authors have advocated using a p value of 0.01 or lower as the standard cut-off value, rather than the traditional 0.05. However, you are still detecting either (a) an extremely rare event or (b) the null is not true. The p-value still does not tell you which one is true.

Others have advocated the use of confidence intervals (CI). Paraphrasing the original definition if we apply a 95% confidence procedure multiple times to a set of data, 95% of the CIs generated will contain the true value of the parameter of interest.[9] However, it is mostly interpreted as an interval which has a 95% probability of containing the true value of the parameter. It is also considered that the CI width is a measure of uncertainty and that the interval contains the "likely" values of the parameter.[10] However, Morey et al.[11] have pointed out that none of these properties of CIs are proven. They advocate the use of Bayesian credible intervals. This carries us into territories which are not within the scope of this article.

Other Problems in Practice

In addition to the intrinsic problems of p-values outlined above, there are a large number of behavioral and sociocultural problems associated with NHST. Examples include the use of simultaneous multiple hypothesis testing with selective reporting of only those which are "statistically significant"; p-hacking, a process of data dredging, applying different tests to the same data, choosing one-sided or two-sided tests, all to achieve "significance"; and publication bias on the part of the authors, reviewers and editors to favor publication of only those articles which achieve significance.

The Path Ahead

As we saw, a large proportion of the literature which is based on statistical significance is meaningless. Basing health care decisions on such fragile foundations is a disservice to our patients, ourselves and above all to our science.

Authors, reviewers and editors need to pay much more attention to the process and methodology of research. Is the research question formulated well? How relevant is the research question? Is the design of the study good? Are the processes of randomization and concealment of allocation designed, documented and implemented properly? If the trial is blinded, is the procedure of blinding well designed, documented and implemented? What are the outcomes of interest? Are they relevant, hard or soft, surrogate or true? Is the process of measurement standardized, the observers trained, the process monitored for errors? Once the data are gathered, how are they handled? Are all data accounted for, without discarding some data from analysis? Are the questions to be addressed and the analyses to be performed prespecified? If so, have the protocols been followed? Are all the analyses done documented, without any selective omission? If any of these are inadequate, any amount of sophisticated statistical analysis is not going to yield us the truth.

If you still perform NHST, Colquhoun[2] has a set of recommendations, which I paraphrase below:
1. All NHST assume random allocation of treatments. Hence, NHST should not be applied to any observational studies.
2. Never use the word "significant" in the paper.
3. Just state the p-value, and give the effect size and confidence intervals. But be aware the 95% confidence intervals may be misleadingly narrow.
4. Observation of a p-value close to 0.05 (from either direction) means nothing more than the question is "worth another look".
5. Do some rough calculations of the sample size required to show a worthwhile effect.

He also advocates the use of a threshold p value of 0.001, but I strongly disagree with that recommendation.

Gelman advocates a move from NHST to Bayesian interaction model building and verification.[12] A statistical hypothesis is much more specific than a scientific hypothesis. A rejection of the null hypothesis in the former can occur due to violation of technical assumptions, without there actually being an effect. There is always measurement error. This can be large enough to cause you to reject the null hypothesis. Treatment effects vary. The same measurement on the same person can be different at different times or in a different environment. This is to a large extent due to interaction with a number of other variables. Despite this, when we test out hypotheses, we compare to the non-meaningful comparison point of zero effect. Once we truly accept that treatment effects vary, we move away from the goal of establishing a general scientific truth from a small experiment and move toward modelling variation, situation-dependent traits and dynamic relations. "We move away from is-it-there-or-is-it-not-there to a more helpful, contextually informed perspective."

Whether one follows Bayesian predictive modelling or not, the following general recommendations will improve the quality of our research.

1. Analyze all your data. Use all data to provide yourself and your readers with all the relevant information.
2. Present all your comparisons. The readers have a right to know if the researchers trawled through everything and selected only the best results for presentation, or if they followed an arbitrary decision pathway of what to look for. This can be done in the form of a big table or graph instead of several paragraphs of text. This will require more effort from the readers too.
3. Make your data public. If a question is worth studying, giving other researchers access speeds up the rate of progress. Patient confidentiality can be preserved by anonymizing the data.

CONCLUSION

In summary, NHST using p-values has a huge number of drawbacks and does not produce definitive evidence, nor provide predictive models. A Bayesian or non-Bayesian predictive model building utilizing prior information we already have, is a better option. However, good analysis is no substitute for good data collection. Small sample studies of small effects will only tell us that we do not have enough information to draw any conclusions. Presenting data more fully and increasing data availability should help all types of analyses.

ACKNOWLEDGMENT

For serving as a sounding board and for catching at least two major mistakes, I wish to thank my wife, Prof. Sandhya Yaddanapudi.

REFERENCES

1. Fisher RA. The arrangement of field experiments. J Min Agric. 1926;33:503-13.
2. Colquhoun D. An investigation of the false discovery rate and the misinterpretation of p-values. R Soc Open Sci. 2014;1:140216.
3. Sellke T, Bayarri MJ, Berger JO. Calibration of p-values for testing precise null hypotheses. Am Stat. 2001;55:62-71.
4. Bahadur RR. Rates of convergence of estimates and test statistics. Ann Math Statist. 1966;37:303-24.
5. Dean AG, Sullivan KM, Soe MM. OpenEpi: Open Source Epidemiologic Statistics for Public Health, 3.03. www.OpenEpi.com, updated 2014/09/22, accessed 2017/07/11.
6. Bartolucci AA, Tendera M, Howard G. Meta-analysis of multiple primary prevention trials of cardiovascular events using aspirin. Am J Cardiol. 2011;107:1796-801.
7. Ioannidis JPA. Contradicted and initially stronger effects in highly cited clinical research. JAMA. 2005;294:218-28.
8. Ioannidis JPA. Why most discovered true associations are inflated. Epidemiology 2008;19:640-8.
9. Neyman J. Outline of a theory of statistical estimation based on the classical theory of probability. Philos Trans R Soc London, Ser A. 1937;236:333-80.
10. Masson MEJ, Loftus GR. Using confidence intervals for graphically based data interpretation. Can J Exp Psychol. 2003;57:203-20.
11. Morey RD, Hoekstra R, Rouder JN, et al. The fallacy of placing confidence in confidence intervals. Psychon Bull Rev. 2016;23:103-23.
12. Gelman A. The connection between varying treatment effects and the crisis of unreplicable research: a Bayesian perspective. J Manag. 2015;41:632-43.

CHAPTER 4

Remifentanil for Labor Analgesia

Preet Mohinder Singh, Anuradha Borle

KEY POINTS

- ❏ Epidural analgesia remains the gold standard in terms of analgesic efficacy for labor analgesia, however, intravenous remifentanil is also a viable and effective alternative.
- ❏ Remifentanil undergoes rapid metabolism in the maternal blood and further metabolism in the newborn, thus adverse effects on the neonate are minimal.
- ❏ Patient controlled analgesia technique after proper patient education to appropriately time the remifentanil bolus can achieve near complete pain relief.
- ❏ Vigilant monitoring is a must when remifentanil is used for labor analgesia. Appropriately trained paramedical staff can enhance patient safety and analgesic efficacy by adjusting drug delivery rate, as and when needed.
- ❏ Clinical adoption rate of remifentanil is still low due to lack of universal availability and higher costs related to drug patent issues.

INTRODUCTION

"Soft molecule" is a term used for rapidly metabolized/less stable molecules. For clinical anesthesiologists, this has attracted much attention over the last decade by virtue of its organ independent yet reliable metabolic potential.[1] Soft molecules are typically "ester compounds" that undergo rapid cleavage by various esterases present in abundance in the body.[2] The prototype molecule that paved the way for such development is remifentanil. Remifentanil is a potent, short-acting synthetic opioid with a short half-life. Chemically it has an ester linkage which undergoes rapid hydrolysis by non-specific tissue and plasma esterases making its elimination organ independent, thus making it a perfect "soft molecule". Most often one would opt to use such drugs in patients where organ functions are compromised. As a corollary, their use can also be prioritized in patients where organ functions are not yet fully mature or developed. Any systemic drug administered intravenously to laboring mother is likely to have some degree of fetal transference. Thus, opioid "soft molecule" remifentanil by virtue of organ independent and predictable metabolism becomes an intuitive choice for use in labor analgesia.

The ideal choice for labor analgesia has eluded many since many decades. The problem in southeast Asian region extends beyond an agent/method of choice. On the first-place people need awareness on possibilities for analgesia during labor. In our own survey in Indian villages, we found very poor public awareness on the scope of labor analgesia.[3] Establishing the need for labor analgesia is beyond the purview of this chapter, however, we would focus on how remifentanil is a viable and practical choice for this indication.

INTRAVENOUS OPIOIDS AND LABOR ANALGESIA

Neonatal brain has enhanced sensitivity to the apneic effects of systemic opioids.[4] An ideal intravenous opioid is expected to result in optimal analgesia without altering the pattern of uterine contractions and fetal cardiography. In addition, its effect on the respiratory pattern of both mother and fetus should be minimal allowing the administration to be continued until the end of the expulsion phase. Opioids being lipid soluble drugs are bound to have maternofetal transference. So, analgesic opioid administered to the parturient is likely to have effects on the newborn. The trick here is to find the best agent that can have least of these effects. One of the initial opioids tried for labor analgesia was fentanyl. Early studies reported that the plasma site concentrations in non-pregnant patients for equivalent dose fentanyl were higher. This led to a belief that pregnancy enhanced the opioid metabolism. Such reduced concentrations in non-pregnant patients was later demonstrated for almost all opioids. It was later established that rather than specific enhancement in metabolism, it was the increased volume of distribution (related to plasma expansion during pregnancy) that attributed to the decreased concentration in the parturient. Before, clinicians resorted to remifentanil, the reported demerits with other opioids include:

a. *Fentanyl:* It has very high lipid solubility and a high protein binding capacity. This compounded by high potency (800 times more potent than meperidine) seemed like an attractive choice, further a peak of action 3 to 4 minutes after a bolus could help coincide with uterine contraction. However, trials have demonstrated several adverse effects in the neonate, with a high incidence of naloxone requirement at birth, low neurobehavioral scores up to 7 days after birth and an adverse dose dependent impact on the capacity to breastfeed soon after the birth.[5]

b. *Meperidine:* It has been a popular choice in the developing world for labor analgesia in view of its low cost. It however, has been consistently shown to have poor analgesic efficacy.[5] The analgesic benefits demonstrated in early studies may actually be rated to its sedation rather than direct analgesic activity. A well conducted meta-analysis also demonstrated lower fetal pH in parturients receiving meperidine for labor analgesia thus posing questions on newborns safety.[6]

c. *Alfentanil:* Only a few studies have evaluated the use of alfentanil in labor analgesia. The comparisons demonstrated poor analgesic profile[7] and also more pronounced fetal effects when compared to meperidine.[8]

Remifentanil: The Ideal Choice

Remifentanil, was introduced in the market in early 1990s but was never tried in laboring women initially. For more than one decade, the properties of remifentanil were explored in trials of surgical anesthesia, sedation and perioperative analgesia in non-obstetric populations. It was only in 1998 when it was first used in obstetric anesthesia.[9] This was after extensive study of drug's pharmacokinetic profile in pregnant patients and neonates. Remifentanil clearly scores over other available opioids in the further discussed aspects.

Maternofetal Transference

Volikas et al. studied the maternofetal transference of remifentanil by measuring real-time concentrations. The concentration ratio of remifentanil in the umbilical cord/uterine artery was reported to be around 0.88. This meant that the drug did rapidly traverse the placenta into the fetal circulation. Further evaluation of concentration ratios in umbilical artery and umbilical vein showed a ratio of only 0.29. This rapid decline in concentration ratio was very promising and suggested significant rapid metabolism and redistribution.[10]

Metabolism

Hill et al. in their pharmacokinetic evaluation of remifentanil reported its plasma clearance to be nearly doubled in pregnant patients. This was attributed to the increased concentration of plasma esterases with pregnancy.[11] Clinically this finding translates into the fact that rapid maternal metabolism would mean smaller fetal transmission and thus diminished fetal effects.

Maternal Side Effects Profile

Opioid use in the perioperative period has been associated with increased incidence of postoperative nausea vomiting. Blair et al. in one of the early studies reported that by virtue of its short half-life (nearly 4 minutes) remifentanil does not accentuate the incidence of postoperative nausea vomiting in laboring women.[12] Thus, giving it further edge over other systemic opioids.

Absence of Acute Tolerance

One of the rare reported side effects with the use of opioid infusions is development of acute tolerance and increased dose requirements. Attributing to rapid metabolism and minimal interaction with hepatic enzyme induction such phenomena has not been reported with remifentanil. Thus, patients in labor and even after delivery can receive remifentanil infusions for extended durations without requiring potentially dangerous dose escalations. Another aspect that deserves a special mention here is that since hepatic enzyme induction/inhibition does not alter remifentanil kinetics. Parturient receiving other drugs are unlikely to require dosing alterations for remifentanil.

Minimal Alterations in Cardiotocography (CTG)

Transient variability in the CTG tracing has been reported, but these effects are much less frequent than the ones observed with the systemic administration of other opioids.[13]

No Developmental Side Effects on Neonatal Brain

Anesthetic drug related apoptosis in the newborn brain has derived much attention recently. Trials show that agents with GABA or NMDA blocking activity may be associated with induction of caspase enzyme in the newborn brain that triggers long-term developmental adverse effects.[14] Pethidine in addition to mu opioid effect may have addition activity and can be associated with possibility of brain cell apoptosis. Remifentanil being a pure and short acting mu opioid agonist has not been reported to be associated with such phenomena.[15]

No Active Metabolite

Remifentanil is rapidly metabolized to an inactive metabolite (remifentanil acid) by plasma and tissue esterases. Absence of active metabolite allows for prolonged infusions during labor without any possibility of residual clinical effect.

LABOR EPIDURAL—THE GOLD STANDARD VERSUS REMIFENTANIL

The ease of administration of remifentanil beats the expertise needed for the use of epidural analgesia. Although many hospitals globally use epidural analgesia as the gold standard for labor, it has many limitations. Epidural analgesia may not be best option for women with an absolute or relative contraindication that include the following:

Parturient Receiving Thromboprophylaxis

Irrespective of the cause for the need of thromboprophylaxis managing epidural in such patients is always challenging. One has to space out the drug delivery for thromboprophylaxis to insert or even remove the epidural catheter. Despite all the cautions, patient may still remain at a higher risk of epidural hematoma development. In some cases, it may not be practical to stop thromboprophylaxis at all. In such patients, remifentanil automatically gets preference.

Patients with Congenital Bleeding Tendencies

This subgroup includes patients with bleeding disorders like Von Willebrand's disease, hemophilia, thromboasthenia etc. Patients remain at a higher risk of epidural hematoma and epidural should be avoided in these patients.

Patients with Certain Cardiac Defects

Certain cardiac valvular lesions with fixed cardiac output are relative contraindication to epidural use. Epidural local anesthetic induced vasodilatation can lead to hemodynamic compromise in stenotic lesions involving mitral or aortic valve. In such situations, intravenous remifentanil emerges as relatively safer option.

Spinal Abnormalities

It is not uncommon to see pregnant patients with spinal dysraphism or scoliosis. In such patients, epidural placement is neither safe nor easy. Patients with scoliosis may have unpredictable local anesthetic spread in the epidural space leading to patchy analgesic effect. In such situations, it may be wise to prophylactically switch to intravenous remifentanil for labor analgesia.

Suspected Infections

It is not advised to perform a central neuraxial puncture in any parturient with suspected bloodstream or central nervous system infection. In such situations, intravenous analgesics are the preferred choice.

Patient Preference

Despite good preoperative counseling some group of patients would insist on avoiding needle puncture in the back. In such patients, epidural analgesia is an absolute contraindication.

Based on the analgesic efficacy evidence, there is no denying to the fact that labor epidural remains the gold standard. However, in the above situations one would prefer intravenous analgesia (with remifentanil) over epidural technique.

COMPARATIVE ANALGESIC POTENTIAL

Remifentanil versus Central Neuraxial Analgesia

Numerous trials and multiple meta-analysis have concluded upon the analgesic superiority of central neuraxial blocks over intravenous remifentanil.[16,17] The most recent meta-analysis reported that after 2 hours of initiation of epidural labor analgesia, pain scores remained lower by 3 units (on a numeric pain scale of 0 to 10) in comparison to intravenous remifentanil.[17] Similar analgesic superiority was proved for combined spinal epidural (CSE) technique in a recent Cochrane review.[18,19] Freeman et al. performed a large multicenter randomized controlled trial comparing labor epidural to intravenous remifentanil. Interestingly, they concluded that although epidural was superior in terms of quantified pain relief, the patient satisfaction was comparable after labor.[20] This could partly be related to sedation in addition to analgesia caused by remifentanil whereas local anesthetic based epidural techniques have no sedating potential. Thus, patient anxiety is also alleviated with the use of remifentanil. Despite exhaustive literature on safety of epidural in labor and no reported increase in cesarean section rates, conventional obstetricians are still concerned with theoretical risks of increased cesarean sections occurring with possible motor block during epidural analgesia. Remifentanil is free of such concerns and generates more confidence towards normal labor.

Nitrous Oxide and Remifentanil

Nitrous oxide by virtue of its rapid onset and offset is still used as a labor analgesic in some parts of the world. Volmanen et al. demonstrated that remifentanil administered via an intravenous infusion was nearly three time more effective than Entonox in laboring women.[21] Many clinicians also advocate the use of remifentanil in combination with nitrous oxide for higher analgesic efficacy.[22]

Remifentanil versus Fentanyl

Trials comparing fentanyl to remifentanil have shown equivocal results in terms of analgesic potential. However, there are many other clinical parameters assessed during these trials that establish remifentanil's superiority. Higher number of women opted to shift to labor epidural over intravenous fentanyl (compared to ones receiving remifentanil). More neonates in the fentanyl group required resuscitation compared with those receiving remifentanil.[23,24] These trials also conclude that higher level of vigilance for transient hypoxic episodes may be required with remifentanil use.

Remifentanil versus Meperidine

Meperidine has lower analgesic potency than remifentanil and the time to peak action is also delayed. So, after an intravenous bolus the peak action overshoots the uterine contraction. Further multiple doses repeated over time are likely to have residual action in view of long metabolic half-life and generation of an active metabolite (nor-meperidine). Lower cost however is the only factor that favors the use of meperidine in the developing world.[23]

SAFETY CONCERNS WITH THE USE OF REMIFENTANIL

Multiple trials report the possibility of higher incidence of hypoxic events with the use of remifentanil infusions.[25] These episodes are usually transient and self-limiting often without a clinical consequence. Recently, Bonner et al. reported patient mortality related to cardiorespiratory arrest in a patient administered remifentanil for labor analgesia. Their experience led to formulation of many safety precautions that must be adopted while remifentanil infusion is used for labor and delivery.[26,27] Based upon the available literature,[22] the basic safety requirements to be ensured while using remifentanil for labor analgesia are summed up in Table 1.

REMIFENTANIL INFUSION REGIMENS: CLINICAL PEARLS

The use of remifentanil during labor makes use of many protocols and technologies with marked variations and individual choices. The evidence for the administration methods described below is derived from primarily European trials, where remifentanil for labor is a popular choice already.

Continuous Infusion

This is one of the simplest administration technique used for remifentanil. A continuous baseline infusion can be initiated at a rate of 0.025 µgm/kg/min and gradually stepped up to a maximum of 0.15 µgm/kg/min based upon patient's analgesic response and sedation. At this infusion rate, maternal and neonatal side effects are expected to be minimal.[28] This regimen is associated with minimal adverse effects and is not patient dependent unlike patient controlled analgesia (PCA), this may however be not as efficacious as PCA.[29]

Table 1: Safety protocol for using remifentanil during labor analgesia	
Patient selection	• Informed/written consent – with detailed explanation to the patient • Dedicated intravenous cannula for remifentanil infusion • No additional opioid during and 4 hours prior to the initiation of infusion
Infusion protocols	• Bolus not more than 40µ (details administration techniques described in text)
Continuous monitoring	• One to one nursing-trained labor room nurse • Pulse oximetry and heart rate monitoring
Periodic review every half hour	• Pain quantification • Respiratory rate • Sedation scores
Alarm—call for help protocol	• Respiratory rate lower than 8 breaths/minute • Pulse oximeter saturation lower than 90% • Not arousable patient (excessive sedation)
Trained anesthesiologist must be available in the vicinity of labor room	

PCA Bolus without Baseline Infusion

This is a patient dependent protocol and educating patient prior to initiation is a pre-requisite. The pharmacokinetics of remifentanil play a vital role in success of this protocol. The peak action of remifentanil is attained in around 2-3 minutes, however uterine contractions typically last for 80-90 seconds. Thus, if the bolus is administered at the initiation of contraction, the peak pain of contraction and remifentanil peak action will not coincide. Thus, patient must be instructed to initiate the drug bolus before an anticipated contraction. Blair et al. demonstrated that IV PCA bolus ranging from 0.25 to 0.5 µgm/kg with a lockout interval of 2-3 minutes can safely reduce labor pain in most of the parturient. (Total bolus not more than 40 µgm.)[12]

Baseline Infusion and PCA Bolus

Many clinicians have tried different baseline infusion rates supplementing the above described PCA bolus settings. A well-studied protocol includes a constant regimen using a baseline infusion at 0.025 to 0.1 µgm/kg/min with a reoccurring bolus of 0.25 µgm/kg. The use of baseline infusion can increase the analgesic efficacy but maternofetal safety can be compromised.[30]

Target Controlled Infusions (TCI)

Computerized drug delivery systems have shown promising results in out of operating room settings.[31] In a recent innovative trial, Schwarz et al. evaluated TCI model for remifentanil in parturient. Remifentanil TCI was started at the rate of 1 ng/mL and titrated in 0.5 ng/mL increments to the lowest effective dose.[32] They reported increased neonatal and maternal respiratory complications with TCI use. This may be related to the fact that TCI modeling yet needs to be modified to pharmacokinetic alterations related to pregnancy. At the time of writing, this protocol is relatively new and in more or less for investigational purposes only.

Having described the above regimens choosing one over the other is difficult. It is suggested that one should adopt any of the above regimen based upon the hospital protocols and available paramedical support. Logical modifications in the above suggested doses can help tinker the drug delivery best suited to one's own population for best yet safe outcomes.

LIMITATIONS OF REMIFENTANIL FOR LABOR ANALGESIA

For our readers in southeast Asia the biggest practical limitation is availability of remifentanil for this indication. Further cost factor also plays a critical role when it is to be evaluated against labor epidural. Thus a "cost performance ratio" is a major hurdle in its regular use. From our own experience, the Drug controller of India (DCI) has not approved remifentanil for use in labor analgesia and this discourages trials for Indian population. Although, many global studies have evaluated remifentanil and adopted it in clinical practice, the approval in by DCI is still pending.

Further, population in the subcontinent need education on possibilities of alleviating labor pain. People assume it to be a natural process and thus refrain from getting treatment. We agree that "Labor is a natural process but suffering due to it, is not". Thus, public education via media sources can help adopt labor analgesic techniques, be it epidural or remifentanil.[3]

Whatever said and done, remifentanil remains to be a drug with potential to cause life threatening complications. Although, fetal transmission is small but how relevant it is clinically still needs to be correctly addressed. By the time newborn is assessed after delivery for opioid side effects, remifentanil is mostly metabolized (as the delivery and assessment process take more than 4 minutes—the half-life of remifentanil). Recently, Hill et al. cast doubts on possibility of clinically relevant adverse events. They reported the use of remifentanil in anesthesia for ex-utero intrapartum treatment procedures (EXIT procedures) and cesarean sections using higher doses than the ones used for analgesia. They reported the occurrence of fetal immobility and a decrease in variability of fetal heartbeat.[11]

The pharmacokinetic profile of remifentanil also poses unique challenges. As already described in the PCA section, the patient needs to be aware of optimal timing of initiation of remifentanil bolus. Patient coherence to attain peak drug action during the peak contraction time also is a challenge.

CONCLUSION

There is enough evidence in favor of using remifentanil to prevent labor pain. The analgesic efficacy and ease of administration are liable to make it a popular choice. Close vigilant monitoring is critical to the use of remifentanil during labor for analgesia. Remifentanil PCA is an important advancement in the obstetric anesthesia armamentarium. In addition, remifentanil has the potential to become the method of choice for preventing labor pain in many hospitals and especially for parturients who want to avoid neuraxial analgesia or when its use is contraindicated.

REFERENCES

1. Goudra BG, Singh PM. Remimazolam: the future of its sedative potential. Saudi J Anaesth. 2014;8:388-91.
2. Chitilian HV, Eckenhoff RG, Raines DE. Anesthetic drug development: novel drugs and new approaches. Surg Neurol Int. 2013;4:S2-10.
3. Singh PM, Kumar A, Trikha A. Rural perspective about anesthesia and anesthesiologist: a cross-sectional study. J Anaesthesiol Clin Pharmacol. 2013;29:228.
4. Bosch GE van den, White T, El Marroun H, et al. Prematurity, opioid exposure and neonatal pain: do they affect the developing brain? Neonatology. 2015;108:8-15.
5. Evron S, Ezri T. Options for systemic labor analgesia. Curr Opin Anaesthesiol. 2007;20:181-5.
6. Olofsson C, Ekblom A, Ekman-Ordeberg G, et al. Lack of analgesic effect of systemically administered morphine or pethidine on labour pain. Brit J Obstet Gynaecol. 1996;103:968-72.
7. Reynolds F, Sharma SK, Seed PT. Analgesia in labour and fetal acid-base balance: a meta-analysis comparing epidural with systemic opioid analgesia. Brit J Obstet Gynaecol. 2002;109:1344-53.
8. Morley-Forster PK, Reid DW, Vandeberghe H. A comparison of patient-controlled analgesia fentanyl and alfentanil for labour analgesia. Can J Anaesth. 2000;47:113-9.
9. Kan RE, Hughes SC, Rosen MA, et al. Intravenous remifentanil: placental transfer, maternal and neonatal effects. Anesthesiology. 1998;88:1467-74.
10. Volikas I, Butwick A, Wilkinson C, et al. Maternal and neonatal side-effects of remifentanil patient-controlled analgesia in labour. Br J Anaesth. 2005;95:504-9.

11. Hill D. Remifentanil patient-controlled analgesia should be routinely available for use in labour. Int J Obstet Anesth. 2008;17:336-9.
12. Blair JM, Hill DA, Fee JP. Patient-controlled analgesia for labour using remifentanil: a feasibility study. Br J Anaesth. 2001;87:415-20.
13. Volmanen P, Akural EI, Raudaskoski T, et al. Remifentanil in obstetric analgesia: a dose-finding study. Anesth Analg. 2002;94:913-7.
14. Lei X, Guo Q, Zhang J. Mechanistic insights into neurotoxicity induced by anesthetics in the developing brain. Int J Mol Sci. 2012;13:6772-99.
15. Roelants F, De Franceschi E, Veyckemans F, et al. Patient-controlled intravenous analgesia using remifentanil in the parturient. Can J Anaesth. 2001;48:175-8.
16. Schnabel A, Hahn N, Broscheit J, et al. Remifentanil for labour analgesia: a meta-analysis of randomised controlled trials. Eur J Anaesthesiol. 2012;29:177-85.
17. Liu Z-Q, Chen X-B, Li H-B, et al. A comparison of remifentanil parturient-controlled intravenous analgesia with epidural analgesia: a meta-analysis of randomized controlled trials. Anesth Analg. 2014;118:598-603.
18. Simmons SW, Cyna AM, Dennis AT, et al. Combined spinal-epidural versus epidural analgesia in labour. Cochrane Database Syst Rev. 2007;3:CD003401.
19. Simmons SW, Taghizadeh N, Dennis AT, et al. Combined spinal-epidural versus epidural analgesia in labour. Cochrane Database Syst Rev. 2012;10:CD003401.
20. Freeman LM, Bloemenkamp KW, Franssen MT, et al. Patient controlled analgesia with remifentanil versus epidural analgesia in labour: randomised multicentre equivalence trial. BMJ. 2015;350:h846.
21. Volmanen P, Akural E, Raudaskoski T, et al. Comparison of remifentanil and nitrous oxide in labour analgesia. Acta Anaesthesiol Scand. 2005;49:453-8.
22. Hinova A, Fernando R. Systemic remifentanil for labor analgesia. Anesth Analg. 2009;109:1925-9.
23. Douma MR, Verwey RA, Kam-Endtz CE, et al. Obstetric analgesia: a comparison of patient-controlled meperidine, remifentanil, and fentanyl in labour. Brit J Anaesth. 2010;104:209-15.
24. Marwah R, Hassan S, Carvalho JCA, et al. Remifentanil versus fentanyl for intravenous patient-controlled labour analgesia: an observational study. Can J Anaesth 2012;59:246-54.
25. Devabhakthuni S. Efficacy and safety of remifentanil as an alternative labor analgesic. Clin Med Insights Womens Health. 2013;6:37-49.
26. Bonner JC, McClymont W. Respiratory arrest in an obstetric patient using remifentanil patient-controlled analgesia. Anaesthesia. 2012;67:538-40.
27. Singh P. Remifentanil — was it only respiratory arrest? Anaesthesia. 2012;67:1044.
28. D'Onofrio P, Novelli AMM, Mecacci F, et al. The efficacy and safety of continuous intravenous administration of remifentanil for birth pain relief: an open study of 205 parturients. Anesth Analg. 2009;109:1922-4.
29. Shen MK, Wu ZF, Zhu AB, et al. Remifentanil for labour analgesia: a double-blinded, randomised controlled trial of maternal and neonatal effects of patient-controlled analgesia versus continuous infusion. Anaesthesia. 2013;68:236-44.
30. Balki M, Kasodekar S, Dhumne S, et al. Remifentanil patient-controlled analgesia for labour: optimizing drug delivery regimens. Can J Anaesth. 2007;54:626-33.
31. Singh PM, Borle A, Goudra BG. Use of computer-assisted drug therapy outside the operating room. Curr Opin Anaesthesiol. 2016;29:506-11.
32. Schwarz GL, Volmanen P, Albrechtsen S, et al. Remifentanil target-controlled infusion during second stage labour in high-risk parturients: a case series. Acta Anaesthesiol Scand. 2013;57:802-8.

CHAPTER 5

Low Flow Anesthesia: Revisited and Reiterated

Asha Tyagi, Rashmi Salhotra

KEY POINTS

- Reduction of fresh gas flows utilized during general anesthesia provides a scope for containment of healthcare cost. Additionally, it helps in reducing the global pollution levels and improving the heat and humidity levels of the inhaled gases which are otherwise cold and dry.
- There are many definitions of low flow anesthesia, however, the key concept is that at least 50% of the expired gases are rebreathed after carbon dioxide removal and fresh flow rate used is less than the patient's minute ventilation.
- The essential equipment to deliver low flow anesthesia is a circle system with a soda lime absorber, an anesthesia machine capable of delivering reduced flows without any significant leaks, a flow compensated vaporizer for delivery of the anesthetic agent, and oxygen and carbon dioxide analyzers.
- The conduct of low flow anesthesia can be divided into three phases: initiation (where there is 'wash-in' of volatile anesthetic along with denitrogenation), maintenance, and termination (where there is 'wash-out' of the volatile anesthestic agent).
- Understanding of time constant and uptake mechanics of anesthetic gases and agents is central to implementing low flow anesthesia safely.
- The concerns with the use of sevoflurane and production of compound A in low flow anesthesia have been more theoretical than real. It is, in fact, one of the better suited agents for this technique based on its pharmacological profile.
- With the use of modern anesthesia machines, vaporizers inside the circuit and respiratory gas monitoring systems, low flow anesthesia can be conducted with great safety in the hands of experienced anesthesiologists.

INTRODUCTION

The term "low flow anesthesia" was introduced by Foldes in 1952 for an anesthetic technique performed with a fresh gas flow rate of 1 liter/min.[1] The evolution of "low flow" anesthesia can be explained by a logically driven need to decrease the flow rates of gases used during anesthesia. Buying and supplying gases involves a cost, as for all drugs. Several studies have now conclusively proven that low fresh gas flow rates are associated with significantly lower consumption and cost of inhalational agents, besides the saving in carrier gases such as oxygen, nitrous oxide and air. Lower flow rates would also favor environmental concerns by decreasing the pollution inside operating rooms.

The use of the semi-open or open anesthesia breathing system entails an obligatory loss of the gases to the environment. This stems from using a minimum fresh gas flow to avoid rebreathing and consequent build-up of carbon dioxide in the breathing system and its inhalation by the patient. With the advent of absorptive elements such as caustic potash followed by soda lime, lowering of gas flows became a clinical reality in anesthesia. The "Waters-to-and-fro" canister was simple but voluminous equipment that contained soda lime for carbon dioxide absorption, while the inhaled and exhaled gases passed through it in reverse directions. It had the disadvantage of potential for dust inhalation into patient's airways. In case of soda lime exhaustion the entire canister could pose as a dead space.

The use of a circle system wherein the inspiratory and expiratory gases follow dedicated paths in a circular motion, with a canister containing soda lime for carbon dioxide absorption circumvented the disadvantages associated with Water's canister. The first circle system for delivering closed system anesthesia is credited to Brian Sword.

Low flow anesthesia appears to have been variably defined at several volumes ≤ 4 liters/minute. Baum defined it as a flow rate that forces at least 50% of the expired gases to be redelivered to the patient, albeit after carbon dioxide removal.[2] In clinical practice it mostly implies the use of a flow rate less than the patient's minute ventilation, or less than 2 liters/minute.[2]

In ideal situations, with a completely closed anesthetic delivery system the flow of gases can be dropped to a minimum level wherein only the volumes taken up by the patient are replaced (metabolic flow). Since this is more or less an extreme scenario wherein there are no leaks anywhere in the anesthesia delivery system thus being completely closed, it is difficult to be practiced in most real life clinical situations.

A useful classification of low flow anesthesia based on the volumes used includes the extremely reduced metabolic flow (250 mL/min); minimal flow (250–500 mL/min); low flow (500–1000 mL/min); medium flow (1–2 liter/min); or high flow (2–4 liter/min).[3]

BASIC PHYSIOLOGIC CONCEPTS RELEVANT TO APPLICATION OF LOW FLOW ANESTHESIA

Uptake of Anesthetic Agents and Gases

As the fresh gas flow rates are decreased, the fraction of rebreathed gas increases making mandatory a greater precision on anesthetic agent or gas delivery. Considering that a mixture of oxygen, nitrous oxide and volatile anesthetic agent is to be delivered during low flow anesthesia, the aim would be to ensure adequate replacement of the three constituents matching their uptake by the patient. The uptake of each of these three constituents is different and can be approximated.

The distinction between uptake of the three constituents is that for oxygen it is fairly constant during anesthesia, unlike for nitrous oxide and anesthetic agent. Uptake of oxygen can be given by Brody's formula wherein it equals 10 × weight in $kg^{3/4}$ (mL/min).

The uptake of nitrous oxide depends largely on the concentration gradient between the alveoli and venous blood. Uptake is thus very rapid initially when there is no nitrous oxide in venous blood while alveolar concentrations build up fast with inhalation, and it then slows down with time. Severinghaus formula represents uptake of nitrous oxide as $1000 \times t^{-1/2}$ (mL/min).

The uptake of volatile anesthetic agents is also rapid initially but is affected by a number of factors including desired concentration and solubility as well as the cardiac output. According to Lowe's formula the uptake of anesthetic agent can be calculated as the product: $f \times MAC \times \lambda B/G \times Q \times t^{-1/2}$ (mL/min).

Concept of Time Constant

To understand the time required for attaining desired anesthetic agent or gas concentration in the breathing system and consequently patient's alveoli, concept of "time constant" needs to be recalled. For low flow anesthesia, time constant is a measure of the time taken for alterations of the fresh-gas composition to lead to corresponding alterations of the gas composition within the breathing system.[4] As a numerical value, the time constant describes the speed of any exponential process. The concept is thus applicable to the wash-in or wash-out of the anesthetic agent or the gas, being exponential in nature.

As per the concept of a time constant, at the end of one time constant, the concentration of the anesthetic agent or gas in the system will have reached 63% of final value. After two time constants, it will have reached 86.5%, and after three about 95% of the alteration in the agent's fresh gas concentration will have taken place.

Based on the calculation formula given by Conway[4] time constant (T) is proportional to the volume of the system including the anesthetic circuit and the lungs (VS); and inversely proportional to the difference between the amount of anesthetic agent delivered into the breathing system (VD) and the individual uptake (VU) at a particular time.

i.e. T = VS / (VD – VU)

When the vaporizer is switched on initially, the VD will be directly proportional to the fresh gas flow. Since T is inversely proportional to VD, this implies that the time constant is inversely proportional to the flow rate itself. Thus, higher the fresh gas flow rate, shorter is the time constant; and lower the flow rate longer is the time constant. The clinical implication of the inverse relationship between flow rate and time constant results in a considerable time delay between altering anesthetic gas composition at site of delivery and producing corresponding change within the breathing system when low flows are used.

The time constant, additionally, will also be affected by solubility of the anesthetic agent since it affects the VU, i.e. uptake. Time constant will be more prolonged when the individual anesthetic uptake or solubility of the anesthetic agent is higher. The prolonged time constants must be taken into account whenever the anesthetic concentration is changed during low flow anesthesia.

PHASES OF LOW FLOW ANESTHESIA IN CLINICAL PRACTICE

Three distinct phases of low flow anesthesia with differing concerns and principles can be delineated including induction, maintenance and termination.

Induction Phase

During induction, there are certain factors that retard the attainment of adequate anesthetic agent or gas concentration in the alveoli.

Firstly, there is a rapid and large uptake of nitrous oxide as well as anesthetic agent at beginning of anesthesia, making alveolar concentrations so much harder to be achieved. Secondly, lowered flow rates will make the time required for wash-in of the agents or gases slower than with higher flows (prolonged time constant). Lastly, the presence of nitrogen in the lung volume and breathing system also poses as a hindrance in attaining adequate anesthetic concentration. The uptake of anesthetic agent or gas from the lung being large in the beginning causes the concentration of the insoluble nitrogen to increase, diluting the alveolar concentration of anesthetic agent even further.

It is thus always advisable to denitrogenate the breathing system and functional residual capacity of the lungs. Assuming this volume to be a 6-7 liters and 3 liters respectively, each would yield a total of 10 liters to be denitrogenated. Also, time constant can be expressed as a function of the volume of system divided by gas flow rate, since delivered anesthetic agent depends on the flow rate in beginning. This implies that at a flow rate of 1 liter/min, the time constant to denitrogenate 10 liters of volume and make it equilibrate with the composition of fresh gas being would be $10/1 = 10$ minutes. Thus, three time constants, i.e. almost 30 minutes would be needed to denitrogenate the volume to 95% at a flow of 1 liter/minute. This makes use of low flows undesirable at beginning of induction.

Keeping these requirements in mind, following modifications in technique are suggested for induction.

- **Initial period of high flow:** Use of high flows for a short period of time reduces the time constant and thus the required inhaled concentration of anesthetic agent and denitrogenation is attained faster. It remains the commonest method of induction during low flow anesthesia. The use of a fresh gas flow of 10 liters/minute and 2MAC of anesthetic agent concentration has been advocated.[5] The only disadvantage is that it uses high flows which offsets the advantage of economy but the higher flows are used only for a very short period of time. This is also known as 'loading' the circuit.[6] Another recommendation is to use a flow equalling minute ventilation and 3MAC concentration of anesthetic agent;[6] or a flow of 4 liters/minute for 10-20 minutes to achieve anesthetic agent and gas equilibrium between the breathing system and delivered concentrations.[7] The precise time of high flow is best monitored by attainment of desired gas concentration, adequate depth of anesthesia and complete denitrogenation.[7]

- **Larger concentrations of inhaled anesthetic with reduced flows:** If the flow rates are kept lowered from the beginning, using larger concentrations of the anesthetic agent can help achieve desired alveolar concentration rapidly despite the rapid uptake. Usually, 400-500 mL of vapor of anesthetic agent is required over first 10 minutes of anesthesia. This translates to $400-500/10 = 40-50$ mL vapor per minute. At a flow rate of 1 liter/minute, 50 mL vapor would be delivered at a raised vaporizer output of 5%. Thus an initial high concentration for 10 minutes may be required at lowered flows, followed by decrease in the vaporizer output concentration. However, the effect of rapid uptake of nitrous oxide cannot be overcome by this technique. There will be a deficiency of gas volume in the system.

Such an alternative method of using low flow anesthesia mandates using rates as low as 1/10th of the patient's minute ventilation right from the beginning to the end of the anesthetic procedure aiming to minimize the consumption of inhalational agent.[8] This was proposed with desflurane after performing induction with intravenous propofol. The flow rates of 10 mL/kg/min were initiated and the desflurane vaporizer set to its maximum output value of 18%. Once the end-tidal desflurane concentration reached 6–7%, vaporizer setting was reduced to 10%. After some time, an increase in the end-tidal desflurane concentration was seen, indicating the end of the high uptake phase. The vaporizer was then set at 1–2% above the end-tidal value to maintain the desired desflurane concentration. The authors concluded that despite maintaining low FGF rates from the beginning, it was easy to maintain the end-tidal concentration of desflurane in the desired range. The alternative method of low flow technique has also been used successfully with sevoflurane.[9]

- **Injection of anesthetic agent into breathing system:** An alternative technique for delivery of precise quantity of anesthetic agent includes the injection of liquid anesthetic directly into the circuit. However, though this technique allows rapid changes in concentration of delivered anesthetic, concerns exist regarding its safety, particularly with controlled ventilation, since dangerously high anesthetic concentrations may be rapidly achieved.[10]

The induction phase can be thus shortened by increasing the initial high fresh gas flow rate, or selecting an anesthetic agent with low blood solubility and correspondingly low uptake like sevoflurane or desflurane, or increasing the initial delivery of the anesthetic agent by setting a high concentration on the vaporizer, or going for stepwise gradual reduction in the flow rate, e.g. reducing the flow to 2 L/min after the initial 5 minutes, to 1 L/min after 10 min and, finally, to 0.5 L/min after 15 minutes.[7]

Maintenance Phase

For maintenance of anesthesia using low flow technique the emphasis remains on avoiding a hypoxic mixture, ensuring adequate depth by titrating anesthetic agent and being aware of methods to rapidly change the anesthetic agent or gas concentrations.

- **Avoiding hypoxic mixture:** Administration of hypoxic mixture is to be continuously guarded against during low flow technique. At high gas flows, the oxygen concentration in the fresh gas is similar to that in the breathing system. Once the flows are lowered, the fraction of expired/rebreathed air in the breathing system increases thus lowering the oxygen concentration. The precise concentration will depend upon quantum of reduction of flow, and individual oxygen consumption. In addition, since nitrous oxide uptake is rapid in the beginning and decreases with time, its concentration in the breathing system will also rise with time and affect the relative oxygen concentration. After 60 min of anesthesia with 50% nitrous oxide in oxygen, uptake of nitrous oxide is only 130 mL/min, while oxygen uptake remains constant at about 200–250 mL/min.[11] Also, nitrogen can accumulate in a low-flow system as it is excreted from blood, unless high fresh-gas flows have been used initially.

   Since inspired oxygen concentration in breathing system is flow dependent, while the percentage of oxygen should be increased to 40–50% with low flows it should be 50–60% with minimal flows.[7] Another recommended technique is to alter the oxygen percentage with time wherein oxygen and nitrous oxide are used in volumes of 400 mL and 600 mL for initial 20 minutes following a period of denitrogenation with high flows. After 20 minutes of maintenance with low flows, volume of oxygen is increased and nitrous oxide decreased (500 mL each) since the uptake of nitrous oxide would have fallen thus increasing its concentration and lowering inspired oxygen in the breathing system.[6] In clinical practice it is known that due to all the above influences, the inspired oxygen concentration in the breathing system varies continuously and hence its monitoring is highly recommended.[7]

- **Adjusting delivery of anesthetic agent:** Another goal during maintenance with low flow technique is to ensure an adequate depth of anesthesia by titrating delivery of the volatile anesthetic agent. The uptake of anesthetic agent is initially more rapid and depends on its potency, solubility and cardiac output.

  Similar to difference in inspired oxygen concentration and that in delivered fresh gas with reduction of flows, the concentration of anesthetic agent also varies. Due to anesthetic agent uptake its concentration in breathing system is less than that set on vaporizer. As flow rates are lowered and the rebreathing fraction in breathing system increases, the concentration of anesthetic agent is diluted secondary to ongoing uptake. As a result the vaporizer setting has to be considerably higher than intended inspired concentration during induction, and lower during termination.

  Another concern during maintenance phase is that whatever change is intended in inspired anesthetic agent or gas takes longer to implement than with high flows. This is because of the increase in time constant as a consequence of lowered flows. To rapidly change the inspired anesthetic agent or gas concentration transient increase in gas flows can be used till a new equilibrium is attained.[7]

  Adequate dosing of anesthetic agent was more difficult and unpredictable with the earlier vaporizer-inside-circle system. With the use of low fresh-gas flows and a vaporizer inside the circuit, the concentration of the volatile anesthetic agent delivered to the patient could reach up to five times that set on the vaporizer after only a few minutes.[12] Also the older vaporizers used outside the circle systems which were not flow compensated could also deliver higher concentrations than that set on the dial. The modern day vaporizers are flow compensated and have overcome these limitations.

- **Avoiding leaks in the system:** Any leaks in the system have to be guarded against since the effect on gas volume loss may become significant. A potential source of gas loss is side-stream gas analyzers that may entrain 100–200 mL/min. These can be returned to the expiratory limb of the breathing system to minimize loss especially with minimal or metabolic flows.[10]

Termination Phase

During termination of low flow technique for emergence of the patient, the primary concern is the increased duration required for wash-out of the anesthetic agent and gas. This is because of the long time constant due to lowered flows. The time required will depend upon the extent of flow reduction used and duration of anesthesia.

Intuitively it appears that less soluble agents such as sevoflurane and desflurane will be washed-out of the body earlier with more rapid recovery. However, if the low flows are continued the washed-out agent will merely recirculate in the breathing system and be inspired again. The variations in recovery profile due to agent solubility will manifest only with high gas flows. Thus in clinical practice recovery profile with agents of differing solubility is largely similar when using low flows.[7]

With minimal flows being used, the vaporizer can be switched off 10 minutes prior to expected end of surgery. If the duration of anesthesia was prolonged, the vaporizer may be switched off even earlier. End of procedure requires a brief duration of high flows to eliminate the nitrous oxide as well.

Another method for expediting emergence is the use of activated charcoal to adsorb the anesthetic agent while nitrous oxide is washed out at the very end using high flows.[13] A separate charcoal containing canister is required for this, through which the gases are diverted at end of surgery.[14]

USE OF NITROUS OXIDE DURING LOW FLOW TECHNIQUE

The disadvantages of nitrous oxide are known and remain irrespective of the flow rates used.[15] Enthusiasts for use of nitrous oxide with low flows emphasize on the use of closed system eliminating the threat of environmental pollution, and using its advantageous effects such as decrease in opioid and anesthetic agent requirement as well as faster induction. However, using air instead of nitrous oxide for low flow technique makes the conduct safe and easy, and also circumvents the disadvantages seen with nitrous oxide.

EQUIPMENT AND MONITORING REQUIREMENTS

To conduct low flow anesthesia, certain mandatory requirements should be met. The most obvious would be a carbon dioxide absorber present in the breathing system. The anesthesia machine flow meters should have graduations showing the low flow range and small alterations in flow of the carrier gases, preferably with a minimum of 50 mL/min and graduations of 10 mL/min to enable extreme reductions.

The rebreathing system should not have a leak greater than 100 mL/min.[6,14] The ventilator should be fresh gas flow compensated, i.e. able to deliver the tidal volume irrespective of the flow rates being used. There are various modalities such as fresh gas decoupling valve or closed loop feedback system for achieving the same.[7]

Monitoring of inspiratory oxygen and end-tidal carbon dioxide are also a must, more so than with high flows. Changes in inspired oxygen can be caused by individual oxygen consumption, and any deleterious effect will be more pronounced at low flows. It should be remembered that while carbon dioxide build up in a system could be slow at high flows the effect will be fast at low flows. With the use of low flow technique the capnograph curves may not show the typical waveform, with slightly ascending expiratory plateau due to contamination of inspired gas with expired gas.

Monitoring of the volatile anesthetic agent concentration is also recommended. The delivered concentration is different from that in the breathing system, depending on the fresh gas flow used. The lower the flow, greater the discrepancy between the two. Minute ventilation as well as airway pressure monitoring is highly desirable. If at any stage the volume supplied into the breathing system is lesser than taken up by the patient, minute ventilation as well as airway pressures will fall. The vaporizer should be able to deliver accurate concentrations at low flows also, a feature that most modern day vaporizers possess.

SEVOFLURANE, COMPOUND A AND NEPHROTOXICITY

Sevoflurane interacts with carbon dioxide absorbents and forms fluoromethyl-2-2-difluoro-1-(trifluoromethyl) vinyl ether, commonly referred to as compound A. Compound A has been the subject of intense research and controversy after it was initially suggested that it could cause renal injury in rats.[16] This and other studies suggested a threshold for renal injury of compound A levels of 25-50 ppm or more.[17,18] Subsequently, numerous studies in surgical patients as well as human volunteers have attempted to evaluate possible renal injury following sevoflurane anesthesia as a result of compound A formation. It is now noted that there are marked differences between human and rat renal biochemistry.[19] It therefore appears that compound A is of theoretical concern and academic interest only; and to date, no significant clinical renal toxicity has been associated with the use of sevoflurane. It is therefore now generally believed that compound A is considerably safe in humans at the concentrations typically found during LFA with sevoflurane.[19]

The specific concern about compound A had led the Food and Drugs Administration (regulatory body for the USA) to set a 1 liter/min lower limit for flow rate during sevoflurane anesthesia with a 2 MAC-hour exposure limit for rates between 1 and 2 liter/min. In December 1997, this was revised to 1 liter/min while no restriction was ever imposed in the UK.[19]

ACCUMULATION OF TRACE GASES WITH LOW FLOW ANESTHESIA

Trace gases may accumulate during low flow anesthesia. These could include those with low solubility such as methane, nitrogen and hydrogen; or those with high solubility such as acetone, ethanol or carbon monoxide. Gases with low solubility are relatively innocuous and can be flushed with intermittent high flows, but those with high solubility cannot be simply flushed out. Therefore, it has been recommended that patients with pre-existing comorbidities should receive a fresh gas flow of at least 1 liter/min. Acetone and ethanol concentrations do not reach harmful levels with these flows and carbon monoxide does not seem to accumulate in large amounts.[20,21]

ADVANTAGES OF LOW FLOW ANESTHESIA

Economic

Baum[22] theorized that if all anesthetists in Germany and the United Kingdom were to switch to using low flows (1 liter/min) instead of high flows (4 liter/min), then, over an average year, the reduction in consumption of inhalational agent in these two countries alone could be projected to include 33,000 liters of liquid isoflurane and 46,000 liters of liquid enflurane, in addition to 350 million liters of oxygen and 1000 million liters of nitrous oxide.

Preservation of Heat and Humidity

Appropriate humidification and warming of anesthetic gases can have a significant impact on the function and integrity of tracheal mucosa. During anesthesia, the absolute humidity of the inspired gas mixture should range between 17 and 30 mg H_2O/L and its temperature should range between 28 and 32°C. These values can be achieved with the use of low flow anesthesia.[22]

Environmental Concerns

Concerns exist about the operating room exposure to anesthetic agents and environmental pollution. Chlorinated hydrocarbons are broken down by ultraviolet radiation releasing chlorine atoms, which deplete the protective ozone layer. While chlorinated hydrocarbons anesthetics contribute only around 0.01% of the global release of chlorofluorocarbons, reduction of unnecessary waste of anesthetic gases could reduce this further. Nitrous oxide depletes ozone through nitric oxide production, and also reflects heat back to the earth, contributing directly to global warming. Using low flow anesthesia could reduce the wastage of nitrous oxide as well.[23] The concentration of anesthetic gases in the vicinity of the anesthesia machine is found to be 40–150% higher with high flow anesthesia as compared with anesthesia practiced with rates of 1.5 liters/min.

RISKS ASSOCIATED WITH LOW-FLOW ANESTHESIA

Low flow anesthesia had lost its popularity due to certain risks associated with its inappropriate use. These can include accidental hypoxia, over- or underdosage of volatile anesthetics, hypercapnia or accumulation of potentially toxic trace gases. However, with the advent of sophisticated equipment and a thorough understanding of the uptake kinetics of anesthetic gases it remains an efficacious technique in the armamentarium of the anesthesiologists.[2]

WHY A NEED TO REVISIT LOW FLOW ANESTHESIA?

The concepts involved in low flow anesthesia are well evidenced. It is known to be associated with economical and environmental advantages along with indirect benefits of improved pulmonary dynamics of the anesthetic gases, increased mucociliary clearance, maintained body temperature and reduced fluid loss.[24] However, the relevance of revisiting it remains since it has been noted that continued and persistent education and advocacy of low flow technique is required to continue reaping its benefits.[25]

CONCLUSION

The clinical application of low flow anesthesia requires a thorough understanding of pharmacology and uptake of inhalational anesthetic agents and gases. The concept of wash-in and wash out of the inhalational anesthetic agents are key to its practice. The modern anesthesia machines and the anesthetic agents like sevoflurane and desflurane, which are less soluble, are best suited to the conduct of low flow anesthesia. It is important to have an oxygen analyzer which would guard against the delivery of hypoxic mixture to the patient as the flows are reduced. Monitoring of carbon dioxide levels in the inspired air is useful to guard against hypercarbia and detect the absorber exhaustion. The technique has the advantages of economy, less pollution and preservation of heat and humidity.

REFERENCES

1. Foldes FF, Ceravolo AJ, Carpenter SL. The administration of nitrous oxide- oxygen anesthesia in closed systems. Ann Surg. 1952;136:978-81.
2. Baum JA, Aitkenhead AR. Low-flow anesthesia. Anesthesia. 1995;50:37-44.
3. Baker AB. Back to basics—a simplified non-mathematical approach to low flow techniques in anesthesia. Anaesth Intensive Care. 1994;22:394-5.
4. Conway M. Closed and low-flow systems. Theoretical considerations. Acta Anaesthesiological Belgica. 1984;34:257-63.
5. Mapleson W. The theoretical ideal fresh gas flow sequence at the start of low flow anesthesia. Anesthesia. 1998;53:264-72.
6. Low Flow Anesthesia-revisited [Internet]. Available from www.isapondicherry.in/sites/default/files/. Accessed on 25.5.17.
7. Low Flow Anesthesia [Internet]. Available from https://www.draeger.com/Products/Content/m-644-. Accessed on 2.6.17.
8. Ponz L, Saenz J, Garcia J, Iraeta H. An alternative method for low flow anesthesia with Desflurane: A-956. Eur J Anaesth. 2006;23:246.
9. Tyagi A, Venkateswaran V, Jain AK, et al. Cost analysis of three techniques of administering sevoflurane. Anesthesiol Res Pract. 2014;2014:459432.
10. Baum JA. Technical requirements for anesthesia management with reduced fresh gas flow. In: Baum JA (Ed). Low Flow Anesthesia: The Theory and Practice of Low Flow, Minimal Flow and Closed System Anesthesia. Oxford: Butterworth Heinemann; 1996. pp. 87-128.
11. Conway CM. Anesthetic breathing systems. In: Scurr C, Feldman F (Eds). Scientific Foundations of Anesthesia, 3rd edn. London: William Heinemann; 1982. pp. 557-66.
12. Mapleson W. The concentration of anesthetics in closed circuits: theoretical study. Br J Anaesth. 1960;32:298-309.
13. Jantzen JP. More on black and white granules in the closed circuit. Anesthesiology 1988;69:437-8.
14. Low flow anesthesia [Internet]. Available from www.isakanyakumari.com/CASCO2012/CME/I%20A%2010.pdf. Accessed on 8.6.17.
15. Joshi GP, Pennant JH, Kehlet H. Evaluation of nitrous oxide in the gas mixture for anesthesia (ENIGMA) studies: the tale of two large pragmatic randomized controlled trials. Anesth Analg. 2017;124:2077-9.
16. Morio M, Fujii K, Satoh N, et al. Reaction of sevoflurane and its degradation products woth soda lime. Toxicity of the byproducts. Anesthesiology. 1992;77:1155-64.
17. Gonsowski CT, Latser MJ, Eger EI 2nd, et al. Toxicity of compound A in rats. Effect of a 3-hour administration. Anesthesiology. 1994;80:556-65.
18. Keller KA, Callan C, Prokocimer P, et al. Inhalation toxicity study of a haloalkene degradant of sevoflurane, compound A (PIFE) in Sprague-Dawley rats. Anesthesiology. 1995;83:1220-32.
19. Nunn G. Low-flow anesthesia. Contin Educ Anaesth Crit Care Pain. 2008;8:1-4.
20. Strauss JM, Hausdorfer J. Accumulation of acetone in blood during long-term anesthesia with closed system. Br J Anaesth. 1993;70:363-4.

21. Strauss JM, Bannasch W, Hausdorfer J, et al. Die Entwicklung von Carboxyhemoglobin wahrend Langzeitnarkosen im geschlossenen Kreissystem. Anaesthesist. 1991; 40:324-7.
22. Baum JA. Advantages of rebreathing. In: Baum JA (Ed). Low Flow Anesthesia: The Theory and Practice of Low Flow, Minimal Flow and Closed System Anesthesia. Oxford: Butterworth Heinemann; 1996. pp. 70-84.
23. Logan M, Farmer JG. Anesthesia and the ozone layer. Br J Anaesth. 1989;63:645-7.
24. Hönemann C, Hagemann O, Doll D. Inhalational anesthesia with low fresh gas flow. Indian J Anaesth. 2013;57:345-50.
25. Ryu HG, Lee JH, Lee KK, et al. The effect of low fresh gas flow rate on sevoflurane consumption. Korean J Anesthesiol. 2011;60:75-7.

CHAPTER 6

Local Anesthetic Systemic Toxicity

Nishkarsh Gupta, Anju Gupta

KEY POINTS

- Local anesthetic induced systemic toxicity (LAST) is a grave complication of regional anesthesia which can be rapidly fatal and refractory to resuscitation.
- Best bet in preventing LAST occurrence is in being prepared, sensible and vigilant.
- High index of suspicion should be maintained for LAST in any patient with altered mental status, seizure or cardiovascular symptoms following a regional blockade.
- Indication of lipid emulsion (LE) use in a patient with suspected LAST depends on its clinical severity and rate of progression.
- Early use of LE is now being recommended after management of airway, so as to prevent progression of LAST to cardiovascular collapse rather than treat it once it has set in.
- Use of ultrasonography guidance for regional blocks has shown encouraging evidence in reduction in incidence of LAST and should be a rule rather than exception in years to follow.

INTRODUCTION

Local anesthetic (LA) drugs have a vast safety record when used in appropriate dosages and routes.[1-3] However, they have the propensity to cause adverse reactions which can range from mild nonspecific symptoms to severe life-threatening systemic toxicity. Increased plasma levels due to inadvertent intravascular injection or use of high dose in normal anatomic site can lead to cardiac arrest in an otherwise healthy patient which can be refractory to standard resuscitative measures.[1,2] Fortunately, local-anesthetic systemic toxicity (LAST) is rare and usually limited to mild nonspecific symptoms.[1] Nevertheless, LAST continues to be of serious concern as it can be rapidly fatal depending on the rate of rise of plasma concentration of the LA. Last decade has seen increasing awareness of this complication and there has been focus on the treatment of LAST. This chapter intends to provide an overview of LAST and its treatment with lipid emulsion.

INCIDENCE

Clinical evidence suggests that LAST from the use LAs is rare.[1,4-6] A series involving 20,000 patients having peripheral nerve blocks, reported low incidence of LAST with majority of cases manifesting only mild symptoms, and only one case progressing to cardiac arrest.[4] Another large surveillance report of French anesthesiologists also reported a low incidence of seizures (0 to 25 in 10,000), and no episode of cardiac arrest due to LAST.[5] LA toxicity may occur in 2.5 to

20 per 10,000 peripheral nerve blocks[5,6] and about 1.2–11 per 10,000 epidurals.[5,7] Notwithstanding, analysis of closed malpractice claims in the United States from 1980 to 1999, revealed that epidural anesthesia (primarily obstetrical) was responsible for all the cases of death or brain damage due to unintentional intravenous injection of LA.[8]

PATHOPHYSIOLOGY

Local anesthetics block the voltage gated sodium channels and thus inhibit the generation and propagation of nerve impulses. The degree of nerve blockade depends on both drug concentration and its volume.[1,2,9] LA exists as ionized and unionized form (which crosses the cell membrane) in the plasma. The relative proportion of the two fractions depends on their pKa.[9] Agents with a pKa value near 7.4 permits more LA in the lipid soluble unionized form to enter the cell. Another important physiochemical property of LA compounds is their hydrophobicity which is expressed as octanol-buffer partition coefficient and is proportional to the bulk of alkyl substituents on its aromatic ring and tertiary amine.[9,10] High lipophilicity increases the potency and the duration of block.

Barring lignocaine, all the other amide LAs have an asymmetric carbon atom and exist as enantiomers, i.e. stereoisomers differing in the arrangement at the asymmetric or chiral carbon atom. Though structurally identical, these molecules have different affinity at various effector sites. In particular, the dose required to cause lethality is 78% greater with levobupivacaine compared to its R-(+) enantiomer.[9] Occurrence of LAST after injection depends on many factors including dose and concentration of LA, lipophilicity of LA, site of injection, plasma protein binding, and patient risk factors (Table 1).[1-3,9-11] Although maximum permissible

Table 1: Causes and risk factors of LAST	
Factors affecting occurrence of LAST	
Drug	Potency (lipophilicity) Dose (volume and concentration) Rate of injection Stereoselectivity (racemic mixture/pure enantiomer)[13] Intrinsic vasoconstrictor action Addition of vasoconstrictor (epinephrine/phenylephrine)[9]
Site of blockade	Decreasing toxicity from head to foot Intercostal > caudal and epidural > brachial plexus > femoral and sciatic nerve block[9,10,12]
Patient risk factors	Extremes of age Pregnancy Respiratory/metabolic acidosis
	Hypoxia Hyperkalemia Drug interaction (class I antiarrhythmics, beta-blockers, calcium channel blockers) Genetic predisposition Cardiac disease Renal disease Hepatic disease

doses have been recommended for all LAs, systemic LA levels may vary considerably, depending on site of injection and the particular drug. When 1000 mg lignocaine is injected subcutaneously, it results in similar plasma concentration as its half dose injected epidurally or one third injected via intercostal route.[12] LA toxicity can be potentiated by certain patient factors (extremes of age, acidosis, hypoxia, cardiovascular disease, liver disease, hypoproteinemia), concomitantly administered drugs (lignocaine, phenytoin, beta-blockers, sodium channel blockers) and mitochondriopathies.[9,10,12]

SIGNS AND SYMPTOMS

Injection of toxic amounts of LA drug systemically can manifest as either central nervous system or cardiovascular symptoms. LAST may present immediately (within 60 s) due to intravascular injection of LA with direct access to the brain. A late presentation (after 1–5 mins) may occur due to intermittent intravascular injection, lower extremity injection, or delayed tissue absorption.[14]

Central Nervous System Toxicity

Local anesthetics can readily cross the blood-brain barrier and the potential for central nervous system (CNS) toxicity correlates directly with the potency of LAs. At low plasma concentration, mild subjective symptoms appear, such as light-headedness, dizziness, disorientation and drowsiness. Circumoral and tongue numbness and metallic taste in mouth are the earliest indication of CNS toxicity.[6,14,15] Sensory system disturbances like visual and auditory symptoms (difficulty in focusing and tinnitus) may also occur. With increasing plasma concentration, CNS excitatory symptoms including shivering, nystagmus, muscular twitching, and tremors of facial muscles and distal parts of the extremities predominate. Eventually, generalized tonic clonic convulsions may occur. However, if sedatives drugs have been coadministered, CNS depression can occur without a preceding excitatory phase.[3,14,15] This can lead to masking of the valuable initial warning signs and direct progression to cardiovascular toxicity.

CNS excitation is purported to be the result of blockade of inhibitory pathways in the cerebral cortex by LAs, thus allowing facilitatory neurons to function unopposed.[6,15] Uncontrolled convulsions can lead to acidosis (both respiratory and metabolic) which further potentiates CNS toxicity. Increased $PaCO_2$ enhances cerebral blood flow and thereby, LA delivery to the brain.[2,6,15] Also, decreased intracellular pH due to neuronal diffusion of CO_2 facilitates conversion of the unionized LA to the protonated form which cannot diffuse out and hence aggravate CNS toxicity.[2,15] Hence, in case of LAST, it is of utmost importance to promptly assist ventilation and circulation as needed to prevent hypercapnia, acidosis and hypoxemia.

Cardiovascular Toxicity of Local Anesthetics

Cardiovascular toxicity of LAs usually heralds at a plasma concentration far exceeding that for CNS toxicity but the underlying pathophysiology has not been fully elucidated. LAs exert their cardiotoxicity primarily by a dose-dependent blockage of sodium channels (cardiac myocyte-specific voltage-gated sodium channel), which decreases the rate of depolarization in the conducting tissues of

Purkinje fibers and ventricular muscle.[16,17] This leads to a prolonged PR interval and QRS complex. Higher concentrations of LAs depress spontaneous pacemaker activity in the sinus node and lead to sinus bradycardia and arrest. LAs have also been shown to antagonize the intracellular calcium and potassium currents.[17] Apart from these direct cardiac effects, action on the brainstem leading to impaired arterial baroreceptor reflex attenuates the heart rate response to changes in systemic blood pressure.[16,17] Lastly, individuals with L-carnitine deficiency exhibit an increased susceptibility to LA associated cardiac toxicity, suggesting that they also affect mitochondrial function and fatty acid metabolism.[18] LAs also have a biphasic effect on blood vessels causing direct vasoconstriction at low plasma levels and vasodilation at higher levels.[19] The potential for cardiovascular toxicity, like that for CNS toxicity, correlates closely with their lipid solubility.

Comparative Cardiovascular Toxicity (CC/CNS Ratio)

Ratio of doses required for irreversible cardiovascular collapse (CC) and for CNS toxicity is the CC/CNS ratio. This ratio is much lower for bupivacaine (3.7 ± 0.5) than for lignocaine (7.1 ± 1.1).[2,9,14] So, fatal ventricular arrhythmias are more common with bupivacaine than with lignocaine. In fact, in experimental studies, similar doses of high potency LAs caused severe ventricular arrhythmias without any significant depression in myocardial contractility whereas lower potency LAs led to a negative inotropic effect without any arrhythmia.[15] Pregnant patients have a lower CC/CNS ratio for bupivacaine (2.7 ± 0.4) and hence are prone for its cardiotoxic effects.[2,15]

Bupivacaine has most potent cardiotoxic effects due to its several unique features:
- It has an inherently greater affinity for binding resting and inactivated sodium channels. It has the most prominent effect on the rapid phase of depolarization in Purkinje fibers and ventricular muscle.[16]
- All LAs bind sodium channels during cardiac systole and dissociate during diastole. The dissociation of bupivacaine during diastole occurs more slowly, particularly at high heart rates.[17] This prevents a complete recovery and leads to its accumulation.
- Bupivacaine also leads to more pronounced inhibition on cardiac sarcolemmal calcium and sodium current and calcium release from the sarcoplasmic reticulum.[1,16,17] This may explain the increased myocardial depression and atrioventricular block with bupivacaine.

Newer potent long-acting agents levobupivacaine (S enantiomer of bupivacaine) exhibits 30 to 40% less cardiotoxicity than bupivacaine in equal doses because these are much less potent in blocking inactivated voltage-gated sodium channels.[9,13] Similarly, presence of the propyl side chain of ropivacaine renders it less cardio-depressive than the larger butyl side chain of bupivacaine.[13] However, ropivacaine is 40–50% less potent as compared to bupivacaine.[13] In fact, animal studies have shown that in equipotent doses, risk of CNS toxicity is similar with both.[20] However, ropivacaine may still be preferred over bupivacaine in view of the slower kinetics of the latter, leading to prolonged sodium channel blockade and hence toxicity.[17]

MANAGEMENT OF LAST

A famous saying by Benzamin franklin *"An ounce of prevention is worth a pound of cure"* is very relevant to LAST. Favorable outcome for a case of LAST relies on being "prepared", being "sensible", being "vigilant" and appropriate timely treatment.[14]

- *Being prepared* means the facilities where significant amounts of local anesthetic doses are frequently used should establish a plan for management of LAST and maintain a LA toxicity kit with instruction on its use at a strategic location easily accessible to everyone.
- *Being sensible* means strictly implementing the risk reduction strategies (as have been described in Table 2), so as to prevent the occurrence of LAST.

Test Dose–Use and Interpretation

The commonly used test dose of 3 mL of lidocaine 1.5% with epinephrine 1:200000, detects intrathecal (detectable sensory block) or intravenous (increase in systolic blood pressure and heart rate) within 1-2 minutes of injection. In adults, epinephrine 10–15 µg/mL has been found to be 80% sensitive in detecting intravascular injection.[14,23] The positive response is increase in heart rate (HR) by more than 10 beats/minute or increase of systolic blood pressure (SBP) more than 15 mm Hg.[14] However, its usefulness is limited in elderly, obstetric patients, sedated or anesthetized patients and in those taking beta-blockers.[22,23] Despite its limitation, use of test dose remains the most reliable marker for detecting intravascular injection.[11,14,22] In pregnant patients injection of epinephrine is not the best test (low positive predictive value) and has significant side effects

---

Table 2: Risk reduction strategies for LAST [11,14,21,22]

1. Maximum recommended dose should be calculated for each patient and lowest possible dose of the LA which can effectively produce the desired block should be used. When two different LA are used together additive toxicity of the two should be kept in mind.
2. Incremental fractionated dosing must always be practiced for all patients. Drug should be slowly injected in small aliquots (0.1–0.2 mL/kg) with frequent aspiration, followed by pauses of at least one arm brain circulation time (15–30 s) while monitoring for any symptoms of toxicity. Continuous ECG monitoring (for changes in QRS complex, heart rate, or rhythm) may help in terminating injection of LA before a lethal dose is administered.
3. Use of imaging techniques (ultrasound guidance/fluoroscopy) whenever feasible.
4. Newer less cardiotoxic enantiomers ropivacaine and levobupivacaine should be used especially where higher doses or continuous infusions are required.
5. Continuous infusion of LAs is safer than intermittent boluses, if a catheter is used.
6. Test dose containing a pharmacological marker (epinephrine, isoprenaline, fentanyl, etc.) should always be used.
7. LAST can have delayed manifestation (after 15 mins). So, patients receiving regional blocks with LA should be closely monitored for minimum of 30 mins postinjection.
8. LA toxicity kit containing 20% LE 500 mL, infusion set, 50 mL syringe, and instruction card on its use should always be kept in areas where LA is being injected in significant amount.
9. An epidural test dose should be given to rule out accidental intravenous or intrathecal catheter placement.

(decreased uteroplacental blood flow after IV or epidural injection). So, other drugs like fentanyl 100 µg may be preferred as a test dose. Intrathecal placement of fentanyl may lead to drowsiness in parturients.[11]

In children, the recommended test dose volume is 0.1 mL/kg of an LA solution containing of 5 µg/mL epinephrine.[14,22] Various factors affect the reliability of test dose in children including:[22]

- Drugs and dosage for general anesthesia
- Higher baseline heart rates in children
- Altered reactivity of pediatric cardiovascular system to epinephrine
- Technique of general anesthesia
- Use of premedication
- LA used.

In young children anesthetized with sevoflurane, intravascular injection of a test dose containing 2.5-5 µg/mL leads to an early onset (20-40 seconds) of increased T wave amplitude.[24] This is followed by an increase of HR by more than 10 beats per minute along with a transient 15 mm Hg increase in SBP. Under total intravenous anesthesia, rise in diastolic blood pressure within 1-2 minutes of injection was found to be more sensitive.[25]

- *Being vigilant* implies monitoring every patient during and after the LA injection to allow early recognition of systemic toxicity. Standard American Society of Anesthesiologists (ASA) monitoring should always be used in every patient receiving LAs even, if surgery is being done under pure regional block. Monitoring should be extended to postoperative period for short procedures as LAST can occur up to 30 minutes after injection.[26] Communication should be maintained with the patient during and after injection to allow early detection of impending LAST. If immediate alteration in mental status of the patient is noticed, termination of injection will prevent fatal amounts of LA to be delivered to the patient. Presence of any kind of neurological or cardiovascular symptoms following a regional block should prompt suspicion of LAST.[22] Need for sedation should be carefully considered in all patients undergoing regional anesthesia as even minimal sedation may hamper with patient's reporting of symptoms pertinent to LAST and thus, its early recognition.
- *Early treatment*: An animal report in 1962 had first suggested the efficacy of LE in hastening recovery from barbiturate-coma.[27] Nonetheless, the credit for its application to LA toxicity goes to Dr Guy Weinberg MD who incidentally discovered that pretreatment of rats with LE led to remarkable increase in the fatal dose of bupivacaine by 50%.[28] He had also documented that animals treated with LE following bupivacaine toxicity had better hemodynamics and survival as compared to use of vasopressors or cardiac message for resuscitation.[29,30] Because of the potential lethal nature of LAST, randomized controlled trial to study the efficacy of LE on human subjects is not ethically feasible. Hence, we would have to rely on animal studies and case reports to investigate the effectiveness of lipid rescue in LAST. Moreover, usefulness of case reports is negated by publication bias as the reports with successful outcome are more likely to be published.

Rosenblatt et al. in 2006 reported the first clinical case of successful resuscitation with LE in a patient with refractory bupivacaine toxicity.[31] Following this report, several case reports described its efficacy for treatment of various other amide LAs.[32-35] Literature does not recommend any one formulation of LE as superior to another, but 20% intralipid is the most commonly used LE in this regard. Propofol is understandably not an appropriate substitute for LE since it has lower lipid content (10%) and its negative inotropic effects are counterproductive in a patient who is likely to have hemodynamic instability.[36]

Earlier, LE was used in patients with refractory LAST after conventional cardiopulmonary resuscitation had failed, but recent literature supports its early use at the first sign of CVS involvement, prolonged seizure activity, or with rapid progression of symptomatology.[33,37-39] Nevertheless, ACLS protocol including ensuring patent airway, oxygenation and ventilation, and performing chest compressions) still take a priority to prevent hypercapnia, acidosis and hypoxemia which can further aggravate the toxicity.[9,14,21,40] Contrary to conventional resuscitation protocol, during ACLS for LAST, smaller doses of epinephrine (<1 mcg/kg) are recommended as it has been found to reduce efficacy of lipid rescue and impair resuscitation in animal studies.[41] LAs being lipid soluble are sequestered in local tissues and can be slowly released in the blood later. Thus, severe CNS and CVS symptoms may recur in a patient with LAST and observation should be extended for at least for 12 hours after the episode.[1,11,14] ASRA guidelines for treatment of LAST have been mentioned in Table 3.

THEORIES OF MECHANISM OF LE EFFECTIVENESS IN LAST

- **Theory of "Lipid Sink":** This theory holds that lipophilic LAs preferably partition into the lipemic plasma compartment created by LE in a 1:12 ratio thereby reducing their concentration in the plasma and making them unavailable for interaction at the target sites.[42] Weinberg et al. documented increased bupivacaine clearance from isolated rat hearts when LE was infused is in sync with present theory.[43] In humans, this theory was favored by a case in which a patient suffering from severe refractory cardiovascular toxicity due to bupropion and lamotrigine, had favorable outcome with LE treatment.[44] His blood samples post lipid infusion showed a fall in lipophilic bupropion levels while same was not true for other nonlipophilic drug lamotrigine. Lipid infusion is now being proposed as an antidote for lipophilic toxidromes when conventional treatment proves futile.[26] However, the only human trial on the role of intralipid as an antidote to bupivacaine failed to establish a lipid sink effect and therefore, evidence is still unclear in this regard.[45]
- **Metabolic theory:** Lipids are energy substrate for myocardium and thus, LE enhances myocardial substrate supply and raises its high energy phosphate content.[46] It thereby acts at cellular level to counter the metabolic inhibitory effect that bupivacaine.
- **Ionotropic theory:** Increased serum triglyceride levels due to LE infusion is thought to increase cellular calcium influx via action on calcium ion channels.[47,48] This may reverse the myocardial depression induced by bupivacaine which is said to have pronounced action on calcium channels of heart.[9]
- **Other theories:** Other less favored theories are that LE has a direct action within the tissue where lipid components interact and oppose bupivacaine molecules in the cardiac muscle.[15,36] One school of thought is that LE might act through nitric oxide pathways and counter bupivacaine's inhibitory cardiovascular effects.[36]

Table 3: ASRA guidelines in local anesthetics systemic toxicity (LAST) management[14]

1. Prompt and effective airway management to prevent hypoxia and acidosis.
2. Benzodiazepines are preferred for treatment of seizures but propofol or thiopental are acceptable alternatives.
3. Propofol should be avoided in high doses for seizure control in patients with CV compromise as it may further depress cardiac function. In such cases suxamethonium or other neuromuscular relaxants in low doses should be considered.
4. If case of cardiac arrest, standard ACLS with the following modifications should be initiated:
   - Epinephrine should be used in small incremental doses (beginning with 10–100 μg boluses)
   - Vasopressin is not recommended as substitute to epinephrine
   - Calcium channel blockers and β-adrenergic receptor blockers should be avoided
   - Amiodarone is preferred for treatment of ventricular arrhythmias; lignocaine is contraindicated.
5. LE treatment:
   - May be administered soon after recognition of LAST, but airway management is the initial priority.

   Dose:
   i. 1.5 mL/kg (lean body weight) 20% LE as bolus
   ii. 0.25 mL/kg per minute of infusion, continued for at least 10 mins after hemodynamic stability achieved
   iii. If still unstable, consider repeat bolus and doubling infusion to 0.5 mL/kg per minute
   iv. Approximately 10 mL/kg is the recommended upper limit for LE for initial 30 mins.
6. Propofol should not be used instead of LE.
7. In case of LAST refractory to LE and vasopressor therapy, prompt institution of CPB should be done. The closest facility capable of providing it should be notified early when CV compromise is first identified during an episode of LAST as its initiation can take significant amount of time.

Adverse Effects of LEs as an Antidote

Lipid emulsions have remarkable safety record as an antidote for LA toxicity. Despite its vast data on effectiveness in case of multitude of toxidromes, the reported adverse effects are limited to increased serum amylase enzyme in a patient[49] and an instance of acute lung injury[44] where direct causality could not be proved. Most of the proposed risks of LE are theoretical and usually not a concern with its short term administration as in case of LAST. Some of them include:[9,36]

- Increased risk of infection as LE impairs reticuloendothelial system and inflammatory responses.
- Thrombophlebitis with peripheral intravenous administration.
- Allergic reactions including anaphylaxis due to egg lecithin and soya bean oil.
- With macroparticles (> 5 μm in size) fat emboli may develop.
- Altered consciousness, lethargy and seizures in children.
- Risk of pulmonary hypertension (infusion rates > 100 mL/kg/h).
- Interference with extracorporeal membrane oxygenator circuits.
- Intracranial pressure may be raised in patient with traumatic brain injury.

LAST IN PEDIATRIC PATIENTS

Local anesthetics bind predominantly to alpha-1 acid glycoprotein and red cells but also to human serum albumin with a lower affinity.[41] During first 6-9 months of age, AGP concentration is lower and reaches adult levels after first year of life. Also, hepatic clearance of amide LAs is less in the first year of life. Especially, CYP1A2 enzyme which metabolizes lignocaine and ropivacaine is immature till 4-7 years of life.[3,9] This predisposes infants to LA toxicity.[1,2,3,9] However, increased hematocrit and volume of distribution protects them to some extent.

LAs mainly act by preventing fast inward sodium channels from opening. This LA induced block has two components: tonic (concentration dependent) and phasic (frequency dependent). The phasic block intensifies as the rate impulse increases. Hence, in newborn and infants, the higher heart rates predispose them to bupivacaine induced phasic block.[3,9] Also, higher cardiac output and regional blood flow in young children leads to faster LA systemic absorption and higher peak plasma concentrations.[3] Hence, epinephrine is commonly used to enhance duration of regional and central blocks along with LA agents in children. The usual concentration of epinephrine recommended is 1:200,000 but concerns of reduced spinal cord blood flow have prompted a reduction in this concentration to half in infants less than 6 months by many.[3,22]

Nerve blocks in this population are rarely used as sole anesthesia technique and use of general anesthesia masks the initial neurological signs of LA toxicity. Hence, LAST may manifest directly as cardiovascular collapse in children.[3,14,22] In combination with GA, low concentration of LA (0.2-0.25% of bupivacaine, levobupivacaine and ropivacaine) should be used in minimum effective volume for desirable regional block. Maximum dose of these LAs should be limited to 2-2.5 mg/kg (caudal block), 1.2-1.7 mg/kg (thoracic epidural) and 0.5 mg/kg (peripheral nerve blocks).[1,3,9] Even lower concentrations (0.625-1.25%) are recommended for continuous infusion of LAs (maximum recommended rate is 0.2 mg/kg/h for neonates, 0.3 mg/kg/h in 1-6 months old infants and 0.4 mg/kg for older children).[1,3,11,9] Ropivacaine and levobupivacaine are safer in children because of their decreased cardiotoxicity risk. Ventricular conduction blockade is the main manifestation of cardiotoxicity. ECG changes can be QRS widening, bradycardia, and Torsades de pointes which can degenerate into ventricular fibrillation or asystole. Treatment is the institution of standard basic and advanced pediatric life support with an emphasis on adequate oxygenation and ventilation. Adrenaline is used in small incremental doses of 2-4 mcg/kg.[2,15,18] Defibrillation is performed in the dose of 2-4 joules/kg. The recommended dose of LE in pediatric patients is 20% intralipid 5 mL/kg intravenously as bolus.[15,18,50] This can be repeated up to maximum of 10-12 mL/kg, if hemodynamic stability is not achieved. Maintenance infusion is usually not recommended in children.[15,18] Rather, they are kept under close observation for recurrence of symptoms of toxicity.

RECENT ADVANCES IN THE TREATMENT OF LAST

Use of lipid rescue in LAST is now considered a standard of care. Recently, electrophoresis studies comparing commercially available intralipid with liposome vesicle dispersions have found that the dispersion preparations had increased interaction with LAs and hence, may be more suitable alternative in future.[51] Extracorporeal cardiopulmonary support was also reported as lifesaving in some cases of refractory bupivacaine toxicity.[52] Rapid-response extracorporeal membrane oxygenator is increasingly being used in some advanced setups for this purpose. Ultrasonography has shown promising results in reducing LA toxicity.[4,53,54] Recent statistics suggest a reduction of LAST across its clinical continuum by 65% [level of evidence (LOE) III] with its application.[4] This is because visualized procedure avoids vessels in the path of injection. There is a strong literature backing (LOE Ia) on a reduction in the incidence of unintended vascular puncture (a surrogate outcome for LAST) with USG guidance as compared to use of peripheral nerve stimulator.[53] The use of ultrasound guidance was reported to reduce the incidence of LAST from more than 1:1000, to 1:1600 in a series of more than 20,000 patients.[54] Others have reported a reduction in incidence of seizures with use of ultrasound for nerve blocks.[4] These encouraging results should not deter practitioners from maintaining a high level of vigilance as incidence of serious LAST still remains at approximately 2.6 per 10,000 ultrasound guided blocks.[55]

CONCLUSION

Local-anesthetic systemic toxicity is a rare but grave complication of LA use. It can be prevented by vigilant monitoring, having risk reduction strategies in place and a plan to tackle such an event. In recent times, LE is being hailed as a one stop solution for treatment of LAST and is being recommended by various guidelines in this regard. Stocking of intralipid should be mandatory at every site where LAs are being used in doses sufficient to risk LAST. Widespread adoption of ultrasonography for regional anesthesia, use of less toxic LAs and awareness of safety guidelines has ensured that the incidence of LAST remains on a decreasing trend.

REFERENCES

1. Mulroy MF. Systemic toxicity and cardiotoxicity from local anesthetics: incidence and preventive measures. Reg Anesth Pain Med. 2012;27:556-61.
2. Dillane D, Finucane BT. Local anesthetic systemic toxicity. Can J Anesth. 2010;57:368-80.
3. Berde CB. Toxicity of local anesthetics in infants and children. Pediatr. 1993;122(5): S14-S20.
4. Barrington M, Kluger R. Ultrasound guidance reduces the risk of local anesthetic systemic toxicity following peripheral nerve blockade. Reg Anesth Pain Med. 2010;35: 152-61.
5. Auroy Y, Benhamou D, Bargues L, et al. Major complications of regional anesthesia in France. The SOS Regional Anesthesia Hotline Service. Anesthesiology. 2002;97:1274-80.
6. Brown DL, Ransom DM, Hall JA, et al. Regional anesthesia and local anesthetic-induced systemic toxicity: seizure frequency and accompanying cardiovascular changes. Anesth Analg. 1995;81:321-8.
7. Tanaka K, Watanabe R, Harada T, et al. Extensive application of epidural anesthesia and analgesia in a university hospital: incidence of complications related to technique. Reg Anesth. 1993;18:34-8.
8. Lee LA, Posner KL, Domino KB, et al. Injuries associated with regional anesthesia in 1980s and 1990s: A closed claim analysis. Anesthesiology 1994;101:143.

9. Mather LE, Copeland SE, Ladd LA. Acute toxicity of local anesthetics: underlying pharmacokinetic and pharmacodynamic concepts. Reg Anesth Pain Med. 2005;30:553-66.
10. Lirk P, Picardi, Hollmann MW. Local anesthetics: 10 essentials. Eur J Anaesthesiol. 2014;31:575-85.
11. Mulroy MF, Hejtmanek MR. Prevention of local anesthetic toxicity. Reg Anesth Pain Med. 2010;35:175-8.
12. Rosenberg PH, Veering BT, Urmey WF. Maximum recommended doses of local anesthetics: a multifactorial concept. Regional Anesthesia and Pain Medicine. 2004;29: 564-75.
13. Casati A, Putzu M. Bupivacaine, levobupivacaine and ropivacaine: are they clinically different? Best Pract Res Clin Anaesthesiol. 2005;19:247-68.
14. Neal JM, Bernards CM, Butterworth JF, et al. ASRA practice advisory on local anesthetic systemic toxicity. Regional Anesthesia and Pain Medicine. 2010;35(2):152-61.
15. Wolfe MF, Butterworth JF. Local anesthetic systemic toxicity: update on mechanisms and treatment. Curr opin Anaesthesiol. 2011;24:561-6.
16. Block A, Covina B. Effect of local anesthetic agents on cardiac conduction and contractility. Reg Anesth. 1982;6:55.
17. Clarkson CW, Hondeghem LM. Mechanism for bupivacaine-induced depression of cardiac conduction: fast block of sodium channels during action potential with slow recovery from block during diastole. Anaesthesiology. 1985;62:396-405.
18. Wong GK, Joo DT, McDonnell C. Lipid resuscitation in a carnitine deficient child following intravascular migration of an epidural catheter. Anesthesia. 2010;65(2):192-5.
19. Newton DJ, McLeod GA, Khan F, et al. Vasoactive characteristics of bupivacaine and levobupivacaine with and without adjuvant epinephrine in peripheral human skin. Bri J Anesthesia. 2005;94(5):662-7.
20. Hermanides J, Hollmann MW, Stevens MF, et al. Failed epidural: causes and management. Br J Anaesth. 2012;109:144-54.
21. Griffiths WH, Picard J, Weinberg G. Guidelines for the Management of Severe Local-Anesthetic Toxicity: The Association of Anaesthestists of Great Britain and Ireland. Available from URL: http://www.aagbi.org/publications/guidelines/docs/latoxicity07.pdf.
22. Ivani G, Suresh S, Ecoffey C, et al. The European Society of Regional Anesthesia and Pain Therapy and the American Society of Regional Anesthesia and Pain Medicine Joint Committee Practice Advisory on Controversial Topics in Pediatric Regional Anesthesia. Regional Anesthesia and Pain Medicine. 2015,40(5):526-32.
23. Moore DC, Batra MS. The components of an effective test dose prior to epidural block. Anesthesiology. 1981;55(6):693-6.
24. Desparmet J, Mateo L, Eccoffey C, et al. Efficacy of an epidural test dose in children anesthetized with halothane. Anesthesiology. 1990;72:249-51.
25. Polaner DM, Zuk J, Luong K, et al. Positive intravascular test dose criteria in children during total intravenous anesthesia and remifentanyl are different than during inhaled anesthesia. Anesth Analg. 2010;110:41-5.
26. Cave G, Harvey M. Intravenous lipid emulsion as antidote beyond local anesthetic toxicity: a systematic review. Acad Emerg Med. 2009;16:815-24.
27. Russell R, Westfall B. Alleviation of barbiturate depression by fat emulsion. Anesth Analg. 1962;41:582-5.
28. Weinberg GL, VadeBoncouer T, Ramaraju GA, et al. Pretreatment or resuscitation with a lipid infusion shifts the dose-response to bupivacaine-induced asystole in rats. Anesthesiology. 1998;88(4):1071-5.
29. Weinberg GL, Di Gregorio G, Ripper R, et al. Resuscitation with lipid versus epinephrine in a rat model of Bupivacaine overdose. Anesthesiology. 2008;108(5):907-13.

30. Weinberg G, Ripper R, Feinstein DL, et al. Lipid emulsion infusion rescues dogs from bupivacaine-induced cardiac toxicity. Regional Anesthesia and Pain Medicine. 2003;28(3):198-202.
31. Rosenblatt M, Abel M, Fischer G, et al. Successful use of a 20% lipid emulsion to resuscitate a patient after a presumed bupivacaine-related cardiac arrest. Anestheiology. 2006;105:217-8.
32. Sonsino D, Fischler M. Immediate intravenous lipid infusion in the successful resuscitation of ropivacaine induced cardiac arrest after infraclavicular brachial plexus block. Reg Anesth Pain Med. 2009;34:276-7.
33. Charbonneau H, Marcou T, Mazoit J, et al. Early use of lipid emulsion to treat incipient mepivacaine intoxication. Reg Anesth Pain Med. 2009;34:277.
34. Foxall G, McCahon R, Lamb J, et al. Levobupivacaine induced seizures and cardiovascular collapse treated with intralipid. Anesthesia. 2007;62:516-8.
35. Dix SK, Rosner GF, Nayar M, et al. Intractable cardiac arrest due to lignocaine toxicity successfully resuscitated with lipid emulsion. Critical Care Medicine. 2011;39(4):872-4.
36. Weinberg GL. Treatment of local anesthetic systemic toxicity (LAST). Regional Anesthesia and Pain Medicine. 2010;35(2):188-93.
37. Weinberg GL. Intravenous lipid emulsion: why wait to save a life? Emergency Medicine Australasia. 2011;23(2):113-5.
38. Markowitz S, Neal JM. Immediate lipid emulsion therapy in the successful treatment of bupivacaine systemic toxicity. Regional Anesthesia and Pain Medicine. 2009;34(3):276.
39. Litz RJ, Roessel T, Heller AR, et al. Reversal of central nervous system and cardiac toxicity after local anesthetic intoxication by lipid emulsion injection. Anesthesia and Analgesia. 2008;106(5):1575-7.
40. Vanden Hoel TL, Morrison LJ, Shuster M. Cardiac arrest in special situations. Circulation. 2010;122:S829-61.
41. Di Gregorio G, Schwartz D, Ripper R, et al. Lipid emulsion is superior to vasopressin in a rodent model of resuscitation from toxin-induced cardiac arrest. Critical Care Medicine. 2009;37(3):993-9.
42. Weinberg G, Lin B, Zheng S, et al. Partitioning effect in lipid resuscitation: further evidence for the lipid sink. Critical Care Medicine. 2010;38(11):2268-9.
43. Weinberg GL, Ripper R, Murphy P, et al. Lipid infusion accelerates removal of bupivacaine and recovery from bupivacaine toxicity in the isolated rat heart. Regional Anesthesia and Pain Medicine. 2006;31(4):296-303.
44. Sirianni A, Osterhoudt K, Calello D, et al. Use of Intralipid in the resuscitation of a patient with prolonged cardiovascular collapse after overdose of bupropion and lamotrigine. Ann Emerg Med. 2007;51:412-5.
45. Litonius E, Tarkkila P, Neuvonen PJ, et al. Effect of intravenous lipid emulsion on bupivacaine plasma concentrations in humans. Anesthesia. 2012;67:600-5.
46. Silveira LR, Hirabara SM, Alberici LC, et al. Effect of lipid infusion on metabolism and force of rat skeletal muscles during intense contractions. Cellular Physiology and Biochemistry. 2007;20(1-4):213-26.
47. Fettiplace M, Ripper R, Lis K, et al. Rapid cardiotonic effects of lipid emulsion infusion. Crit Care Med. 2013;41:e156-e62.
48. Coat M, Pennec JP, Guillouet M, et al. Haemodynamic effects of intralipid after local anesthetics intoxication may be due to a direct effect of fatty acids on myocardial voltage-dependent calcium channels. Annales Francaises d'Anesthesie et de Reanimation. 2010;29(9):p661.
49. Marwick P, Levin A, Coetzee A. Recurrence of cardiotoxicity after lipid rescue from bupivacaine induced cardiac arrest. Anesth Analg. 2009;108:1344-6.

50. Shah S, Gopalakrishnan S, Apuya J, et al. Use of Intralipid in an infant with impending cardiovascular collapse due to local anesthetic toxicity. J Anesth. 2009;23:439-1.
51. Lokajova J, Laine J, Puukilainen E, et al. Liposomes for entrapping local anesthetics: a liposome electrokinetic chromatographic study. Electrophoresis. 2010;31(9):1540-9.
52. Froehle M, Haas NA, Kirchner G, et al. ECMO for Cardiac Rescue after Accidental Intravenous Mepivacaine Application. Case Reports in Pediatrics; 2012, Article ID 491692, 5 pages.
53. Orebaugh SL, Kentor ML, Williams BA. Adverse outcomes associated with nerve stimulator guided and ultrasound guided peripheral nerve blocks by supervised trainees: update of a single-site database. Reg Anesth Pain Med. 2012;37:577-82.
54. Sites BD, Tanzer AH, Herrick MD, et al. Incidence of local anesthetic systemic toxicity and neurologic symptoms associated with 12,688 ultrasound-guided nerve blocks. An analysis from a prospective clinical registry. Reg Anesth Pain Med. 2012;37:478-82.
55. Neal JM. Ultrasound-guided regional anesthesia and patient safety: update of evidence. based analysis. Reg Anesth Pain Med. 2016;41:275-88.

CHAPTER 7

Videolaryngoscopy: Current Perspectives

Chand Sahai, Bimla Sharma

KEY POINTS

- The importance of videolaryngoscopy has recently been recognized in the DAS 2015 guidelines.
- The guidelines state that all anesthesiologists should be trained in videolaryngoscopy and a videolaryngoscope (VL) must be available to them in the operation theatre.
- The VLs provide a better view and increased field of vision than the traditional laryngoscopy and those with angulated blades have the ability to look around the corner.
- Less force is required when using a VL as direct line of sight not required.
- Videolaryngoscope plays a stellar role in teaching and training.
- Different types of VLs are available, each with unique features. Familiarity with the device is needed by following the manufacturers advice to avoid complications.
- Good view with angulated blade VLs does not necessarily translate into easy endotracheal ingress since one is seeing an indirect image. Preforming the endotracheal tube with a stylet helps access the glottic opening.

INTRODUCTION

Endotracheal intubation is considered the gold standard for securing the airway, a mandatory skill not only for anesthesiologists in the operating environment, but for personnel working in high-tension areas like the intensive care unit and out of hospital settings. Though with the increasing use of extraglottic devices, especially those which offer some protection against pulmonary aspiration, the use of tracheal tube has declined.[1] However, the tracheal tube still offers the single most important advantage of preventing pulmonary aspiration and is indicated in head and neck, upper abdominal, thoracic and laparoscopic and prolonged surgery lasting more than 2 hours duration. Patients with chronic obstructive pulmonary disease where high inflation pressures are required and also those requiring postoperative ventilation, are mostly managed with the tracheal tube as the airway device of choice. Difficult endotracheal intubation or problematic airway management may not be infrequent and may result in severe complications in close to 1/22,000, and death or brain damage in 1:150,000 anesthetics. These complications are the main cause of anesthesia-related injury, possibly leading to major morbidity and mortality.[2,3] It is imperative that the anesthesiologist is well versed with the anatomy of the patient's airway and relevant comorbidities and therapy (post-radiation or postoperative scarring) which could compromise the same, using the methods available to assess the possibility of running into a difficult situation at the time of intubating the trachea.

NEED FOR VIDEOLARYNGOSCOPES

The gold standard for safe placement of an endotracheal tube is observing its passage between the vocal cords. For direct laryngoscopy (DL), alignment of the oral, pharyngeal, and laryngeal axes is necessary to view the glottis, but line-of-sight visualization may be impossible for some patients secondary to anatomic factors, and due to these limitations, DL may fail.[4] Flexible fiberoptic laryngoscopy is considered the gold standard for difficult intubation; however the device is not quickly available outside the operating room or available to paramedical personnel. During intubation, the fiberoptic scope is introduced into the trachea and the endotracheal tube (ETT) is blindly railroaded over it. Blind ETT advancement may prove challenging, stressful, and even occasionally injurious. Despite careful airway evaluation, DL and fiberoptic intubation failure cannot always be predicted.[5,6]

Videoscopy has made inroads into our daily life especially in the field of information technology. Our surgical colleagues have been using video technology since the 1980s but the anesthetists have employed this innovation much later, in the field of airway management.

VIDEOLARYNGOSCOPES

The advent of the video camera chip led to the development of the videolaryngoscope (VL), one that has contributed to the safety of the airway in a variety of situations. VLs are rigid devices that allow indirect laryngoscopy, or visualization of the vocal cords and related airway structures without a direct line of sight. The micro video camera attached to the VL is placed on the tip of the laryngoscope blade, which transmit the laryngoscopic view to an external monitor, allowing the operator to perform tracheal intubation while watching the video screen instead of looking through the small opening of the mouth. They are fundamentally retraction devices with illumination and optical elements. VLs come into the category of "Devices for difficult endotracheal intubation" for adult and pediatric population.[7] As the images are displayed on a monitor and a line of sight is not necessary, there is less cervical manipulation. The display monitor is valuable for the enlarged view of the real time endotracheal intubation and can thus be used as a teaching aid where the instructor can guide the trainee through the development of this core competency, step-by-step, shortening the learning curve.

CLASSIFICATION

Based on the blade shape there are three main types of VLs (Flowchart 1): (a) the standard or Macintosh blade type, (b) angulated blade type and (c) anatomically shaped with a guide channel.[7] There are some VLs where the blade is in the Miller style, but this is available only in the pediatric sizes.[8]

Macintosh Type

So called because the VL has a blade, which is similar to the standard Macintosh blade, the difference being the inclusion of a digital camera at the tip of the blade. The technique of insertion of a VL with Macintosh blade resembles the standard direct laryngoscopic technique. Here the glottis may be viewed either directly or on the video monitor screen.[9,10] The ETT is inserted as it is when using DL, with or

Flowchart 1: Taxonomy of videolaryngoscopes.

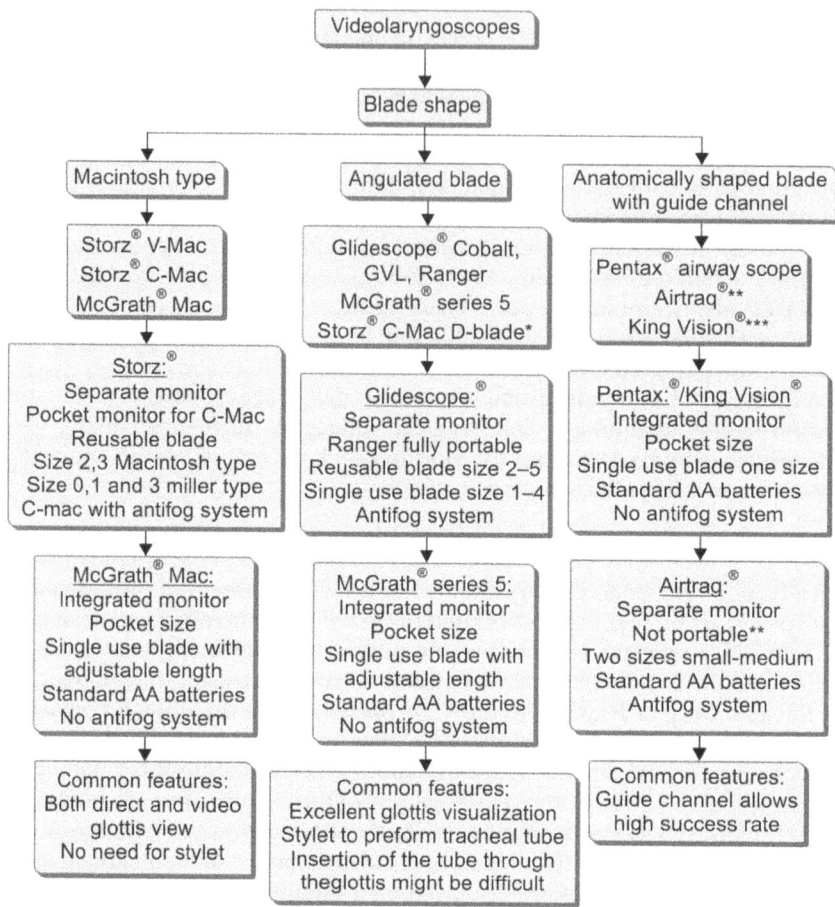

(*D-BLADE = C-MAC's specific characteristics but has the same common features as other angulated blades; **Although not a video-laryngoscope *per se*, the Airtraq can be used with a clip-on camera and a wireless recorder; ***King Vision = same features as Pentax-AWS but equipped with an anti-fog system).
Source: From Paolini JB, Donati F, Drolet P. Review article: Videolaryngoscopy: another tool for difficult intubation or a new paradigm in airway management? Can J Anesth. 2013;60:184-91 with permission.

without a stylet. The V-MAC (Karl Storz, Tuttlingen, Germany), its newer version, the C-MAC (Karl Storz, Tuttlingen, Germany), and the McGRATH MAC (Aircraft Medical, Edinburgh, UK) are examples of this category.

Angulated Blade Type

The VLs with angulated blades have sharper curves than the Macintosh blade. This blade curvature allows a look "around the corner" to produce a clear image of the glottis on the video screen with minimal flexion or extension of the patient's head and neck, however direct visualization is generally not feasible.[9,10] They are normally introduced in the middle of the oral cavity without tongue displacement. The blade glides along the palate and the posterior pharynx until its tip reaches the vallecula or the posterior aspect of the epiglottis, if it obscures the glottis.[9] Unlike the devices which have a Macintosh type blade, the ETT would also need to be introduced "around the corner": a technique that involves placing a stylet into the ETT and shaping the assembly to resemble the far end of a hockey stick about 60 degree angle to match the blade curvature. The hyperangulated VLs (The GlideScope video-laryngoscope (GVL) (Verathon Medical, Bothell, WA, USA), the C-MAC D-BLADE (Karl Storz, Tuttlingen, Germany), and the McGRATH Series 5 (Aircraft Medical, Edinburgh, UK) provide good glottic views but it still may be difficult to maneuver the ETT into the target opening.

Tube Channel Type

These VLs have an anatomically shaped blade with an angle resembling the older Bullard™ or WuScope fiberoptic laryngoscopes and have a guide channel for directing the tracheal tube to the glottis. These VLs have handle-mounted screens, e.g. Pentax-AWS Airway Scope; Hoya Corporation, Tokyo, Japan) and the King Vision (King Systems; Noblesville, USA). Though the Airtraq (Teleflex Medical SRL; Varedo, MB, Italy) has a guide channel it uses an optical system for glottic viewing instead of a camera to relay the images.[9] In this group, the ETT is placed in the VLs guide channel, and this assembly is inserted in the midline of the patient's mouth, without lateral tongue displacement and advanced slowly until the epiglottis is seen.[9] The tip of the blade is directed posterior to the epiglottis, to elevate it and thus visualize the vocal cords. To avoid difficulty with tracheal tube insertion, it is vital to keep the glottic opening in the center of the monitor. The tube is then directed into the trachea via the guide channel. Even though the clinicians are more comfortable with Macintosh-type and angulated blade-type VLs as they provide an experience resembling traditional DL, studies suggest that the skills needed to use devices equipped with a tube channel are easily mastered by experienced and novice laryngoscopists alike.[11,12]

Despite their different shapes and characteristics, there is little information regarding which VL design could be more advantageous in various clinical situations. Figure 1 shows the difference in the curvatures of the blades of the Macintosh and the C-MAC D laryngoscopes.

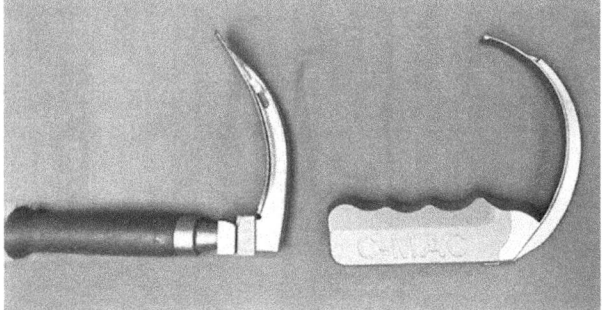

Fig. 1: The Macintosh laryngoscope (left) and the C-MAC videolaryngoscope with D-blade (right) showing the difference in the blade curvature.
Courtesy: Dr Chand Sahai, Department of Anesthesia, Pain and Perioperative Medicine, Sir Ganga Ram Hospital, New Delhi, India.

ADVANTAGES OF VIDEOLARYNGOSCOPY

The VL has a number of advantages. It provides a better view than that offered by direct laryngoscopy, even using a Macintosh type blade, the difference in the larger field of vision being afforded by the position of the light source at the tip of the blade. For the difficult airways, VLs have the extra curved blades which have the ability to 'see around the corner', stretching the field of vision so that a structure not visible on direct laryngoscopy is easily seen or requires minimal neck or head manipulation for the same. This has been explained in detail by Van Zundert et al.[13] that in DL the distance between the vocal cords and the laryngoscopist's eye is approximately 30 to 40 cm and this means the angle of view is a mere 15°; however in VL there is a mere 2 to 3 cm between VL tip and the larynx, so the angle of view increases to 60°. With the D blade of the C-MAC, the view is supposed to be 80° however this is restricted by the tip of the blade to around 60°. This is clearly shown in the image of the light field by a Macintosh blade and a C-MAC D blade (Fig. 2).

Another advantage is that the better view requires less force when using a VL so there is reduced trauma to the soft tissues and the teeth. The incidence of postoperative sore throat is also reduced.

The VL is useful when rapid sequence intubation is required and in patients who are at risk of hypoxia. On occasion, incidental vocal cord malignancy has been diagnosed at the time of videolaryngoscopy and finally the VL can digitally record and store the tracheal intubation, which can be used for training purposes. The authors have been routinely using VL for evaluation of vocal cord movements following thyroid, parathyroid or anterior cervical spine surgery.

DISADVANTAGES OF VIDEOLARYNGOSCOPY

One of the earliest drawbacks of the VL has been its high cost factor, but with the development of newer camera technologies it is possible that cheaper and better models would emerge. With the VL, it takes a little longer to intubate, there is loss of depth perception, fogging occurs in some VLs and in field situations, some VLs might not be effective because of sun glare.

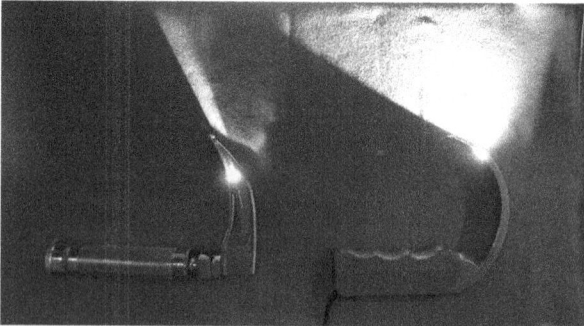

Fig. 2: The Macintosh laryngoscope (left) and the C-MAC videolaryngoscope with D-blade (right) showing the difference in the field of illumination.
Courtesy: Dr Chand Sahai, Department of Anesthesia, Pain and Perioperative Medicine, Sir Ganga Ram Hospital, New Delhi, India.

The wide variety of VLs with differing specifications and blade positioning can pose a problem of choice. Also, a great view does not always translate into an easy intubation, for one is literally looking around the corner and introducing an endotracheal tube with a preshaped stylet within the glottic opening needs practice. Oral trauma is also a possibility, if the VL is not introduced into the mouth under direct vision, the same is true for the endotracheal tube. The mouth opening needs to be adequate for VL insertion. At present no comparative studies are available for the choice of VL for a specific situation, or evidence of its usefulness as a rescue device.

VLs are described as devices that could help to reduce peri-intubation complications, e.g. reducing the force required to visualize the glottis would reduce the number of intubation attempts.[14,15] But videolaryngoscopy may fail when there is a limited mouth opening, a large tongue, a tumor in the oropharynx or laryngospasm, when vision is blurred (by fogging, secretions, blood, or vomitus), or when cricoid pressure is being applied.[10,16,17]

SCOPE OF VIDEOLARYNGOSCOPES

Failed and Difficult Airway

According to the 2003 difficult airway guidelines, a difficult airway is defined as the clinical situation in which a conventionally trained anesthesiologist experiences difficulty with facemask ventilation of the upper airway, difficulty with tracheal intubation, or both.[18] Since the 2003 guidelines, changes have been made in this definition: in addition to the face mask and tracheal tube, the 2013 ASA Difficult Airway Management Algorithm includes the supraglottic airway in definitions related to difficulties in ventilation and placement.[19]

Apart from the danger of causing morbidity and even mortality, a mismanaged difficult airway has legal implications. The closed claims of the 1980s revealed that respiratory events (inadequate ventilation, difficult endotracheal intubation and esophageal intubation) resulting from difficult airways were the single most important source of anesthesia liability.[20] Since the introduction of capnography, esophageal intubations have been drastically reduced but difficult intubations remained a potential hazard in 27% of adverse events between 1991 and 2007.[21] In the USA and UK in as much 10 to 15% of anesthesia airway related claims, aspiration is the reason for litigation.[22,23] Pulse oximetry has become a standard of care in the operation theatre with resultant decrease in the incidence of inadequate oxygenation and ventilation.[24] However, the same results have not been obtained in out of operating room locations due to over sedation and lack of appropriate monitoring.[25-27]

Videolaryngoscopy has become a recognized technique to improve the glottic view when conventional laryngoscopy has failed.[28-32] It has been included in the difficult airway revised 2013 guidelines as an initial approach to intubation (awake or following induction of general anesthesia) and following failed intubation in which face mask ventilation is adequate.[33] The new Difficult Airway Society (DAS) guidelines have focused on the first attempt, being the best attempt at laryngoscopy since several incidents relating to airway complications following problems at intubation have been reported in the 4th National Audit Project (NAP 4).[34] Plan A should maximize the likelihood of successful intubation at the first attempt, or failing that, limit the number and duration of attempts at laryngoscopy, to prevent airway trauma and progression into a "can't intubate, can't oxygenate" (CICO) scenario.[2]

Special Role in Pediatrics

The pediatric age group including the neonates is also subject to difficult airways and situations where knowing how to quickly and efficiently intubate the trachea could avoid a life-threatening airway emergency. In addition to anatomical difference of the pediatric airway from their adult counterpart, their pulmonary reserve is low and the oxygen consumption is high. All these factors combine to impede adequate visualization of the airway making a successful pediatric endotracheal intubation difficult. The rapid rate of desaturation in children means that the time to tracheal intubation is more critical than obtaining a good view of the glottis, since this does not guarantee an easy endotracheal intubation. Times of 30 seconds or less are recommended for this, in fact the Neonatal Resuscitation Guidelines limit the intubation attempt to 30 seconds.[35] This is because improper intubation attempts could result in airway trauma, hypoxia and hemodynamic instability.[36] It is imperative that the visibility of airway structures be improved, something that the pediatric videolaryngoscopes are capable of. A study in manikins in a cardiac arrest scenario found that pediatric VLs do not improve the time to intubation while a recent Cochrane analysis on use of VLs in neonatal resuscitation found insufficient evidence to make a case for or against the use of VLs for endotracheal intubation.[37,38] Most of the pediatric VLs have been introduced as a scaled down version of the adult VLs. Various sizes are available in pediatric VLs: GlideScope® (Verathon Medical Devices), DCI Video Intubation Systems (Karl-Storz Endoscope), TruView PCD (Truphatek), Airtraq (Prodol) and McGrath Series 5 (Aircraft Medical Ltd.) C-MAC Miller type blade (C-MAC® Miller Pediatric Video Laryngoscope). As in the case of adult VLs the pediatric videolaryngoscopes are not all the same, each has its own unique features and clinical applications and the designs continue to evolve.

Videolaryngoscopy and Obese Patients

As in the pediatric populations, many factors need to be considered in the obese patients presenting for surgery. Both physiology and anatomy is altered in these individuals, making for difficult facemask ventilation and tracheal intubation. The changes seen are an increase in the airway resistance, reduction in chest wall elasticity and a raised diaphragm. Fat deposition in the pharyngeal wall increases the incidence of pharyngeal collapse, short thick neck all of which impede optimal patient positioning for glottic view resulting in difficult intubation. Increased BMI is related to difficult intubation. BMI of more than 50 and neck circumference of more than 42 cm are independent predictors of difficult intubation in the obese.[39-41]

There have been several reports of use of VLs in obese patients. Intubation via the C-MAC Storz video laryngoscope improved the glottic view in 86 morbidly obese.[42] Another study using VLs (GlideScope, Storz V-Mac and McGrath) found reduced intubation time, number of attempts and necessity of using adjuncts when the C-Mac was used.[43] Others have advised that the VL be employed routinely for the morbidly obese patient.[44]

Videolaryngoscope in the Obstetric Patient

Eighty percent of the mortality following cesarean delivery is attributable to difficult airway management.[45] Despite the advancement of airway techniques the incidence of failed intubation in the obstetric population remains unchanged.[46] Though VL use in obstetrics is infrequent, there have been some studies using various VLs in cesarean sections.[47-51] The 2015 guidelines on difficult and failed intubation in obstetrics recommend that the VL be available as an alternative to direct laryngoscopy.[52]

Role of Videolaryngoscopes in the Intensive Care Unit

Intubation employing a videolaryngoscope may take longer due to several reasons such as lack of experience, problematic tube advancement, and the diversion of the operator's attention between the VL monitor and the insertion of the tube in to the patient's trachea,[53-55] a lag period that an ICU patient with critical respiratory reserve can ill afford. The ASA is strongly in favor of using the VL in the scenario of difficult intubation.[33] In addition, the VLs have been used in ICU for patients with high-grade Cormack and Lehane requiring tracheal tube exchange via airway exchange catheters by providing improved glottic image.[56] The devices have been similarly useful while extubating patients with difficult airway. Videolaryngoscopes have also been used to aid the insertion of percutaneous tracheostomies in the ICU.[57,58]

Teaching Skills

One of the best properties of the VL is the stellar role it can play in training postgraduate students the art of tracheal intubation. The instructor can view the minutiae of a trainee performing intubation, from blade insertion and position, real time tube insertion and point out relevant anatomical landmarks too. This is possible only with VLs which have remote screens, where not only the instructor and trainee but the entire OT personnel can view the tracheal intubation. The assistant who is also looking at the monitor can adjust the pressure, force and direction, if the larynx needs to be pushed into a better position. In direct laryngoscopy only the intubator sees the larynx but with the VL it can be a team effort which results in successful tracheal intubation.

Direct laryngoscopy is still considered the gold standard of airway management, acquiring proficiency in the skill has a variable learning curve, needs experience and regular practice. Aligning the three axes to have an adequate line of sight subjects the patient to head extension, neck flexion, manipulation of the laryngeal inlet from without to obtain a better view; lifting forces could be 35-50 N. These stressful features can result in pharyngeal, laryngeal and/or dental injury; adverse events in patients who have poorly controlled hemodynamics, even displacement of fracture in cervical injuries or instability.[59-61]

Though a difficult airway, be it a result of difficult mask ventilation or inability to achieve an adequate view of the glottis, has been tackled by appropriate patient positioning and the direct laryngoscopic methods aided by adjuncts like the stylet, bougie and change of blade size, etc. success is not a certainty and more equipment was needed in the anesthesiologists armamentarium. A retrospective analysis by Aziz et al. on 1,427 patients in whom one of five alternate rescue devices were employed when direct laryngoscopy had failed, it was found

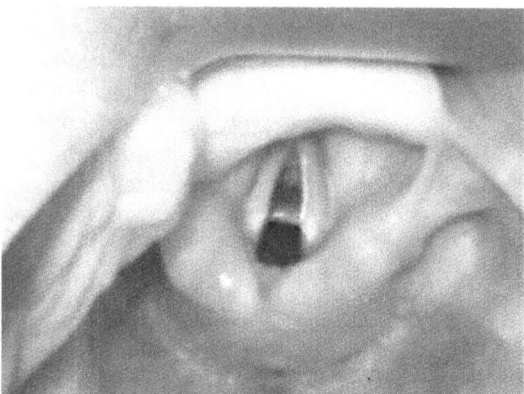

Fig. 3: Kovacs' sign showing the cricoid ring visible through the vocal cords.
Courtesy: Dr Chand Sahai, Department of Anesthesia, Pain and Perioperative Medicine, Sir Ganga Ram Hospital, New Delhi, India.

that the videolaryngoscope had the highest success rate of 92% in securing the airway, even a fiberoptic bronchoscope was only 78%.[62]

Tackling the difficult airway with a hyper-angulated blade requires a sound knowledge of its shape and the various tips and tricks that have been employed such as the Kovacs sign (Fig. 3).[63,64] In this sign the cricoid ring is visible through the vocal cords and means that the VL blade is too close to the glottic inlet and will make for a steep angle which will be difficult to negotiate with the ETT. Withdrawal of the blade will reduce the angle and provide more room between blade tip and glottis and ease the introduction of the ETT.

A meta-analysis published in 2005 looked at 35 high quality studies which examined more than 50,000 adults with apparently normal airway anatomy where there was no larynx seen in 5.8% of cases on laryngoscopy.[65] This study and others emphasize that the prediction of difficult airway is hardly an exact science.

Several factors contribute to a difficult airway and there is no one way to predict difficulty and no single apparatus to ensure that the trachea is safely intubated preferably on the first attempt. To date airway assessment remains unsatisfactory and one may be confronted by an airway that appeared to pose no problem for the intubator but turned out to be difficult at the time of tracheal intubation. So, over the years of development of airway management many techniques as well as a wide variety of equipment in the airway armamentarium have emerged to tackle the issue of difficult airway.

COMPLICATIONS OF VIDEOLARYNGOSCOPES

Complications may occur whenever the airway is instrumented. Injuries of teeth, soft tissues of the pharynx and hypopharynx, vocal cords, and trachea have been described with video laryngoscopy.[66-69] In a large multicenter trial, pharyngeal injury occurred in 1% of 1,100 patients with predictors of difficult laryngoscopy who were randomly assigned to intubation with the Glidescope or the C-MAC D-blade.[68] There was no difference in the rate of complications between the two devices.

Majority of injuries are caused by inappropriate use of VLs, and these can be avoided by directly watching the insertion and advancement of the laryngoscope and the endotracheal tube (rather than looking at the monitor) until the tip passes beyond the soft palate or camera. The risk of trauma has also been attributed to a videolaryngoscope "blind spot". This refers to the inability to see the tip of the ETT in the hypopharynx after direct vision is lost and before the tip can be viewed indirectly through the videodisplay.[69,70]

SAFETY OF VIDEOLARYNGOSCOPES

Initially the VLs were considered as rescue tools to manage the difficult airway and this thinking limited their use to making an appearance only in failed airway scenarios. Now they are being considered as first line to airway management by the present stress on maximizing first attempt success rate. This has been supported by a study by Silverberg[71] where patients undergoing urgent ETI were randomized to Glidescope videolaryngoscopy or direct laryngoscopy as the primary intubation device. The Glidescope was used with 100% success rate as a rescue device for failed DLs and of these in 82% of cases first attempt success rate of ETI was achieved. There was no significant difference in the complication (desaturation, hypotension, etc.) rates of the two devices.

Another feature contributing to safety of the various VLs is the strict adherence to the manufacturer's instructions for use. Many of the injuries caused by the use of VLs have been the direct result of ignoring the steps in the visualization and endotracheal intubation, whether the DL style introduction of laryngoscope blade in the right corner of the mouth to sweep the tongue to the left or introduction in the middle of the tongue as in the C-MAC D blade.

FUTURE RECOMMENDATIONS

Tracheal intubation is a two-stage process. In the first part, the glottis is viewed using the direct laryngoscope or the videolaryngoscope, the latter excelling in this as it projects a clear and enlarged image on the monitor. All laryngoscopy systems direct or indirect are designed to improve the stage of visualization and not the stage of tracheal tube introduction. The two stages need to be merged, and the only currently available equipment, which can provide both, is the flexible bronchoscope. The best approach presently appears to be a combined one wherein the flexible bronchoscope is combined with a Macintosh laryngoscope or a videolaryngoscope. The results from the combined approach are promising.[72,73] Future research needs to focus on forging a link between visualization and intubation so that the two processes flow smoothly from one to the next as a single movement.

CONCLUSION

One of the core skills of a practicing anesthesiologist is successful airway management, which is the main bastion of our specialty. The fall out of a failure to intubate could be laryngeal spasm, bronchospasm, bleeding due to trauma resulting from multiple attempts at securing the airway, hypoxia, hypercarbia, dysrhythmias, brain damage and even death. As of now there is no one solution to the difficulties posed by an airway not amenable to adequate oxygenation and ventilation, be it due to difficult facemask ventilation, glottic visualization or endotracheal intubation. There are many devices available to tackle the problem, each unique in its own way. This distinctiveness may be an advantage in some difficult airway scenarios but useless in others. The device chosen in a particular situation depends on patient habitus, comorbidities, surgical procedure, experience of the operator responsible for airway control and the need to use a combination of devices and techniques. In this smorgasbord of airway devices, the videolaryngoscope has a definite role to play in ensuring patient safety by being the means to a quick, safe airway control. The clinician should be well versed in the use of the device chosen for difficult intubation, by using it in routine airway management.

REFERENCES

1. Cook TM, Woodall N, Frerk C. Results of the first phase of NAP4: census. Major complications for airway management in the UK: results of the Fourth National Audit Project of the Royal College of Anaesthesists and the Difficult Airway Society. 2011;4:24-8.
2. Cook TM, Woodall N, Frerk C. Major complications for airway management in the UK: results of the Fourth National Audit Project of the Royal College of Anaesthesists and the Difficult Airway Society. Part 1: Anaesthesia. Br J Anaesth. 2011;106:617-31.
3. Peterson GN, Domino KB, Caplan RA, et al. Management of the difficult airway: a closed claims analysis. Anesthesiology. 2005;103:33-9.
4. Adnet F, Baillard C, Borron SW, et al. Randomized study comparing the "sniffing position" with simple head extension for laryngoscopic view in elective surgery patients. Anesthesiology. 2001;95:836-41.
5. Johnson DM, From AM, Smith RB, et al. Endoscopic study of mechanisms of failure of endotracheal tube advancement into the trachea during awake fiberoptic orotracheal intubation. Anesthesiology. 2005;102:910-4.
6. Maktabi MA, Hoffman H, Funk G, et al. Laryngeal trauma during awake fiberoptic intubation. Anesth Analg. 2002;95:1112-4.
7. Gasperi A De. Porta F, Mazza E. Video Laryngoscope: a review of the literature. D Chiumello (Ed). Topical Issues in Anesthesia and Intensive Care. Springer; 2016. pp. 35-54.
8. Paolini JB, Donati F, Drolet P. Video-laryngoscopy: another tool for difficult intubation or a new paradigm in airway management? Can J Anesth. 2013; 60:184-91.
9. Niforopoulou P, Pantazopoulos I, Demestiha T, et al. Videolaryn-goscopes in the adult airway management: a topical review of the literature. Acta Anaesthesiol Scand. 2010;54:1050-61.
10. Asai T. Videolaryngoscopes: do they truly have roles in difficult airways? Anesthesiology. 2012;116:515-7.
11. Baciarello M, Zasa M, Manferdini ME, et al. The learning curve for laryngoscopy: Airtraq versus Macintosh laryngoscopes. J Anesth. 2012;1351-4.
12. Liu L, Tanigawa K, Kusunoki S, et al. Tracheal intubation of a difficult airway using Airway Scope, Airtraq, and Macintosh laryngoscope: a comparative manikin study of inexperienced personnel. Anesth Analg. 2010;110:1049-55.
13. van Zundert A, Pieters B, Doerges V, et al. Videolaryngoscopy allows a better view of the pharynx and larynx than classic laryngoscopy. Br J Anaesth. 2012;109:1014-5.
14. Maassen R, Lee R, van Zundert A, et al. The videolaryngoscope is less traumatic than the classic laryngoscope for a difficult airway in an obese patient. J Anesth. 2009; 23:445-8.

15. Andersen LH, Rovsing L, Olsen KS. GlideScope videolaryngoscope vs Macintosh direct laryngoscope for intubation of morbidly obese patients: a randomized trial. Acta Anaesthesiol Scand. 2011;55:1090-7.
16. Aziz MF, Dillman D, Fu R, et al. Comparative effectiveness of the C-MAC video laryngoscope versus direct laryngoscopy in the setting of the predicted difficult airway. Anesthesiology. 2012;116:629-36.
17. Asai T, Liu EH, Matsumoto S, et al. Use of the Pentax-AWS in 293 patients with difficult airways. Anesthesiology. 2009;110:898-909.
18. American Society of Anesthesiologists Task Force on Management of the Difficult Airway. Practice guidelines for management of the difficult airway: an updated report by the American Society of Anesthesiologists Task Force on Management of the Difficult Airway. Anesthesiology. 2003;98:1269-77.
19. Practice Guidelines for Management of the Difficult Airway: An updated report by the American Society of Anesthesiologists Task Force on management of the difficult airway. Anesthesiology. 2013;118:251-70.
20. Caplan RA, Posner KL, Ward RJ, et al. Adverse respiratory events in anesthesia: a closed claims analysis. Anesthesiology. 1990;72:828-33.
21. Baille R, Posner KL. New trends in adverse respiratory events. ASA Newsletter. 2011; 75:28-9.
22. Domino KB, Posner KL, Caplan RA, et al. Airway injury during anesthesia: a closed claims analysis. Anesthesiology. 1999;91:1703-11.
23. Cook TM, Scott S, Mihai R. Litigation related to airway and respiratory complications of anaesthesia: an analysis of claims against the NHS in England 1995-2007. Anaesthesia. 2010;65:556-63.
24. Cheney FW, Posner KL, Lee LA, et al. Trends in anesthesia-related death and brain damage: a closed claims analysis. Anesthesiology. 2006;105:1081-6.
25. Bhananker SM, Posner KL, Cheney FW, et al. Injury and liability associated with monitored anesthesia care: a closed claims analysis. Anesthesiology. 2006;1045:228-34.
26. Metzner J, Posner KL, Domino KB. The risk and safety of anesthesia at remote locations: the US closed claims analysis. Current Opinion Anaesthesiology. 2009;22:502-8.
27. Metzner J, Posner KL, Lam MS, et al. Closed claims' analysis. Best Pract Res Clin Anaesthesiol. 2011;25:263-76.
28. Cooper RM. Use of a new videolaryngoscope (GlideScope) in the management of a difficult airway. Can J Anaesth. 2003;50:611-3.
29. Cooper RM, Pacey JA, Bishop MJ, et al. Early clinical experience with a new videolaryngoscope (GlideScope) in 728 patients. Can J Anaesth. 2005;52:191-8.
30. Lai HY, Chen IH, Chen A, et al. The use of the GlideScope for tracheal intubation in patients with ankylosing spondylitis. Br J Anaesth. 2006;97:419-22.
31. Kaplan MB, Hagberg CS, Ward DS, et al. Comparison of direct and video-assisted views of the larynx during routine intubation. J Clin Anesth. 2006;18:357-62.
32. Asai T, Shingu K. Use of the videolaryngoscope (letter). Anaesthesia. 2004;59:513-4.
33. Apfelbaum JL, Hagberg CA, Caplan RA, et al. American Society of Anesthesiologists Task Force on Management of the Difficult Airway. Practice guidelines for management of the difficult airway: an updated report by the American Society of Anesthesiologists Task Force on Management of the Difficult Airway. Anesthesiology. 2013;118(2):251-70.
34. Frerk C, Mitchell VS, McNarry AF, et al. Difficult Airways Society 2015 guidelines for the management of unanticipated difficult intubation in adults. Br J Anaesth. 2015;115:827-48.
35. Kattwinkel J. Textbook of Neonatal Resuscitation. 6th Edition. Elk Grove Village: American Academy of Pediatrics and American Heart Association, 2011.
36. Maharaj CH, Costello JF, Higgins BD, et al. Learning and performance of tracheal intubation by novice personnel: a comparison of the Airtraq and Macintosh laryngoscope. Anaesthesia. 2006;61:671-7.

37. Rodriguez-Nunez A, Moure-Gonzales J, Rodriquez-Blanco S, et al. Tracheal intubation of pediatric manikins during ongoing chest compressions. Does Glidescope videolaryngoscope improve pediatric residents' performance? Eur J Pediatr. 2014;173: 1387-90.
38. Lingappan K, Arnold JL, Shaw TL, et al. Videolaryngoscopy vs direct laryngoscopy for tracheal intubation in neonates. Cochrane Database Syst Rev. 2015;2:CD009975.
39. Lundstrøm LH, Moller AM, Rosenstock C, et al. High body mass index is a weak predictor for difficult and failed tracheal intubation: a cohort study of 91,332 consecutive patients scheduled for direct laryngoscopy registered in the Danish Anesthesia database. Anesthesiology. 2009;110:266-74.
40. Riad W, Vaez MN, Raveendran R, et al. Neck circumference as a predictor of difficult intubation and difficult mask ventilation in morbidly obese patients: a prospective observational study. Eur J Anaesthesiol. 2016;33: 244-9.
41. Dixit A, Kulshrestha M, Mathews JJ, et al. Are the obese difficult to intubate? Br J Anaesth. 2014;112:770-1.
42. Maassen R, Lee R, Hermans B, et al. A comparison of three videolaryngoscopes: the Macintosh laryngoscope blade reduces, but does not replace, routine stylet use for intubation in morbidly obese patients. Anesth Analg. 2009; 109:1560-5.
43. Gaszyński T. Clinical experience with the C-MAC videolaryngoscope in morbidly obese patients. Anaesthesiol Intensive The. 2014;46:14-6.
44. Pelosi P, Gregoretti C. Perioperative management of obese patients. Best Pract Res Clin Anaesthesiol. 2010;24:211-25.
45. Lesage S. Cesarean delivery under general anesthesia: continuing professional development. Can J Anesth. 2014;61:489-503.
46. Quinn AC, Milne D, Columb M, et al. Failed tracheal intubation in obstetric anaesthesia: 2-year national case-control study in the UK. Br J Anaesth. 2013;110:74-80.
47. Schonfeld A, Gray K, Lukas N, et al. Videolaryn-goscopy in obstetric anaesthesia. J Obstet Anaesth Crit Care. 2012;2:53.
48. Arici S, Karaman S, Doğru S, et al. The McGrath series 5 video laryngoscope versus the Macintosh laryngoscope: a randomized trial in obstetric patients. Turk J Med Sci. 2014;44:387-92.
49. Ni J, Luo L, Wu L, et al. The Airtraq laryngoscope as a first choice for parturients with an expected difficult airway. Int J Obstet Anesth. 2014;23:94-5.
50. Tonidandel A, Booth J, D'Angelo R, et al. Anesthetist and obstetric outcomes in morbidly obese parturients: a 20-year follow-up retrospective cohort study. Int J Obstet Anesth. 2014;23:357-64.
51. Dinges E, Ortner C, Bollaq L. Osteogenesis imperfect: cesarean deliveries in identical twins. Int J Anesth. 2015;24:64-8.
52. Mushambi MC, Kinsella SM. Obstetric anesthetists'—difficult airway society difficult and failed tracheal intubation guidelines: the way forward for the obstetric airway. Brit J Anest. 2015;115:815-8.
53. Malik MA, Maharaj CH, Harte BH, et al. Comparison of Macintosh, Truview EVO$_2$, Glidescope, and Airwayscope laryngoscope use in patients with cervical spine immobilization. Br J Anaesth. 2008;101:723-30.
54. Sun DA, Warriner CB, Parsons DG, et al. The GlideScope videolaryngoscope: randomized clinical trial in 200 patients. Br J Anaesth. 2005;94:381-469.
55. Enomoto Y, Asai T, Arai T, et al. A new videolaryngoscope, is more effective than the Macintosh laryngoscope for tracheal intubation in patients with restricted neck movements: A randomized comparative study. Br J Anaesth. 2008;100:544-8.
56. Mort TC. Tracheal tube exchange: feasibility of continuous glottic viewing with advanced laryngoscopy assistance. Anesth Analg. 2009;108:1228-31.

57. Jeyadoss J, Nanjappa N, Nemeth D. Awake intubation using Pentax AWS videolaryngoscope after failed fibreoptic intubation in a morbidly obese patient with a massive thyroid tumour and tracheal compression. Anaesth Intensive Care. 2011;39:311-2.
58. Gillies M, Smith J, Langrish C. Positioning the tracheal tube during percutaneous tracheostomy: another use for videolaryngoscopy. Br J Anaesth. 2008;101:129.
59. Leong WL, Lim Y, Sia AT. Palatopharyngeal wall perforation during glidescope intubation. Anaesth Intensive Care. 2008;36:870-4.
60. Chemsian R, Bhananker S, Ramaiah R. Videolaryngoscopy. Int J Crit Illn Inj Sci. 2014; 4:35-41.
61. Thong SY, Lim Y. Video and optic laryngoscopy assisted tracheal intubation–the new era. Anaesth Intensive Care. 2009;37:219-233.
62. Aziz MF, Brambrink AM, Healy DW, et al. Success of intubation rescue techniques after failed direct laryngoscopy in adults: a retrospective comparative analysis from the Multicenter Perioperative Outcomes Group. Anesthesiology. 2016;125:656-66.
63. Levitan RM. Tips for using a hyperangulated video laryngoscope. ACEP Now 2015. http://www.acepnow.com (last accessed on 31st July 2017).
64. Gu Y, Robert J, Kovacs G, et al. A deliberately restricted laryngeal view with the GlideScope® videolaryngoscope is associated with faster and easier tracheal intubation when compared with a full glottic view: a randomized clinical trial. Can J Anaesth. 2016;63(8):928-37.
65. Shiga T, Wajima Z, Inoue T, et al. Predicting difficult intubation in apparently normal patients: a meta-analysis of bedside screening test performance. Anesthesiology. 2005;103(2):429-37.
66. Cooper RM. Complications associated with the use of the GlideScope videolaryngoscope. Can J Anaesth. 2007;54:54.
67. Choo MK, Yeo VS, See JJ. Another complication associated with videolaryngoscopy. Can J Anaesth. 2007;54:322.
68. Aziz MF, Abrons RO, Cattano D, et al. First-attempt intubation success of video laryngoscopy in patients with anticipated difficult direct laryngoscopy: A multicenter randomized controlled trial comparing the C-MAC D-Blade versus the GlideScope in a mixed provider and diverse patient population. Anesth Analg. 2016;122:740.
69. Greer D, Marshall KE, Bevans S, et al. Review of videolaryngoscopy pharyngeal wall injuries. Laryngoscope. 2017;127:349-53.
70. Malik MA, Subramaniam R, Maharaj CH, et al. Randomized controlled trial of the Pentax AWS, Glidescope, and Macintosh laryngoscopes in predicted difficult intubation. Br J Anaesth. 2009;103:761-8.
71. Silverberg MJ, Li N, Acquah SO, et al. Comparison of video laryngoscopy versus direct laryngoscopy during urgent endotracheal intubation: a randomized controlled trial. Crit Care Med. 2015;43(3):636-41.
72. Sgalambro F, Denaro A, Guglielmo M, et al. An algorithm for easy intubation. Combined use of the macintosh laryngoscope and flexible bronchoscope in unexpected difficult intubation. Acts Medica Mediterranea. 2013;29:437.
73. Greib N, Stojeba N, Dow WA, et al. A combined rigid videolaryngoscopy-flexible fibrescopy intubation technique under general anesthesia. Can J Anaesth. 2007;54: 492-3.

CHAPTER 8

Preoxygenation: Physiological Basis, Techniques, Benefits and Potential Risks

Kavita Rani Sharma

KEY POINTS

- Preoxygenation is essential to avoid desaturation during airway management.
- Preoxygenation should be monitored to ensure maximal effectiveness (FeO$_2$ >90%).
- Preoxygenation can be improved by avoiding leaks around the face mask, use of 25° head-up position and use of CPAP/PEEP with or without PSV.
- Apneic oxygenation must be provided in patients at high risk of desaturation.
- Children, pregnant patients, obese, ICU patients and those requiring emergency airway management are at high risk for desaturation.

INTRODUCTION

Preoxygenation is a technique used as a safety measure to prevent oxygen desaturation during various airway management procedures. It essentially does so by increasing the oxygen reserves in the body, which help maintain the oxygen saturation during periods of apnea. Although preoxygenation is being practiced for many years, its role in providing safety against desaturation, especially during management of difficult airway, is increasingly being emphasized over the last two decades. The presence of nitrogen as a large component of alveolar gas was found to be a hindrance in establishing high oxygen tensions in alveoli and hence denitrogenation was recommended by providing high inspired oxygen concentrations during anesthesia to prevent 'suboxygenation' many years back.[1] Over years, preoxygenation became a standard practice as a part of general anesthesia, especially in patients at high risk of developing oxygen desaturation. This likelihood to desaturate was recognized in situations where an extended period of apnea was involved as during rapid sequence induction, and in patients with lower basal oxygen saturation or those with a high oxygen demand. Gradually, with development of unanticipated difficult airway protocols, preoxygenation is being recommended for all patients undergoing airway management during anesthesia. The Difficult Airway Society Guidelines 2015, on management of unanticipated difficult airway in adults, stated that all patients should be optimally positioned and preoxygenated before induction of anesthesia.[2] The ASA Difficult Airway Guidelines[3] recommend administering facemask preoxygenation before initiating management of the difficult airway. An optimum preoxygenation and nasal insufflation of 15 L/min oxygen during apnea is recommended by All India Difficult Airway Association in all patients undergoing airway management.[4]

Preoxygenation is also recommended at emergence from anesthesia. The residual effect of anesthetic agents and opioids may cause hypoventilation. The effects of general anesthesia on lung mechanics decreases functional residual capacity and causes atelectasis, thus contributing to a lower oxygenation as well as a lesser oxygen reserve in the lungs. A compromised airway due to decreased pharyngeal muscle tone, residual neuromuscular blockade or edema due to surgical reasons may also effect the ventilation at emergence. Preoxygenation before the reversal of neuromuscular blockade and tracheal extubation has been recommended in all patients to counter any adverse effects due to these factors by the Difficult Airway Society Guidelines for Extubation.[5] Further, preoxygenation must be done before any airway manipulation procedures such as suctioning or disconnection of airway device from the breathing circuits for any reasons as these lead to an interruption in the desired ventilation.

PHYSIOLOGICAL BASIS OF PREOXYGENATION

Maintenance of hemoglobin oxygen saturation is of utmost importance to maintain tissue oxygenation and prevent hypoxia. Under resting conditions, the hemoglobin is saturated with oxygen present in the functional residual capacity of lungs. This oxygen is in turn replenished through alveolar ventilation, from the oxygen present in inspired gases. The maintenance of this hemoglobin oxygen saturation above the safe 90% depends on the oxygen supply in alveolar ventilation replenishing oxygen store in functional residual capacity, ventilation perfusion characteristics and the body demand of oxygen.

Anesthesia, especially using muscle relaxation, frequently causes apnea. Periods of airway device placement are mostly having apnea. During these periods, tissue oxygenation is maintained by using the oxygen stores in the body. These are small reserves, sufficient for few minutes only, present in the lungs, blood and to some extent in the tissues.

Oxygen Reserves in the Body

The oxygen stores in body provide the oxygen for tissue oxygenation and oppose desaturation in the event of apnea for a short time initially. The main store is in functional residual capacity (FRC). While breathing ambient air, this reserve can be 3000 mL × 0.21 = 630 mL at the most.[6] However, due to presence of humidity and carbon dioxide (CO_2), it is at a much lower value of 400 mL.[7] This is because the oxygen concentration in lungs is not 21% as in room air. The *alveolar oxygen tension* is measured using the "alveolar gas equation".

$$PaO_2 = FiO_2 \times (P_b - 47) - P_aCO_2/R$$

Where PaO_2 is alveolar oxygen tension measured in mm Hg; FiO_2 is the fraction inspired oxygen; Pb is the barometric pressure measured in mm Hg; 47 mm Hg is the vapor pressure of water at body temperature (37°C); $PaCO_2$ is arterial partial pressure of CO_2 used to estimate alveolar CO_2 tension ($PaCO_2$) in mm Hg and R is the respiratory quotient.

The normal value for PaO_2 is 102 mm Hg at sea level. This corresponds to 13.42% oxygen in alveolar gas explaining the 400 mL oxygen in 3000 mL of FRC.

While breathing 100% oxygen, the oxygen reserve in FRC can maximally increase to 2750 mL as the alveolar fraction of oxygen cannot increase beyond 0.95 (not considering humidity).

The second important store is the blood, containing hemoglobin bound and plasma dissolved oxygen. The *oxygen content* is given by

Oxygen content in 1 dL blood = Hb × 1.34 × SaO_2 + 0.003 × PaO_2

Where the oxygen content is in ml; Hb is hemoglobin in gm/dL; 1.34 is actual oxygen carried by one gram of hemoglobin; SaO_2 is hemoglobin saturation; 0.003 is solubility of oxygen in plasma and PaO_2 is arterial partial pressure of oxygen.

With FiO_2 0.21, the oxygen content is 20 mL (15 × 1.34 × 0.98 + 0.3) per 100 mL of blood. The total reserve in blood is 1000 mL. This increases to 1100 mL with 100% inspired oxygen.

The tissues, interstitial fluid, and myoglobin probably account for further storage of 200 mL of oxygen, which increases only minimally with high inspired oxygen.[7] Thus, the oxygen store increases from 1600 mL to around 3900 mL with pure oxygen breathing. This increase of 2300 mL reserve has been confirmed by additional uptake of this volume in physiological studies.[8] The major component of this increase is in the FRC. The increase in oxygen reserve is closely dependent on fraction of inspired oxygen, time for equilibration and FRC.

Oxygen availability is dependent on the stores, shunt fraction, cardiac output and hemoglobin concentration. Also, this entire store is not available for use as a diffusion gradient is required for oxygen to be delivered at tissue level. Anaerobic respiration starts below a certain level and hence desaturation below 90% is unsafe. The ventilation-perfusion distribution and the oxygen consumption decide the duration to which these stores prevent desaturation till safe limits.

OXYGENATION DURING AIRWAY MANAGEMENT

Placement of a definitive airway device is carried out by anesthesiologist and intensivists as a part of airway management during anesthesia, for ensuing ventilator support or protecting the airway against aspiration. Airway devices are also placed during resuscitation in emergency situations. Anesthesia induction using a muscle relaxant involves face mask ventilation during the period the adequate effect of drugs sets in and then a period of apnea during which the airway device is placed till the ventilation is restored through the placed device. This apnea period is the most susceptible period for desaturation. The airway may collapse completely or partially after unconsciousness, compromising movement of respiratory gases or the mask ventilation may be suboptimal. Any factor which decreases the oxygen content in the FRC like airway obstruction, hypoventilation, or which decrease the FRC such as pregnancy, abdominal distention, will decrease the oxygen reserve in the lungs. Anemia will decrease the oxygen reserve in blood. Increased oxygen consumption will deplete the stores rapidly. Prolonged apnea leads to a longer period requiring these reserves. Rapid sequence induction is a special situation where face mask ventilation is avoided after administering a muscle relaxant causing a prolonged apnea situation. A difficult airway may need a longer than usual time to place an airway device. The factors promoting desaturation during airway management/ intubation are summarized in Table 1.

MARKERS OF PREOXYGENATION

Preoxygenation is providing high oxygen content in inspired air so as to replace the nitrogen in the functional residual capacity before performing any airway manipulation such as intubation, extubation or tracheobronchial suctioning.

Table 1: Factors promoting desaturation during airway management

A. Decreased oxygen stores
Airway obstruction
    Complete or partial prior to placement of airway device
Hypoventilation
Decreased FRC
    Obese, children, lung pathologies, abdominal distention, geriatric population, effect of anesthesia, pregnancy
COPD
Anemia
B. Increased oxygen demand
Fever
Children
Pregnancy
Sepsis
C. Increased duration of apnea
Contraindication to mask ventilation—rapid sequence induction
Difficult airway-anticipated or unanticipated
    Difficult mask ventilation
    Difficult intubation
    Failed intubation
    CVCI (can't ventilate, can't intubate)

Preoxygenation may be considered synonymous with denitrogenation. Replacement of nitrogen in FRC with oxygen increases the oxygen reserve and the apnea time without allowing significant arterial hemoglobin desaturation. Patients with a high risk for desaturation must be maximally preoxygenated before any airway procedure where ventilation may be interrupted or compromised[9] which is filling the FRC, blood and tissues with oxygen.

Increase in the fraction of alveolar oxygen (FaO_2) and decreases the fraction of alveolar nitrogen (FaN_2), both being exponential functions, dependent on the time constant. The ratio of alveolar ventilation to FRC decides this constant. The oxygen in FRC increases by 63%, 86%, 95% and 98% after 1, 2, 3 and 4 time constants respectively.[10] Hamilton and Eastwood had recommended decreasing the end tidal nitrogen reserve to less than 5% and increasing end-tidal oxygen to more than 90% for maximal preoxygenation.[1]

The various markers for assessment of efficacy and efficiency of preoxygenation are:

a. Fraction of expired Oxygen (FeO_2) and fraction of expired nitrogen (FeN_2). (Marks efficacy)
b. PaO_2 which reflects PaO_2 in the FRC. (Mark efficacy)
c. Duration of apnea without desaturation (DAWD), as the ultimate aim of preoxygenation is to prevent hemoglobin desaturation. (Marks efficiency)
d. Oxygen Reserve Index which is a novel non-invasive pulse oximeter based nondimensional index[11] which provides clinically important warning of impending desaturation during induction of anesthesia.

DAWD to less than 90% cannot be studied due to safety issues in humans. A computer model was developed and validated to study the hemoglobin desaturation to low levels during apnea.[12] In a healthy 70 kg patient, when FaO_2

Table 2: Factors affecting the efficiency of preoxygenation

1. Inadequate increase in FaO_2
    FiO_2 supplied
    Face mask seal
    Fresh gas flow
    Type of circuit—rebreathing if any
    Duration of breathing
    Alveolar ventilation to FRC ratio
    $PaCO_2$ levels
2. Low FRC
3. Anemia
4. Cardiac output
5. Oxygen demand

progressively decreased from 0.87 (FiO_2 of 1.0) to 0.13 (air), the apnea time to 60% SaO_2 (oxygen saturation of hemoglobin in arterial blood) decreased from 9.9 to 2.8 minutes.[13]

The factors affecting the efficiency of preoxygenation have been summarized in Table 2.

TECHNIQUES OF PREOXYGENATION

Preoxygenation before securing an airway needs a well-fitting face mask. Leaks in a poorly fitting face mask lead to dilution of inspired oxygen by air decreasing the FiO_2 to less than 1.[14] These leaks due to a poorly fitting face mask are frequently encountered in edentulous patients, in the presence of beard, scars, swellings, dressings over face, nasogastric tube or due to inappropriate shape or size of face mask. Leaks lead to suboptimal or failed preoxygenation.

A fresh gas flow sufficient to prevent rebreathing nitrogen is needed to rapidly build up the oxygen concentration in lungs. When using the Mapleson A and the circle systems for preoxygenation, an oxygen flow rate of 5 L/min can adequately preoxygenate the patient within three minutes, while an oxygen flow of 10 L/min is required to achieve a similar fractional end-tidal O_2 concentration with the Mapleson D system.[15] Increasing the FGF to 10 L/min with circle absorber did not offer any advantage with tidal volume breathing as rebreathing of nitrogen was negligible even at 5 L/min.[16] A flow of 10 L/min did increase the DAWD when deep breathing was used.[16] An oxygen flow of 10 L/min can achieve adequate preoxygenation with the Mapleson A (Magill), Mapleson D, and circle anesthesia systems while suboptimal preoxygenation is obtained with oxygen flow at 5 L/min when the 8-deep-breaths in 60 seconds technique is used.[17]

Tidal Volume Breathing

The commonest technique used is spontaneous tidal volume breathing with FiO_2 of 1 for three to five minutes. This technique was proposed by Hamilton and Eastwood in 1955 and is still used as a standard practice.[1] This reduces the FaN_2 to less than 5% in healthy individuals. The FeO_2 at end of 3 min of tidal breathing had been reported from 0.88 to 0.92 by various investigators while PaO_2 rose above 350 mm Hg. The duration of apnea without desaturation (DAWD) to 95% was found to be above 3 min while that to 90% prolonged to more than 9 min.

Breathing pure oxygen beyond 3 min in healthy individuals appears to have little advantage in prolonging DAWD.[16]

Deep Breathing

Deep breathing was studied as an alternative to tidal volume breaths for use in uncooperative patients or when less time is available for preoxygenation. Four vital capacity breaths over a period of 30s were found to attain FeO_2 above 90%[18] and a comparable PaO_2.[19] The DAWD was found to be inferior with four breath method using 5 L/min probably due to nitrogen rebreathing.[16,20]

Eight deep breaths over 60s using 10 L/min flow technique was found to produce PaO_2 higher than 4 breaths over 30s at flow rates of 5 or 10 L/min; and comparable to standard 3 min tidal volume breath preoxygenation. The DAWD was higher with eight breath technique as compared to four breaths or even the 3 min tidal volume technique.[16,21] Rebreathing of nitrogen and the need of a longer than 30s period by tissue and venous compartments for filling up with oxygen may explain the rapid desaturation in 4 breath method.[9] Hyperventilation with a fall in $PaCO_2$ and rise in pH with 60s deep breathing will also contribute to lower oxygen desaturation.[9] Eight deep breaths over 60s has been recommended as a better alternative to 4 deep breath or 3 min tidal volume preoxygenation.[21]

The effectiveness of deep breathing is likely to be better when the breathing is started after a full exhalation and sufficient fresh gas is available to prevent rebreathing of nitrogen. However, maximal exhalation prior to tidal volume breathing slightly steepens the initial rise in FeO_2 during the first minute, but confers no real benefit if maximal preoxygenation is the goal.[22] Maximal exhalation prior to deep breathing for two minutes has no added value in enhancing preoxygenation.[23]

Continuous Positive Airway Pressure/ Positive End-expiratory Pressure

Continuous positive airway pressure (CPAP) and positive end-expiratory pressure (PEEP) maintain the FRC during preoxygenation and mechanical ventilation respectively. The desaturation was delayed with the use of CPAP during preoxygenation followed by mechanical ventilation along with PEEP for 5 minutes before removing the mask and securing the airway.[24]

Pressure Support Ventilation

Pressure support ventilation (PSV) during face mask ventilation has been found to be superior to spontaneous ventilation for preoxygenation in terms of the FeO_2 after 3 min. The mean FeO_2 was 94% as compared to 89% and a greater proportion of subjects reached the FeO_2 above 90% (90–100% vs 65%) with 4-6 cm H_2O PSV and 4 cm H_2O PEEP compared to standard spontaneous breathing with FiO_2 of 1.[25] Noninvasive positive pressure ventilation (NIV) is especially useful for preoxygenation in critically ill patients requiring airway management.[26]

Controlled ventilation or supported ventilation as PSV along with PEEP can also be used in apneic or hypoventilating patients, especially during resuscitation.

Apneic Oxygenation

Oxygenation may be maintained during prolonged apneic periods by providing continuous flow of 100% oxygen into the pharynx after a maximal preoxygenation. This is beneficial during intubation attempts where a prolonged apnea due to airway difficulty is expected or the patient is prone to rapid desaturation because of other reasons. As the consumed volume of oxygen is greater than the volume of CO_2 released in alveoli, there is decrease in the lung volume. This causes passive movement of oxygen, supplied at high flows in the pharynx, maintaining the saturation for prolonged periods. Maximal preoxygenation, delivery of 100% oxygen, upper airway patency and the existence of a high functional residual capacity to body weight ratio are essential for apneic oxygenation to be effective.[10] Although oxygenation can be maintained for prolonged periods, rising CO_2 levels limit the safe duration.[27]

Oropharyngeal or nasopharyngeal catheters can be used to deliver oxygen at flows of 3 L/min, delaying onset of arterial desaturation.[28] Flows of up to 15 L/min have been used for this purpose.[10] Apneic oxygenation has also been found to be useful during laryngoscopy in morbidly obese patients[29] and critically ill patients requiring intubation.[30]

Transnasal High Flow Insufflation

Transnasal humidified rapid insufflation ventilatory exchange (THRIVE) is a new method of delivering high humidified flows of oxygen through a specially designed nasal delivery system. Preoxygenation using high nasal oxygen flow is beneficial during process of intubation.[31,32] It is useful in critically ill patients as well as those with difficult airways. The nasal cannula delivers up to 70 L/min oxygen and works by gaseous mixing and flushing of the dead space.[33] It creates a CPAP, maintains oxygenation and CO_2 levels and prolongs the safe duration of apnea.[34] THRIVE has been recommended for preoxygenation in ICU over the conventional 15 L/min oxygen flow before intubation[35] and in combination with NIV.[36]

Preoxygenation during Emergence/Tracheobronchial Manipulation

Preoxygenation is needed not only during the induction of anesthesia but also before events that may compromise the airway, cause hypoventilation or apnea or predispose an intubated patient to desaturation. Emergence from anesthesia may be associated with residual effect of sedatives, muscle relaxants or post-surgical airway edema compromising the airway or gas exchange. The effects of general anesthesia on the lungs may further cause decreased oxygen reserve. Various perioperative anatomical and physiologic changes that may compromise gas exchange make preoxygenation vital before extubation.[5] Tracheobronchial suctioning or a change of airway device, such as the change of endotracheal tube or tracheostomy tube also mandate that preoxygenation is done maximally before such procedures.

PREOXYGENATION IN SPECIAL SITUATIONS

Pregnancy

Rapid sequence induction causes apneic period to be longer in pregnant patients receiving general anesthesia. Denitrogenation and FeO_2 to 90% attains faster consequent to lower FRC and higher alveolar ventilation.[37] The desaturation after apnea is also rapid as oxygen consumption is high and oxygen reserve in FRC low. The tolerable apnea may be reduced in some patients by up to 60 sec. Both 3 min tidal volume and 8 deep breaths are acceptable for preoxygenation.[38] Oxygen flows during preoxygenation should be kept high (10 L/min) to compensate for the increased minute ventilation.

Pediatrics

The lower FRC and high oxygen consumption lead to a rapid desaturation during apnea in children. The risk of desaturation is higher in children with upper respiratory tract infection.[39] The FeO_2 of 90% is reached in almost all children within 100s with tidal volume breathing whereas it can be reached within 30s with deep breathing.[40] The saturation drops rapidly with apnea.[41] The DAWD to 90% was found to be 96.5s in children less than six months, 160.4s in 2-5 year olds, and 382.4s in 11-18 years old after at least 2 min of spontaneous breathing at FiO_2 1. A novel Oxygen Reserve Index provides a clinically important warning of impending desaturation in pediatric patients during induction of anesthesia.[11] Two minutes of spontaneous tidal volume breathing seems sufficient for maximal preoxygenation in children.[42] THRIVE prolonged the safe apnea time in healthy children but had no effect in improving CO_2 clearance.[43] The potential for cricoid pressure induced obstruction and safe duration of apnea are of concern during rapid sequence anesthesia in children.[44] A modified technique without use of cricoid pressure and gentle bag mask ventilation may be a preferred option.[45]

Chronic Obstructive Pulmonary Disease

The hyperinflation causes FRC to be higher, requiring longer times for denitrogenation. Impairment of gas exchange leads to desaturation even with brief interruption of ventilation. FeO_2 should be monitored to assess the efficacy as periods longer than 5 min of tidal volume breathing may be needed for maximal preoxygenation.[46]

Obesity

The altered pulmonary physiology with a low FRC, closing capacity close or within the tidal volume in supine position and heterogeneity of ventilation perfusion ratio reduces the oxygen stores and increases the time for effective denitrogenation. In addition, the oxygen demand is high. This makes rapid oxygen desaturation likely after anesthesia induction, and more so after apnea.[47-49] Obstructive sleep apnea, if present, can further make mask ventilation difficult. The derecruitment of alveoli continues after general anesthesia. After preoxygenation with standard 3 min tidal volume DAWD was 2.7 min in obese as compared to 6 min in patients with normal BMI.[48] Apneic oxygenation using nasopharyngeal,[49] oropharyngeal or buccal oxygen insufflation[50] is recommended. Oxygen can also be given through the working channel of fiberscope if awake intubation is being planned.

CPAP of 10 cm H_2O during preoxygenation followed by PEEP with pressure support ventilation (PSV) led to a significantly improved PaO_2.[51] CPAP with PSV has been proposed during preoxygenation to prevent atelectasis and maintain oxygenation.[52] The application of NIV before and after general anesthesia is effective in improvement in oxygenation and clearance of carbon dioxide in obese patients.[53] A 25 degree head up position of patient during preoxygenation led to a higher PaO_2 and DAWD as compared to the supine position.[54,55]

Elderly Patients

The oxygen uptake is impaired in the elderly due to a ventilation-perfusion mismatch and increased closing volumes. Although oxygen consumption is decreased, the impaired oxygen uptake results in a rapid desaturation. Tidal volume breathing for 3 or more minutes is needed to effectively increase the body oxygen reserves.

Critically Ill Patients and Emergency Airway Management

Airway management in critically ill patients in intensive care (ICU) or during resuscitation for emergency airway access poses a challenge due to a high risk of desaturation. Lung pathologies such as infection, pulmonary edema, aspiration or trauma decrease the oxygen reserve and impair the ventilation perfusion distribution. The intubation conditions may also be suboptimal due to lack of expertise, equipment, positioning and less available time causing longer apneic times. The oxygen consumption may be higher and cardiac output and oxygen carrying capacity lower. These all factors make these patients more prone to desaturation.

Preoxygenation adds to oxygen reserve and is a must for these patients. Preoxygenation using PSV with PEEP is more effective in reducing arterial desaturation in hypoxemic patients as compared to standard preoxygenation.[56] Noninvasive positive pressure ventilation for preoxygenation has been recommended by AIDAA for critically ill patients requiring tracheal intubation. An apneic oxygenation using nasal cannula at 15 L/min oxygen or high flow nasal oxygen insufflations at 60–70 L/min should be added in these patients to increase the duration of apnea without desaturation.[26] Noninvasive nasal positive pressure ventilation was also useful for optimizing oxygenation during rapid sequence intubation in critically ill emergency patients.[57] Preoxygenation and apneic oxygenation using THRIVE was associated with a low incidence of desaturation during emergency intubation of patients at high risk of hypoxia.[58] As compared to preoxygenation with bag-valve mask (BVM), the efficiency in terms of oxygen saturation was similar and had better oxygenation maintenance during the apneic phase before intubation.[59]

POTENTIAL RISKS OF PREOXYGENATION

Under anesthesia, the decrease in lung volumes due to the supine position, decrease in muscle tone and the change in position and movement of diaphragm cause a tendency for airway closure as the end-expiratory volume approach the closing capacity. Some amount of alelectasis occurs in many patients after general anesthesia. After preoxygenation the rapid absorption of oxygen, as compared to nitrogen, leads to collapse of alveoli and is termed as *absorption atelectasis*.[10] Decreasing the FiO_2 or use of recruitment maneuvers retards the formation of atelectasis. Patients receiving 60–80% oxygen had minimal atelectasis as compared to those receiving 100% oxygen but the time to desaturation also fell with decreasing oxygen concentration.[60] Application of CPAP, PEEP or vital capacity breaths as recruitment maneuvers prevents the atelectasis formation. An oxygen wash-out after preoxygenation and intubation did not prevent atelectasis and it was suggested that a moderate PEEP alone is sufficient to minimize atelectasis and maintain oxygenation in healthy patients.[61]

There may be a delay in diagnosing esophageal intubation after a maximal preoxygenation as the oxygen saturation is maintained for some time with the oxygen reserve. However, this is not a reason to not preoxygenate as the correct placement of endotracheal tube needs to be confirmed by presence of CO_2 in expired air.

Prolonged use of 100% oxygen can cause production of reactive oxygen species associated with lung and retina damage. Short duration of oxygenation as in preoxygenation has not been shown to cause any such effects.

CONCLUSION

Airway management during anesthesia or critical care is often associated with apneic periods with a potential for arterial oxygen desaturation. The body oxygen reserves, which maintain the saturation and provide tissue oxygenation during these periods, may not be sufficient in prolonged apnea or high risk patients. Preoxygenation increases the oxygen reserve in functional residual capacity, blood and tissues by replacing nitrogen with oxygen. It is desirable to maximally preoxygenate all the patients undergoing airway management such as intubation, extubation, change of airway device or tracheobronchial suctioning. An oxygen flow of 5 L/min with tidal volume breathing for three minutes or eight deep breaths at 10 L/min with well fitting face mask using circle absorber circuit are effective ways to preoxygenate. A flow of 10 L/min may be needed with Mapleson A or Bains circuit. Effective preoxygenation is indicated by end-tidal oxygen concentration >90% and end-tidal nitrogen <5%. An efficient preoxygenation increases the duration of apnea without desaturation. The patients requiring emergency airway management, especially rapid sequence intubation, children, patients who are obese, anemic, critically ill or have pulmonary diseases are at high risk of desaturation. Addition of CPAP/PEEP with pressure support ventilation and use of head-up position improve efficacy of preoxygenation. Apneic oxygenation, after maximal preoxygenation, using pharyngeal or buccal oxygen flows from 3–15 L/min during intubation maintains oxygenation for longer periods. High flows using THRIVE has been shown to delay desaturation in high risk patients. The patients at high risk must be maximally preoxygenated and means to improve oxygenation should be added.

REFERENCES

1. Hamilton WK, Eastwood DW. A study of denitrogenation with some inhalation anesthetic systems. Anesthesiology. 1955;16:861-7.
2. Frerk C, Mitchell VS, McNarry AF, et al. Difficult airway society 2015 Guidelines for management of unanticipated difficult intubation in adults. Br J Anaesth. 2015;115: 827-48.
3. Apfelbaum JL, Hagberg CA, Caplan RA, et al. Practice guidelines for management of the difficult airway: an updated report by the American Society of Anesthesiologists Task Force on Management of the Difficult Airway. Anesthesiology. 2013;118(2):251-70.

4. Myatra SN, Shah A, Kundra P, et al. All India Difficult Airway Association 2016 guidelines for the management of unanticipated difficult tracheal intubation in adults. Indian J Anaesth. 2016;12:906-14.
5. Popat M, Mitchell R, Dravid R, et al. Difficult airway society guidelines for the management of tracheal extubation. Anaesthesia. 2012;67:318-40.
6. Bouroche G1, Bourgain JL. Preoxygenation and general anesthesia: a review. Minerva Anestesiol. 2015;81(8):910-20.
7. Rutter TW, Tremper KK. The physiology of oxygen transport and red cell transfusion. In Healy TEJ, Knight PR (Eds). Wylie and Churchill-Davidson's A Practice of Anesthesia. 7th ed. CRC Press, Taylor & Francis Group; 2012. pp. 167-83.
8. Pandit JJ, Duncan T, Robbins PA. Total oxygen uptake with two maximal breathing techniques and the tidal volume breathing technique: a physiologic study of preoxygenation. Anesthesiology. 2003;99:841-6.
9. Benumof JL. Preoxygenation: best method for both efficacy and efficiency. Anesthesiology. 1999;91:603-5.
10. Nimmagadda U, Salem MR, Crystal GJ. Preoxygenation: Physiologic Basis, Benefits, and Potential Risks. Anesth Analg. 2017;124(2):507-17.
11. Szmuk P, Steiner JW, Olomu PN, et al. Oxygen reserve index: a novel noninvasive measure of oxygen reserve: a pilot study. Anesthesiology. 2016;124(4):779-84.
12. Farmery AD, Roe PG. A model to describe the rate of oxyhaemoglobin desaturation during apnoea. Br J Anaesth. 1996;76:284-91.
13. Benumof JL, Dagg R, Benumof R. Critical hemoglobin desaturation will occur before return to an unparalyzed state following 1 mg/kg intravenous succinylcholine. Anesthesiology. 1997;87:979-82.
14. McGowan P, Skinner A. Preoxygenation—the importance of a good face mask seal. Br J Anaesth. 1995;75:777-8.
15. Taha S, El-Khatib M, Siddik-Sayyid S, et al. Preoxygenation with the Mapleson D system requires higher oxygen flows than Mapleson A or circle systems. Can J Anaesth. 2007;54(2):141-5.
16. Nimmagadda U, Chiravuri SD, Salem MR, et al. Preoxygenation with tidal volume and deep breathing techniques: the impact of duration of breathing and fresh gas flow. Anesth Analg. 2001;92:1337-41.
17. Taha SK, El-Khatib MF, Siddik-Sayyid SM, et al. Preoxygenation by 8 deep breaths in 60 seconds using the Mapleson A (Magill), the circle system, or the Mapleson D system. J Clin Anesth. 2009;21(8):574-8.
18. Rooney MJ. Pre-oxygenation: a comparison of two techniques using a Bain system. Anaesthesia. 1994;49:629-32.
19. Gold M, Duarte I, Muravchik S. Arterial oxygenation in conscious patients after 5 minutes and after 30 seconds of oxygen breathing. Anesth Analg. 1981;60:313-5.
20. Gambee AM, Hertzka R, Fisher D. Preoxygenation techniques: comparison of three minutes and four breaths. Anesth Analg. 1987;66:468-70.
21. Baraka AS, Taha SK, Aouad MT, et al. Preoxygenation: comparison of maximal breathing and tidal volume breathing techniques. Anesthesiology. 1999;91:612-16.
22. Baraka AS, Taha SK, El-Khatib MF, et al. Oxygenation using tidal volume breathing after maximal exhalation. Anesth Analg. 2003;97(5):1533-5.
23. Nimmagadda U, Salem MR, Joseph NJ, et al. Efficacy of preoxygenation using tidal volume and deep breathing techniques with and without prior maximal exhalation. Can J Anaesth. 2007;54(6):448-52.
24. Herriger A, Frascarolo P, Spahn DR, et al. The effect of positive airway pressure during pre-oxygenation and induction of anaesthesia upon duration of non-hypoxic apnoea. Anaesthesia. 2004;59:243-47.

25. Tanoubi I, Drolet P, Fortier LP, et al. [Inspiratory support versus spontaneous breathing during preoxygenation in healthy subjects. A randomized, double blind, cross-over trial]. Ann Fr Anesth Reanim. 2010;29:198-203.
26. Myatra SN, Ahmed SM, Kundra P, et al. Republication: All India Difficult Airway Association 2016 Guidelines for Tracheal Intubation in the Intensive Care Unit. Indian J Crit Care Med. 2017;21(3):146-53.
27. Baraka A, Salem MR, Joseph NJ. Critical hemoglobin desaturation can be delayed by apneic diffusion oxygenation. Anesthesiology. 1999;90:332-3.
28. Teller LE, Alexander CM, Frumin MJ, et al. Pharyngeal insufflation of oxygen prevents arterial desaturation during apnea. Anesthesiology. 1988;69:980-2.
29. Ramachandran SK, Cosnowski A, Shanks A, et al. Apneic oxygenation during prolonged laryngoscopy in obese patients: a randomized, controlled trial of nasal oxygen administration. J Clin Anesth. 2010;22:164-8.
30. Russotto V, Cortegiani A, Raineri SM, et al. Respiratory support techniques to avoid desaturation in critically ill patients requiring endotracheal intubation: a systematic review and meta-analysis. J Crit Care. 2017;41:98-106.
31. Barjaktarevic I, Esquinas AM, Johannes J, et al. Preoxygenation with high-flow nasal cannula: benefits of its extended use during the process of intubation. Respir Care. 2017;62(3):390.
32. Ang KS, Green A, Ramaswamy KK, et al. Preoxygenation using the Optiflow™ system. Br J Anaesth. 2017;118(3):463-4.
33. Patel A, Nouraei SA. Transnasal humidified rapid-insufflation ventilatory exchange (THRIVE): a physiological method of increasing apnoea time in patients with difficult airways. Anaesthesia. 2015;70:323-9.
34. Ritchie JE, Williams AB, Gerard C, et al. Evaluation of a humidified nasal high-flow oxygen system, using oxygraphy, capnography and measurement of upper airway pressures. Anaesth Intensive Care. 2011;39:1103-10.
35. Ricard JD. Hazards of intubation in the ICU: role of nasal high flow oxygen therapy for preoxygenation and apneic oxygenation to prevent desaturation. Minerva Anestesiol. 2016;82(10):1098-106.
36. Jaber S, Monnin M, Girard M, et al. Apnoeic oxygenation via high-flow nasal cannula oxygen combined with non-invasive ventilation preoxygenation for intubation in hypoxaemic patients in the intensive care unit: the single-centre, blinded, randomised controlled OPTINIV trial. Intensive Care Med. 2016;42(12):1877-87.
37. Russell GN, Smith CL, Snowdon SL, et al. Preoxygenation and the parturient patient. Anaesthesia. 1987;42:346-51.
38. Chiron B, Laffon M, Ferrandiere M, et al. Standard preoxygenation technique versus two rapid techniques in pregnant patients. Int J Obstet Anest. 2005;14:79.
39. Rolf N, Cote CJ. Frequency and severity of desaturation events during general anesthesia in children with and without upper respiratory infections. J Clin Anesth. 1992;4:200-3.
40. Morrison JE, Jr., Collier E, Friesen RH, et al. Preoxygenation before laryngoscopy in children: how long is enough? Paediatr Anaesth. 1998;8:293-8.
41. Patel R, Lenczyk M, Hannallah RS, et al. Age and the onset of desaturation in apnoeic children. Can J Anaesth. 1994;41:771-4.
42. Xue FS, Tong SY, Wang XL, et al. Study of the optimal duration of preoxygenation in children. J Clin Anesth. 1995;7:93-6.
43. Humphreys S, Lee-Archer P, Reyne G, et al. Transnasal humidified rapid-insufflation ventilatory exchange (THRIVE) in children: a randomized controlled trial. Br J Anaesth. 2017;118(2):232-8.
44. Weiss M, Gerber AC. Rapid sequence induction in children—it's not a matter of time! Paediatr Anaesth. 2008;18:97-9.

45. Priebe HJ. Cricoid force in children. Br J Anaesth. 2010;104:511.
46. Samain E, Biard M, Farah E, et al. Monitoring expired oxygen fraction in preoxygenation of patients with chronic obstructive pulmonary disease. Ann Fr Anesth Reanim. 2002;21:14-9.
47. Berthoud MC, Peacock JE, Reilly CS. Effectiveness of preoxygenation in morbidly obese patients. Br J Anaesth. 1991;67:464-6.
48. Jense HG, Dubin SA, Silverstein PI, et al. Effect of obesity on safe duration of apnea in anesthetized humans. Anesth Analg. 1991;72:89-93.
49. Baraka AS, Taha SK, Siddik-Sayyid SM, et al. Supplementation of pre-oxygenation in morbidly obese patients using nasopharyngeal oxygen insufflation. Anaesthesia. 2007;62:769-73.
50. Heard A, Toner AJ, Evans JR, et al. Apneic oxygenation during prolonged laryngoscopy in obese patients: a randomized, controlled trial of buccal RAE tube oxygen administration. Anesth Analg. 2017;124(4):1162-7.
51. Harbut P, Gozdzik W, Stjernfalt E, et al. Continuous positive airway pressure/pressure support pre-oxygenation of morbidly obese patients. Acta Anaesthesiol Scand. 2014;58:675-80.
52. Coussa M, Proietti S, Schnyder P, et al. Prevention of atelectasis formation during the induction of general anesthesia in morbidly obese patients. Anesth Analg. 2004;98:1491-5.
53. Carron M, Zarantonello F, Tellaroli P, et al. Perioperative noninvasive ventilation in obese patients: a qualitative review and meta-analysis. Surg Obes Relat Dis. 2016;12(3):681-91.
54. Dixon BJ, Dixon JB, Carden JR, et al. Preoxygenation is more effective in the 25 degrees head-up position than in the supine position in severely obese patients: a randomized controlled study. Anesthesiology. 2005;102:1110-5.
55. Altermatt FR, Munoz HR, Delfino AE, et al. Pre-oxygenation in the obese patient: effects of position on tolerance to apnoea. Br J Anaesth. 2005;95:706-9.
56. Baillard C, Fosse JP, Sebbane M, et al. Noninvasive ventilation improves preoxygenation before intubation of hypoxic patients. Am J Respir Crit Care Med. 2006;174:171-7.
57. Kim TH, Hwang SO, Cha YS, et al. The utility of noninvasive nasal positive pressure ventilators for optimizing oxygenation during rapid sequence intubation. Am J Emerg Med. 2016;34(8):1627-30.
58. Doyle AJ, Stolady D, Mariyaselvam M, et al. Preoxygenation and apneic oxygenation using transnasal humidified rapid-insufflation ventilatory exchange for emergency intubation. J Crit Care. 2016;36:8-12.
59. Simon M, Wachs C, Braune S, et al. High-flow nasal cannula versus bag-valve-mask for preoxygenation before intubation in subjects with hypoxemic respiratory failure. Respir Care. 2016;61(9):1160-7.
60. Edmark L, Kostova-Aherdan K, Enlund M, et al. Optimal oxygen concentration during induction of general anesthesia. Anesthesiology. 2003;98:28-33.
61. Östberg E, Auner U, Enlund M, et al. Minimizing atelectasis formation during general anaesthesia-oxygen washout is a non-essential supplement to PEEP. Ups J Med Sci. 2017;24:1-7.

CHAPTER 9

Pulmonary Function Tests and Their Clinical Applications

Susmita Sarangi, Dipali Taneja

KEY POINTS

- Pulmonary function tests (PFTs) are an indispensable tool for clinical evaluation of respiratory health and disease and are frequently used for preoperative evaluation of patients.
- PFTs help in stepwise assessment of postoperative risks of lung resection surgeries.
- Since PFTs are effort dependent, patient's cooperation and understanding of the test is a prerequisite to avoid suboptimal results.
- PFTs are interpreted by comparing the patient's values to predicted values of healthy subjects with similar age, weight, and height.
- A spirogram is a graphic representation of bulk air movement and is typically reported in both absolute and predicted percentage of normal.
- By studying the shape of the volume—time or the flow—volume loop, clinicians can understand the manner in which air is moving into and out of the lungs in specific diseases.
- It is pertinent to categorize the pulmonary function tests based on the pathology being investigated. The respiratory mechanics are best assessed by the static and dynamic lung function tests.
- The gas exchange functions are assessed by measuring Alveolar-arterial PO_2 gradient, diffusion capacity and gas distribution tests.
- Nowadays FeNO is being used as a biomarker for the assessment of airway inflammation and on comparison with conventional tests such as Bronchial provocation test (BPT) or the reversibility of FEV1, measurement of FeNO offer more advantages.

INTRODUCTION

Pulmonary function tests (PFTs) are the conglomeration of series of assessments which are extremely beneficial in clinical evaluation of the respiratory system. Advancement of computer technology has given us the portable and automated devices making them a handy device in assessing the lung function. The purpose of this chapter is to discuss briefly the various tests and their use in distinguishing the types of pulmonary insufficiency and most importantly, their clinical applications and limitations. Since PFT's are effort dependent, patient's cooperation and understanding of the test is a prerequisite to avoid suboptimal results.[1] PFT's are interpreted by comparing the patient's values to predicted values derived from healthy subjects with similar age, weight, and height. It is important to note that the normal predicted values which are programed into the

PFT machines are often based on Caucasian men,[2] and therefore minorities and women may have inaccurate readings. However newer machines have attempted to overcome these errors.

INDICATIONS FOR PULMONARY FUNCTION TESTS

Pulmonary function tests have been indicated for the diagnosis of different types of pulmonary diseases and to assess effectiveness of therapeutic intervention. It helps the clinician to follow response to therapy, determine further treatment goals and in evaluating degree of disability. PFTs are highly indicated in preanesthetic evaluation of patients undergoing any cardiothoracic surgery for risk stratification, for planning anesthesia and for evaluating the need of postoperative ventilator support.

According to the guidelines proposed by GM Tisi (1979), the indications for PFT in a preoperative patient include:[3]
- Age > 70 years
- Obese patients
- Thoracic surgery
- Upper abdominal surgery
- History of cough/smoking
- History of any pulmonary disease.

In 2006 the American College of Physicians (ACP) brought out guidelines for preoperative spirometry. These include:[4]
- Lung resection surgery
- H/o smoking, dyspnea
- Cardiac surgery
- Upper abdominal surgery
- Lower abdominal surgery
- Uncharacterized pulmonary disease (defined as history of pulmonary disease or symptoms and no PFT in last 60 days).

CONTRAINDICATIONS

Performing PFT needs a lot of effort from the patients, hence it is contraindicated in:[1,5]
- Recent ophthalmic or thoracoabdominal surgery
- Thoracic, abdominal and cerebral aneurysms
- Active hemoptysis
- Pneumothorax
- Unstable angina/recent MI within 1 month.

TYPES OF PFTs

It is pertinent to categorize the PFT's based on the pathology being investigated.[6]
I. The respiratory mechanics are best assessed by:[7]
   - Bed side pulmonary function tests
   - Static and dynamic lung function tests.
II. The tests which assess the gas exchange functions involve:
   - Alveolar-arterial PO_2 gradient

- Diffusion capacity
- Gas distribution tests:
  - Single breath nitrogen (N_2) test
  - Multiple breath N_2 test
  - Helium dilution method
  - Radio xenon (Xe) scintigram.

III. The cardiopulmonary interaction can be evaluated both qualitatively and quantitatively.

IV. Miscellaneous PFT's
- Bronchial provocation test
- Split-lung function tests.

ASSESSMENT OF RESPIRATORY MECHANICS

Bed Side Pulmonary Function Tests[8]

As the name suggests these are the easiest tests which can be performed by the patient's bed side to assess pulmonary function.

Respiratory Rate

It is an essential yet frequently undervalued component of PFTs, and is an important evaluator in weaning and extubation protocols. Tachypnea is an indication of increased work of breathing and respiratory muscle fatigue.

Sabrasez Breath Holding Test[9]

In this the patient is asked to take a normal breath and hold it as long as possible. The cardiopulmonary reserve (CPR) is interpreted by the duration of breath held as:
- \>25 seconds indicates a normal CPR
- 15–25 seconds indicates a restricted CPR, and
- <15 seconds shows a very poor cardiopulmonary reserve which is a contraindication for elective surgery.

This test can also be used for rough estimate of vital capacity (VC) as:
- 25–30 seconds = 3500 mL VC
- 20–25 seconds = 3000 mL VC
- 15–20 seconds = 2500 mL VC
- 10–15 seconds = 2000 mL VC
- 05–10 seconds = 1500 mL VC

Schneider's Match Blowing Test[10-12]

This test can be used to measure the maximum breathing capacity (MBC) and forced expiratory volume (FEV1). A lighted match stick is held at a distance of 15 cm or 6 inches away from the patients mouth who is then asked to blow out the flame without pursing his lips, keeping the mouth and match stick at the same level and without allowing any air movement in the room. For interpretation, if the patient is:
- Able to blow out a match: MBC > 60 L/minute, FEV1 > 1.6 L.
- Cannot blow out a match: MBC < 60 L/minute, FEV1 < 1.6 L.

In the *modified match test* the lighted match is kept at 3 distances and the ability to blow out the match stick is indicative of MBC as follows:
- 9" > 150 L/minute
- 6" > 60 L/minute
- 3" > 40 L/minute.

Cough Test[13]
Ability to cough helps to assess the respiratory muscle strength and effectiveness in clearing secretions. For a good effective cough, patient's vital capacity should be more than three times his tidal volume. Cough is ineffective when: FVC <20 mL/kg, FEV1 <15 mL/kg, PEFR < 200 L/minute.

Number Counting Test (Single Breath Counting)[14]
In this test, the patient is asked to take a deep breath, hold it and starts counting till the next breath. It is considered normal, if patient is able to count > 40 and helps to assess his vital capacity.

Wright's Respirometer[15]
This is a compact, lightweight and portable device that has an inferential meter that measures tidal volume and minute volume.

Wright's Peak Flowmeter[16]
This is a hand-held device that is used to measure peak expiratory flow rate (PEFR). The patient is asked to take a deep breath and expire as forcefully and quickly as possible. The flow rate is measured from the dial of the instrument. Though effort dependent, this test is highly reproducible. The PEFR values differ with age, gender and height of an individual and indicate status of large airways. The normal values are:
- Males: 450–700 L/minute
- Females: 350–500 L/minute
- <200 L/minute indicates inadequate cough efficiency.

De-Bono Whistle Blowing Test[17,18]
This measures the PEFR. Patient blows into a wide bore tube at the end of which is a whistle, on the side is a hole with adjustable knob. As patient blows the whistle, the hole is gradually increased till the sound of whistle disappears. The PEFR can be read from the scale at the last position at which the whistle is heard.

Microspirometer[19]
This device measures vital capacity.

In addition to the above, *Bed side pulse oximetry*[20] and *Arterial blood gas (ABG)* are other bedside tests to measure gas exchange and oxygen delivery to the tissues and differentiate between Type I and Type II respiratory failure:
- Type I respiratory failure: PaO_2 less than 8 kPa, normal $PaCO_2$
- Type II respiratory failure: PaO_2 less than 8 kPa, $PaCO_2$ greater than 6.5 kPa.

Though easy to perform, bed side PFTs have certain limitations. During the preanesthetic checkup, they are used as a crude screening method to form an idea of the patient's respiratory reserve. Since there are possibilities of human error, the result should be further evaluated by definitive test.

Static and Dynamic Lung Function Tests

Simple volume based study constitutes the static tests and volume in relation to time constitute the dynamic tests to evaluate the lung mechanics.[21] The lung volumes are static measurements and do not reflect the actual pulmonary function. True tests of ventilation involve a dynamic process of gas flow in and out of lungs with relation to time. Spirometry is the cornerstone of all PFTs and gives the lung volumes.

John Hutchinson invented spirometer in 1840[22] and presently we have fully electronic spirometers. The graph of the respiratory movements made by the spirometer is depicted as a spirogram (Fig. 1). Spirometry measurements involve patient's cooperation. After explaining the procedure, the mouthpiece of the apparatus is put in the patient's mouth ensuring a leak free fitting, and a nose clip is applied to prevent breathing through the nose. The patient inhales completely and rapidly with a pause of <1 second at TLC, thereafter he exhales maximally until no more air can be expelled. The maneuver is repeated at least three times and the best result is noted.[23]

Spirometry is reported in both absolute and as a predicted percentage of normal which vary with gender, age, race, and height. Hence it is important to ensure that reference formulas in a PFT lab are applicable to the patient population being tested.[24] A number of spirometry standards have been developed over the years. According to the American Thoracic Society standardization guidelines[23,25] for acceptability and reproducibility criteria, during spirometry there should be:

- ❏ No cough or glottic closure during the first second of exhalation
- ❏ No variable flow
- ❏ No early termination or cutoff (< 6 sec)
- ❏ No air leak
- ❏ The test should be reproducible without excessive variability. The two largest values for FVC and the two largest values for FEV1 should vary by no more than 0.2 L.

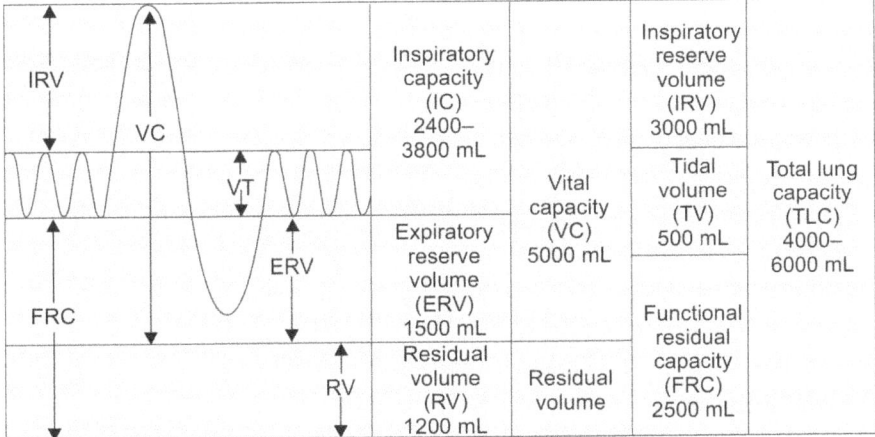

Fig. 1: Standard spirogram showing lung volumes and capacities.

There are four lung volumes and four lung capacities. Lung capacities are the summation of two or more volumes. Lung volumes and capacities reflect the respiratory reserve of the patient, allowing the anesthesiologist to assess the extent to which the patient will tolerate the effects of anesthesia and mechanical ventilation. Postoperative atelectasis can be avoided, if the patient can cough out his airway secretions effectively which is possible when VC is three times the TV. The test has the limitation of not being able to measure the residual volume (RV) and hence also the functional residual capacity (FRC) and total lung capacity (TLC). Definitions and the normal values for different lung volumes and capacities are listed in Tables 1 and 2.[26,27] The same is depicted on a standard spirogram in Figure 1.

Dynamic Lung Function Tests or Forced Spirometry

When flow of gas moving in and out of lung is plotted against time, we get the flow volume loop, and by studying the shape of the loop, clinicians can identify specific diseases.[28] Normal or predicted ranges of values are obtained from large

Table 1: The definitions and normal values of lung volumes

Lung volume	Definition	Values
Tidal volume (TV)	Volume of air inhaled or exhaled with each normal breath	(6–8 mL/kg) or 500 mL
Inspiratory reserve volume (IRV)	The maximal volume of air that can be inhaled over and above a normal inspiration	3000 mL
Expiratory reserve volume (ERV)	The maximal volume of air that can be exhaled after a normal tidal expiration	1500 mL
Residual volume (RV)*	The volume of gas remaining in the lung at the end of a maximal exhalation.	(20–25 mL/kg) or 1200 mL

*RV cannot be measured by spirometry and is calculated by subtracting ERV from FRC (RV = FRC–ERV) or by subtracting vital capacity (VC) from total lung capacity (RV = TLC–VC).

Table 2: The definitions and normal values of lung capacities

Lung capacity	Definition	Value
Total lung capacity (TLC)	The total volume of air in lungs after taking maximum inspiration	4000–6000 L
Vital capacity (VC)	The volume of air exhaled from maximal inspiratory level calculated as TLC-RV	(60–70 mL/kg) 5000 mL
Inspiratory capacity (IC)	The maximum volume of air that can be forcefully inhaled from the end-expiratory tidal position and is calculated as the sum of IRV and TV	2400–3800 mL
Functional residual capacity (FRC)	The volume of air remaining in the lungs at end expiratory tidal position. Sum of RV and ERV	(30–35 mL/kg) 2500 mL

population studies of healthy subjects and are taken from people matched for age sex, height and ethnicity.[24,29]

Forced Vital Capacity (FVC)[29]

The patient makes a maximum inspiratory effort and thereafter exhales as forcefully and rapidly as possible and the exhaled volume of gas is the FVC which is then recorded with respect to time (Fig. 2).[30] The rate of airflow during this rapid, forceful exhalation indirectly reflects the flow resistance properties of the airways. The exhalation should take at least 4 seconds and should not be interrupted by coughing, glottic closure or any mechanical obstruction. Generally, three acceptable tracings are required for analysis, and the values are compared to the percentage of predicted values which are interpreted as follows:

- Normal   80–120%
- Mild reduction   70–79%
- Moderate reduction   50–69%
- Severe reduction   <50%

Forced Expiratory Volume in 1 Sec (FEV1)

FEV1 (*see* Fig. 2) is the volume of air forcefully exhaled during the first second of the FVC maneuver. FEV1 is decreased in both obstructive and restrictive lung disorders.[25] Ratio of FEV1/FVC provides better knowledge on the degree of airway obstruction. FEV1/FVC ratio is reduced in obstructive lung disorders.

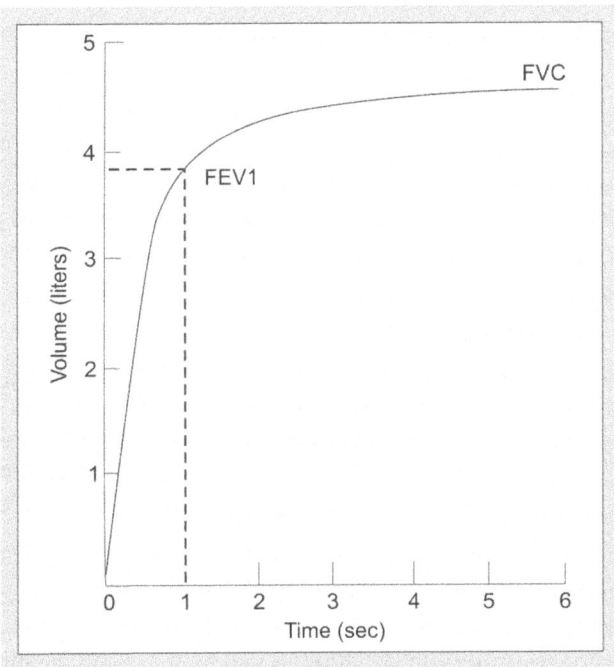

Fig. 2: Forced vital capacity (FVC) and forced expiratory volume in 1 second (FEV1).

Clinical range of FEV1 is as follows:
- Normal   3–4.5 L
- Mild to moderate obstruction   1.5–2.5 L
- Qualifies as handicapped   < 1.0 L
- Disability   0.8 L
- Severe emphysema   0.5 L

When FEV1 is interpreted as of % predicted:[31,32]
- Normal   >75%
- Mild obstruction   60%–75%
- Moderate obstruction   50–59%
- Severe obstruction   <49%

Peak Flow Rate

The maximum flow rate during an FVC maneuver occurs in the initial 0.1 second and is called Peak flow rate.[29] Although it can be estimated by drawing a tangent to the steepest part of the FVC spirogram, the method is subject to large errors.[30] Peak flow is measured conveniently with a handheld flow meter or more accurately with a pneumotachygraph. The peak flow rate in normal adults varies depending on age and height. The normal values are:
- 450–700 L/min in males
- 300–500 L/min in females

Values of <200/L suggest impaired coughing and hence likelihood of postoperative complication.[33,34]

Other forced expiratory flows (FEFs) which can be measured during a FVC maneuver are:[29,35]
- **FEF 200–1200:** It is the flow of air after the initial 200 mL and upto 1200 mL. It indicates PEFR and estimates the function of large airways.
- **FEF 25–75% (Fig. 3):** It is the flow measured over the mid portion of the FVC maneuver. It is independent of patient effort and is an indicator of small airway obstruction. It is a highly variable spirometric index largely because of its dependence on the absolute volume of FVC and on changes in expiratory time with various degree of airway obstruction. Average value of FEF 25–75% in healthy young men is 4.5 to 5 L/sec.

Maximum Voluntary Ventilation (MVV) or Maximum Breathing Capacity (MBC)

Maximum volume of air that can be breathed in and out of the lungs in 1 minute by maximum voluntary effort. The subject is asked to breathe as quickly and as deeply as possible for 12 seconds and the measured volume is extrapolated to 1minute.[37] Periods longer than 15 seconds should not be allowed because prolonged hyperventilation leads to fainting due to excessive lowering of arterial PCO_2 and H^+.[36]

The normal values of MVV are 150–175 L/minute and values <80% denote gross impairment. MVV is markedly decreased in patients with emphysema, airway obstruction and poor respiratory muscle strength.

Clinical analysis of spirometric findings can help in distinguishing between obstructive and restrictive lung diseases (Table 3).[37]

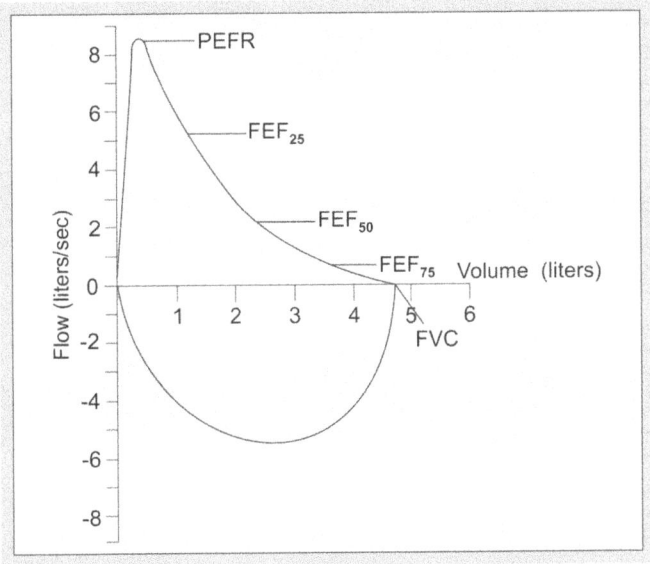

Fig. 3: Flow-volume loop showing peak expiratory flow rate (PEFR) and forced expiratory flow 25–75% (FEF 25–75%).

Table 3: Differences in lung functions between obstructive and restrictive lung disease

	Obstructive	Restrictive
Vital capacity	Normal or decreased	Decreased
Total lung capacity	Normal or increased	Decreased
Residual volume	Increased	Decreased
FEV_1/FVC	Decreased	Normal or increased
Maximum mid expiratory flow rate	Decreased	Normal
Maximum breathing capacity	Decreased	Normal or decreased

Flow Volume Loops

The flow-volume loop is a plot of inspiratory and expiratory flow (on the Y-axis) against volume (on the X-axis) during the performance of maximally forced inspiratory and expiratory maneuvers (Fig. 4). Tracing is obtained when a maximal forced expiration from TLC to RV is followed by maximal forced inspiration back to TLC. The normal expiratory portion of the flow-volume curve is characterized by a rapid rise to the peak flow rate, followed by a nearly linear fall in flow as the patient exhales toward residual volume. The inspiratory curve, in contrast, is a relatively symmetrical, saddle-shaped curve. The flow rate at the midpoint of exhalation (between total lung capacity and residual volume) is normally approximately equivalent to the flow rate at the midpoint of inspiration.[38,39] The initial 1/3rd of the expiratory flow is effort dependent and the final 2/3rd near the RV is effort independent. The Inspiratory curve is entirely effort dependent.

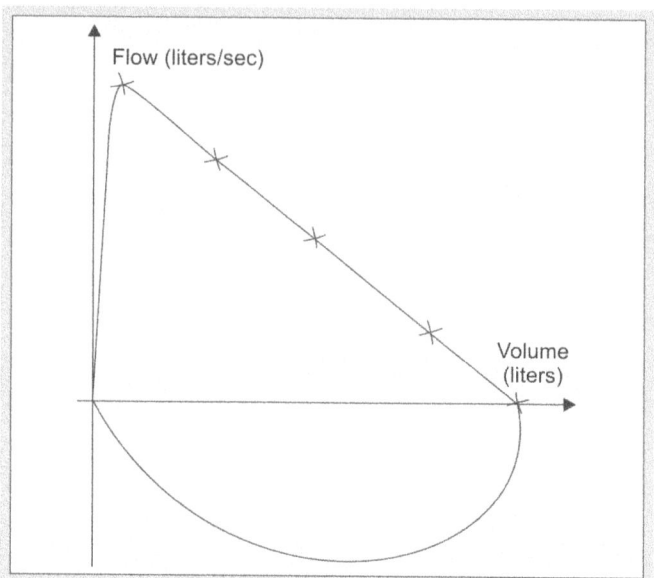

Fig. 4: Normal flow volume loop. It is the graphic analysis of air flow at various lung volumes. Ratio of maximal expiratory flow (MEF)/maximal inspiratory flow (MIF) is mid VC ratio and is normally 1.

Principal advantage of flow volume loops over a typical standard spirometry is that it can identify the anatomical location of the probable obstructive flow. In addition the reversibility of the obstruction in response to bronchodilators can be assessed by comparing the flow volume loops before and after the therapy (Figs. 5 and 6). Changes in the contour of the loop can aid in the diagnosis and localization of airway obstruction and characteristic flow-volume loop patterns are also often found in certain forms of restrictive disease. Flow volume loop in fixed and variable intrathoracic obstruction is depicted in Figures 7 and 8 respectively and that of restrictive lung disease in Figure 9.

Methods of Measuring RV, TLC and FRC

- *Nitrogen washout technique:* The patient breathes 100% oxygen till all the nitrogen in the lungs is washed out. The exhaled volume and its nitrogen concentration is then measured. The difference in nitrogen volume at the initial concentration and at the final exhaled concentration allows a calculation of intrathoracic volume, usually FRC.[40]
- *Helium dilution method:* Using a rebreathing circuit patient breathes from a reservoir containing a known volume and concentration of helium. With each breath, helium in the reservoir gets diluted by the volume of gas in lungs thus enabling calculation of total lung volume (TLC). For example, if 50 mL helium is introduced and the final helium concentration is 1%, then volume of the air in the lungs was 5 L.[41]

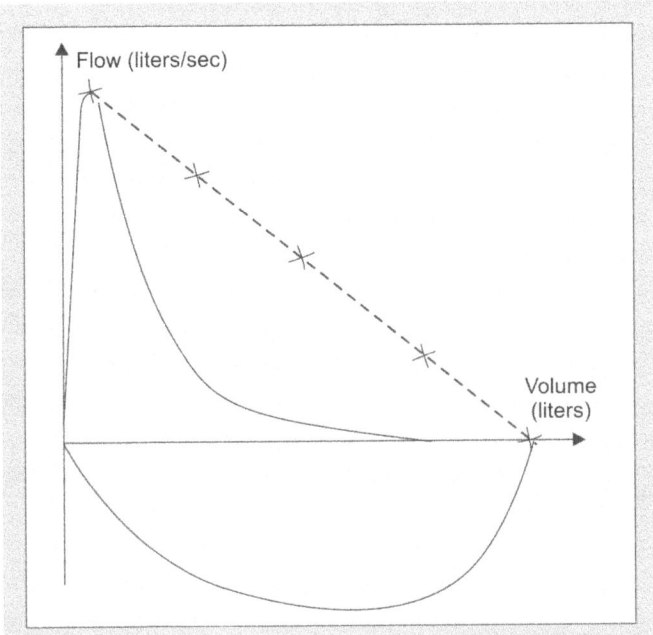

Fig. 5: Flow volume loop in patients with obstructive lung disease (asthma and COPD). The air in the large airways usually can be expired without problems, so PEF may be normal. The small airways are partially blocked, the air will come out slower resulting in a sharp fall in the flow-volume. FEV1 and FEF25–75 will be too low forming a concave F/V loop.[39]

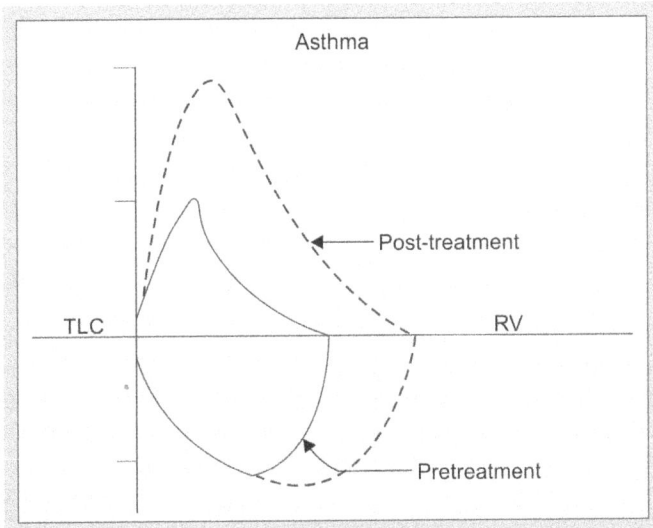

Fig. 6: Reversibility following therapeutic intervention is a characteristic feature of bronchial asthma and not COPD. Following treatment with bronchodilators there is improvement in FEV1 by 12–15% or 200 mL noted on repeating spirometry after 15–30 minutes.[27]

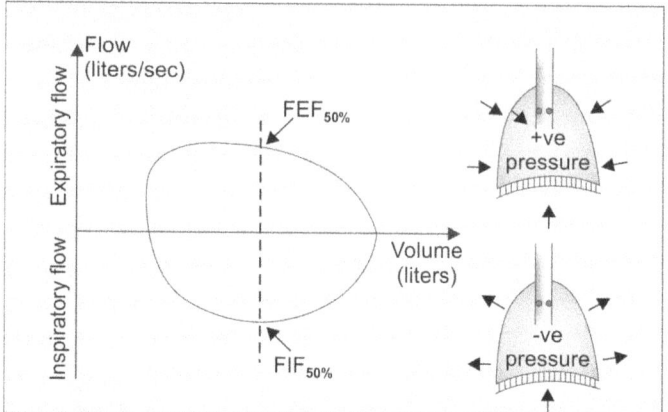

Fig. 7: Fixed airway obstruction occurs in conditions like goiter, endotracheal neoplasm or bronchial stenosis, there is a constant airflow limitation both during inspiration and expiration leading to flattening of both expiratory and inspiratory loop.[29]

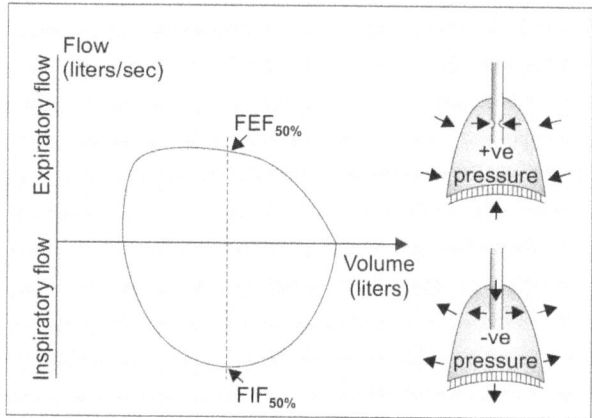

Fig. 8: Variable intrathoracic obstruction occurs in conditions like tracheomalacia and tracheal or bronchial tumors. During forced expiration there is an increase in intrathoracic pressure which decreases airway diameter. The flow volume loop shows a greater reduction in the expiratory phase hence there is flattening of expiratory limb. During inspiration—lower pleural pressure around airway tends to decrease obstruction.

- ❑ *Body plethysmography:* The patient sits inside an airtight box with a known volume, inhales or exhales to a particular volume and then a shutter drops. Patient now makes respiratory efforts against the closed shutter to produce changes in the box pressure proportionate to the volume of air in the chest. As measurements is done at end of expiration, it yields FRC across the breathing tube.[42] Measurements are based on Boyle's law which states that at constant temperature, the volume of a given mass of gas varies inversely with pressure. The advantage of this method over other two methods is that it quantifies noncommunicating gas volumes. Static lung volumes can be measured either by measuring the changes in pressure in a constant volume box or volume

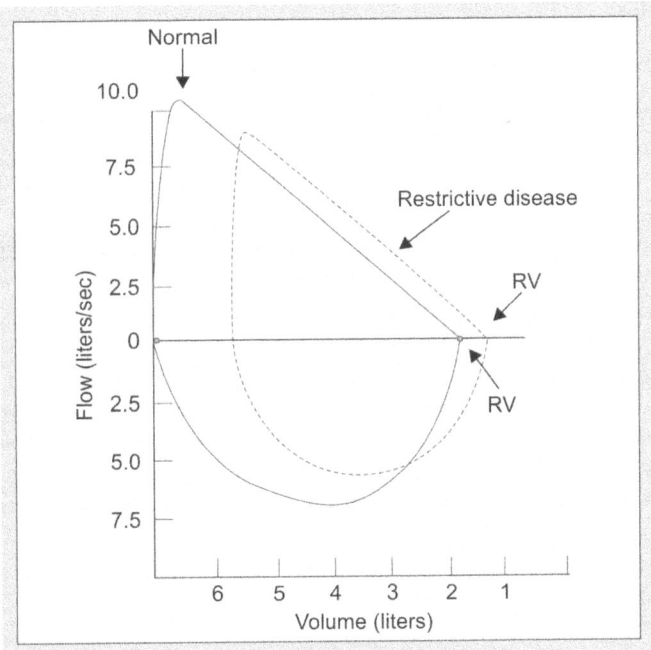

Fig. 9: Flow volume loop in restrictive lung disease due to conditions like interstitial fibrosis, scoliosis, obesity, neuromuscular diseases or following lung resection. The total functional lung volume is low which results in a low FVC, low FRC and low residual volume but FEV1/FVC is often normal. Peak expiratory flow may be preserved or even higher than predicted leading to a tall, narrow and steep flow volume loop in expiratory phase, the curve will descend in a straight line from the PEF to the X-axis.

in a constant pressure box. After the FRC is measured, the measurement of inspiratory capacity, expiratory reserve volume and vital capacity can be done. From these volumes and capacities, the residual volume and total lung capacity can be calculated.[29,41]

TESTS FOR GAS EXCHANGE FUNCTION

The ability of the lung for gas exchange can be assessed by calculating the alveolar-arterial O_2 tension gradient or by assessing the diffusion capacity.[43]

Alveolar-arterial Oxygen Tension Gradient (A-a Gradient)

A-a gradient is a sensitive indicator of detecting V/Q mismatch and indicates the efficiency of gas exchange. Normal value in a young adult at room air is 8 mm Hg to 25 mm Hg and indicates a normal shunt. It increases with age. It distinguishes between true shunt and V/Q mismatch. Increased values indicate shunt, V/Q mismatch, alveolar hypoventilation, or decreased diffusion capacity. Values more than 350 mm Hg are indicative of weaning failure.

A-a gradient PA-a O_2 = PA O_2 – Pa O_2
*PAO_2 = alveolar PO_2 (calculated from the alveolar gas equation)
*PaO_2 = arterial PO_2 (measured in arterial gas)

Formula:

$$\text{A-a gradient} = \left(FiO_2(P_{atm} - P_{H_2O}) - \frac{PaCO_2}{0.8} \right) - PaO_2$$

On room air ($FiO_2 = 0.21$, or 21%), at sea level ($P_{atm} = 760$ mm Hg) assuming 100% humidity in the alveoli ($P_{H_2O} = 47$ mm Hg).

Diffusing Capacity

A test of the diffusing capacity of the lungs for carbon monoxide DLCO, also known as the transfer factor for carbon monoxide (CO) or TLCO, is one of the most clinically valuable tests of lung function. It measures the diffusion of gas across the alveolar membrane which is determined by the surface area and integrity of the alveolar membrane and the pulmonary vascular bed. Normally the value is corrected for the patient's hemoglobin (DLCOc) which gives important information regarding the integrity and function of the alveolar blood membrane. It is measured by a single breath technique where 10% helium and 0.3% carbon monoxide are rapidly inspired, held for 10 seconds and then expired with the measurement of the remaining carbon monoxide. The ten seconds of breath holding required for the DLCO maneuver is easier for most patients to perform than the forced exhalation required for spirometry.[44]

- DLCO = CO mL/min/mm Hg.
- The normal value of DLCO is 20–30 mL/min/mm Hg.

CO is chosen for the test because it has a high affinity for hemoglobin which is approximately 200 times that of O_2, so it does not rapidly build up in plasma. The transfer coefficient (KCO) is DLCOc corrected for alveolar volume. In patients with a pneumonectomy, DLCOc will be reduced due to the loss of approximately half of the surface area of alveolar membrane but KCO will be normal as the remaining lung is normal with normal function of the alveolar blood membrane. Similarly, variation can be seen in diseases that affect the lungs in a heterogeneous manner, e.g. COPD or alpha 1 antitrypsin emphysema. In COPD the upper lobes tend to be preferentially damaged whereas in alpha 1 antitrypsin deficiency the lower lobes are predominantly involved. Therefore, DLCOc will be lower than KCO. Pulmonary emboli should be considered in patients with an isolated reduction in DLCOc without any other obvious respiratory cause.

Intrinsic restrictive diseases, in which the DLCO will be decreased, include:
- Idiopathic pulmonary fibrosis (IPF)
- Sarcoidosis
- Collagen vascular diseases (Wegeners, Goodpastures, etc)
- Amyloidosis.

Extrinsic restrictive diseases, in which the DLCO will be normal, include:
- Obesity
- Scoliosis
- Neuromuscular disease (myasthenia gravis, multiple sclerosis, etc.).

CARDIOPULMONARY EXERCISE TESTING (CPET)

It is used as a preoperative assessment tool. Preoperative risk depends upon the type, site and duration of surgery, apart from associated comorbid diseases in the patients. A VO_2 maximum value of < 15 mL/kg/min and an anaerobic threshold < 11 mL/kg/min are associated with increased perioperative complications.

Functional walk tests utilize an activity that patients are familiar with. They are inexpensive and require little equipment.[45] The most widely employed and investigated of these are the 6-minute walk test (6 MWT) and the incremental shuttle walk test (ISWT).

6-Minute walk test (6 MWT): A subject can walk for 6 minutes in their own maximum pace along a flat level corridor, turning around cones placed at 30 meters/100 feet distances at each end. Median distances covered are 500-600 meters in healthy subjects.[40]

Incremental shuttle walk test (ISWT): Patients walk around cones set at a distance of 9 meters (going around them is covering 10 meters) at speeds that increase every minute by 0.17 meter per second in time to audio signals. As the test progresses, the time allowed for walking the shuttle between beeps decreases. Failure to reach the cone before the next tone or exhaustion will stop the test and total distance walked will then be recorded.[40] A patient with a positive test (6 MWT < 427 meters; AT < 11 mL O_2/kg/minute) is likely to be at high perioperative risk, and a patient with negative test (6 MWT > 563 meters) would be considered low risk. A shuttle walk of 350 m correlates with a VO_2 max of 11 mL/kg/minute.

MISCELLANEOUS PFT'S

Bronchial Provocation Test

Bronchial provocation tests (BPT) are used to assess airway hyper responsiveness by artificially stimulating the airway with agents that can be direct, such as with the use of histamine and methacholine or indirect, such as adenosine monophosphate, exercise, hypertonic saline, eucapnic hyperventilation and mannitol. BPT is a valuable tool for assessing the severity and progression of both asthma and COPD.[46,47]

Split-Lung Function Tests

In the preoperative evaluation of pneumonectomy or lobectomy, split lung function tests are preferred over the global pulmonary function tests. The most conventional split-lung function test is the bronchial balloon occlusion test, in which the segment to be resected is blocked and traditional pulmonary function tests are then repeated and compared to the original. Regional perfusion tests (using IV 133Xe) allows assessing the relative perfusion of each lung. Insoluble, inhaled radioactive-labeled gasses (xenon, 99m-technetium) can be similarly used to conduct regional ventilation tests. The objective is to establish that after pneumonectomy or lobectomy there will be sufficient pulmonary reserve to keep the patient comfortable.

ASSESSMENT OF POSTOPERATIVE RISK IN LUNG RESECTION SURGERIES[48,49]

Stepwise assessment of postoperative risk is the key to the successful outcome of pneumonectomy and lobectomy surgery.

Step 1: Routine PFT's are done and if the following criteria are met, no further workup is necessary and following pneumonectomy, he would be left with at least 1 liter of FEV1 in the residual lung.

FEV1	> 2 liters
FEV1/FVC	> 50%
MVV	> 50% of predicted

Step 2: If the patient does not meet the above criteria on routine PFT, and if the FEV1 volume is less than 2 liter, we need to perform split lung function testing. The best and most current method of estimating split lung function is to perform quantitative V/Q scan. Perfusion scans correlate better with pulmonary function. One can calculate the FEV1 volume of leftover lung by knowing percentage of perfusion to left and right lung. For example:

Preoperative FEV1	1.5 liters
Right lung perfusion	30%
Left lung perfusion	70%

Assessment for lung surgery typically involves prediction of a postoperative FEV1 by using the preoperative FEV1.

Postoperative FEV1 = Preoperative FEV1 × Q% of the remaining lung

If the tumor is in the right lung. Following resection of the right lung, we can estimate 1.5 × 0.7 = 1.05 liters of the left lung to remain. The minimum acceptable predicted postoperative FEV1 is 800 mL. If the predicted postoperative FEV1 volume is less than 800 milliliters the patient is not a candidate for pneumonectomy.

Step 3: If the patient has PPO FEV1 value < 800 mL, and if the surgeon still feels that he has a resectable lesion with a good prognosis, the next evaluation would be to occlude the pulmonary artery (PA) and measure the PA pressure at rest and with exercise. If the PA pressure is elevated at rest or with exercise, the patient is not a candidate for pneumonectomy. The patient obviously has no capillary bed reserve and is not able to tolerate the loss of vascular bed. He will develop cor pulmonale and the expected 5 year survival will be less than 50%. This can also be done on the operating table by clamping the pulmonary artery and measuring PA pressures.

NEWER MEASUREMENTS[50,51]

The presence of endogenous nitric oxide (NO) in the exhaled breath of animals and humans, first described in 1991, lead to a great interest in measuring the fraction of exhaled NO (FeNO) in subjects with asthma and other pulmonary diseases. Recently, FeNO has been used as a biomarker for the assessment of airway inflammation and on comparison with conventional tests, such as BPT or the reversibility of FEV1, measurement of FeNO offer more advantages.

CONCLUSION

The introduction and development of techniques for pulmonary function testing have a long history, and up to the present, it has served as an essential tool for the clinical evaluation of respiratory health and disease. Correct data analysis and a good correlation with clinical findings make these tests a valuable preoperative evaluator. However, in the days to come these techniques and methodology will further improve and new parameters are likely to evolve.

REFERENCES

1. Ranu H, Wilde M, Madden B. Pulmonary function tests. The Ulster Medical Journal. 2011;80(2):84-90.
2. Quanjer PH, Stanojevic S, Cole TJ, et al. Multiethnic reference values for spirometry for the 3-95 year age range: the global lung function 2012 equations: Report of the global lung function initiative (GLI), ERS task force to establish improved lung function reference values. Eur Respira J. 2012;40(6):1324-43.
3. Tisi GM. Preoperative evaluation of pulmonary function. Am Rev respire Dis. 1979; 119(2):293-310.
4. Qaseem A, Snow V, Fitterman N, et al. Risk assessment for and strategies to reduce perioperative pulmonary complications for patients undergoing noncardiothoracic surgery: a guideline from the american college of physicians. Ann Intern Med. 2006; 144:575-80.
5. Cooper BG. An update on contraindications for lung function testing. Thorax Published Online First: 29 July 2010.
6. Marcadet DM. Advancing the frontiers of cardiopulmonary rehabilitation ambulatory chronic heart failure patients in rehabilitation. 2002;Chapter 24:204-9.
7. Gildea TR, McCarthy K. Pulmonary Function Testing. Cleveland clinic. August 2010. www.clevelandclinicmeded.com. Accessed 30.07.2017.
8. Young RC. Practical evaluation of lung function in the physician's office. Journal of the National Medical Association. 1966;58(4):245-9.
9. McMechan FH. The diagnostic and prognostic value of breath-holding test. California State Journal of Medicine. 1922;20(11):377-80.
10. Snider TH, Stevens JP, Wilner FM, et al. Simple Bedside Test of Respiratory Function. JAMA. 1959;170(14):1631-2.
11. Teklu B, Pierson DJ, Fair K, et al. The match test revisited. Blowing out a candle as a screening test for airflow obstruction. J Fam Pract. 1990;31(5):557-8,561-2.
12. Carilli AD, Henderson JR. Estimation of ventilator function by blowing out a match. Am Rev Resp Dis. 1964;89:680-6.
13. Pierce R, Hillman D, Young I, et al. Respiratory function tests and their application. Respirology. 2005;10:S1-S19.
14. Greene BA, Berkowitz S. The preanesthetic induced cough as a method of diagnosis of preoperative bronchitis. Ann Intern Med. 1952;37:723-32.
15. Daykin AP, Nunn GF, Wright BM. The measurement of vital capacity and minute volume with the wright respirometer. Br J Dis Chest. 1978;72:333-5.
16. Vichitvejpaisal P, Nava Kunvichit T, Stitsupamas U, et al. Bedside evaluation of the respiratory function in abdominal surgery with a simplified instrument a controlled study. J Med Assoc Thai. 1990;73(3):145-51.
17. De Bono, EF A whistle for testing lung function. Lancet. 1963;2:1146-7.
18. Cohen, BM A Vest Pocket Ventilation Function Device- the DeBono Whistle. Survey of Anesthesiology: 1966;10(4):332-3.
19. Rytila P, Helin T, Kinnula V. The use of microspirometry in detecting lowered FEV 1 values in current or former cigarette smokers. Prim Care Respir J. 2008;17(4):232-7.
20. Holcomb SS. Monitoring your adult patient with bedside pulse oximetry. Nursing. 2008;38(9):42-4.
21. Barreiro TJ, Perrilo I. An approach to interpreting spirometry. Am Fam Physician. 2004;69(5):1107-15.
22. Spriggs EA. John Hutchinson, the inventor of the spirometer—his north country background, life in London, and scientific achievements. Medical History. 1977;21(4): 357-64.

23. American Thoracic Society: Standardization of Spirometry: Update. Am Eur Respir J 2005;26:319-38.
24. Cheung HJ, Cheung L. Coaching patients during pulmonary function testing: a practical guide. Can J Respir Ther. 2015;51(3):65-8.
25. Laszlo G. Standardisation of lung function testing: helpful guidance from the ATS/ERS Task Force. Thorax. 2006;61(9):744-6.
26. Wanger J, Clausen JL, Coates A, et al. Standardization of the measurement of lung volumes. Eur Respir J. 2005;26:511-22.
27. AARC Clinical Practice Guideline. Static Lung Volumes: 2001 Revision and Update. Respiratory Care. 2001;46(5):531-9.
28. Black LF, Hyatt RE. Maximal respiratory pressures: Normal values and relationship to age and sex. Am Rev Respire Dis. 1971;103:641-50.
29. Thomas JG. Pulmonary function testing. In: Miller RD (Ed). Miller's Anesthesia, 6th ed. Philadelphia: Elsevier Saunders; 2005. pp. 999-1015.
30. Liu CH, Niranjan SC, Clark JW, et al. Airway mechanics, gas exchange, and blood flow in a nonlinear model of the normal human lung. J Appl Physiol. 1998;84(4):1447-69.
31. Mannino DM, Ford ES, Redd SC. Obstructive and restrictive lung disease and functional limitation: data from the third national health and nutrition examination. Journal of Internal Medicine. 2003;254:540-7.
32. Keddissi JI, Elya MK, Farooq SU, et al. Bronchial responsiveness in patients with restrictive spirometry. BioMed Research International. 2013;2013:498205.
33. Lebowitz MD. The use of peak expiratory flow rate measurements in respiratory disease. Pediatr Pulmonol. 1991;11:166-74.
34. Tierney WM, Roesner JF, Seshadri R, et al. Assessing symptoms and peak expiratory flow rate as predictors of asthma exacerbations. Journal of General Internal Medicine. 2004;19:237-42.
35. Wyka KA, Mathews MJ, Rutkowski JA. Pulmonary function testing. Foundations of Respiratory Care. 2nd ed, 2011;Chapter 17:455-81.
36. D'Silva JL, Mendel D. The maximum breathing capacity test. Thorax. 1950;5(4):325-32.
37. Al-Ashkar F, Mehra R, Mazzone PJ. Interpreting pulmonary function tests: Recognize the pattern, and the diagnosis will follow. Cleveland Clinic Journal of Medicine. 2003;70(10):866-81.
38. Karkhanis VS, Desai U, Joshi JM. Flow volume loop as a diagnostic marker. Lung India: Official Organ of Indian Chest Society. 2013;30(2):166-8.
39. Lunn WW, Sheller JR. Flow volume loops in the evaluation of upper airway obstruction. Otolaryngol Clin North Am. 1995;28(4):721-9.
40. Miller RD, Cohen NH, Eriksson LI, et al. Respiratory monitoring. In: Miller's Anesthesia. 8th ed. Philadelphia: Elsevier Saunders. 2015; Chap 5:11541-79.
41. Luo J, Liu D, Chen G, et al. Clinical roles of lung volumes detected by body plethysmography and helium dilution in asthmatic patients: a correlation and diagnosis analysis. Sci Rep. 2017;7:40870.
42. Cotes JE, Chinn DJ, Miller MR. Theory and measurement of respiratory resistance (including whole body plethysmography). In: Lung Function: Physiology, Measurement and Application in Medicine (6th ed). Oxford, UK: Blackwell Publishing Ltd. 2006. pp. 14:150-63.
43. Javaheri S, Sicilian L. Lung function, breathing pattern, and gas exchange in interstitial lung disease. Thorax. 1992;47(2):93-7.
44. Rubinsztajn R, Wrotek K, Krenke R, et al. The interpretation of carbon monoxide diffusing capacity test depending of hemoglobin concentration]. Pneumonol Alergol Pol. 2006;74(1):113-6.

45. ERS Taskforce, Palange P, Ward SA, et al. Recommendations on the use of exercise testing in clinical practice. Eur Respir J. 2007;29(1):185-209.
46. Joos GF, O'Connor B, Anderson SD, et al. Indirect airway challenges. Eur Respir J. 2003; 21:1050-68.
47. Cockcroft D, Davis B. Direct and indirect challenges in the clinical assessment of asthma. Ann Allergy Asthma Immunol. 2009;103(5):369-72.
48. Cukic V. Preoperative prediction of lung function in pneumonectomy by spirometry and lung perfusion scintigraphy. Acta Inform Med. 2012;20(4):221-5.
49. Gould G, Pearce A. Assessment of suitability for lung resection. Contin Educ Anaesth Crit Care Pain. 2006;6(3):97-100.
50. Rao DR, Phipatanakul W. An overview of fractional exhaled nitric oxide and children with asthma. Expert Review of Clinical Immunology. 2016;12(5):521-30.
51. Smith AD, Cowan JO, Brassett KP, et al. Use of exhaled nitric oxide measurements to guide treatment in chronic asthma. N Engl J Med. 2005;352:2163-73.

CHAPTER 10

Neuropathic Pain

Pramod Kumar

KEY POINTS
- While nociceptive pain occurs because of stimulation of nervous system, the neuropathic pain is because of dysfunction of nervous system itself, thus making it a paradox.
- It is a negative pain as it does not indicate any potentially harmful stimuli or disease process while rendering the patient debilitated and disabled.
- Neuropathic pain is associated with paresthesia, dysesthesia, pain and tenderness.
- The various etiological factors for neuropathic pain include trauma, ischemia, infection, metabolic disease and tumor invasion.
- Neuropathic pain is refractory to commonly used analgesics while treatment with gabapentin, opioids and TCA is rather empirical and unsatisfactory.
- Recent trials indicate that lamotrigine, carbamazepine and selective serotonin reuptake inhibitors may be used in patients not responding to routine pharmacotherapy.
- The neurolysis, dorsal column and deep brain stimulation along with neurosurgical procedures have also been used selectively.
- Proper clinical assessment, optimal planning of therapeutic approach and careful monitoring are the keys to successful management.

INTRODUCTION

Neuropathic pain is produced by an injury to the peripheral nerve and/or central nervous system having associated sensory sign and symptoms.[1] Various etiological factors include direct trauma, ischemia, infections, metabolic disease, tumor invasion, surgery, chemotherapy, irradiation, neurotoxins and inherited neuro/degeneration.[2-4] It is associated with (a) spontaneous paresthesia, dysesthesia and pain, (b) pain evoked by movement, and (c) tenderness over partly denervated body part.

TYPES OF NEUROPATHIC PAIN

Neuropathic pain may be classified according to its peripheral or central nervous system involvement (Table 1). Most commonly the following types of neuropathic pain are seen:[3,4]

1. *Traumatic neuropathy* which occurs due to axotomy distal to dorsal root ganglion and is associated with ongoing pain, hyperalgesia.

Table 1: Types of neuropathic pain[4]

Peripheral
- Traumatic neuropathy
- Trigeminal neuralgia
- Diabetic neuropathic pain
- Nerve compression/infiltration by tumors
- Herpetic neuralgia
- Complex regional pain syndrome (CRPS)
- Chemotherapy/Radiotherapy induced neuropathy
- Entrapment neuropathy (carpal tunnel syndrome)
- Radiculopathy
- Phantom limb pain
- Toxic exposure related neuropathies
- Inflammatory demyelinating polyradiculoneuropathy
- Alcoholic polyneuropathy
- HIV sensory neuropathy
- Nutritional deficiency related neuropathies
- Iatrogenic neuralgias (post-mastectomy/thoracotomy pain)
- Idiopathic sensory neuropathy

Central
- Compression myelopathy (spinal canal stenosis)
- HIV myelopathy
- Multiple sclerosis pain
- Ischemic myelopathy
- Pain after stroke
- Pain after spinal cord injury
- Radiation myelopathy
- Syringomyelia
- Parkinson disease pain

2. *Diabetic neuropathy* is length dependent, sometime affecting small fibers only. It is associated with burning pain and paresthesia in the feet.
3. *Trigeminal neuralgia* is due to compression of trigeminal nerve near brain stem and is associated with mechanical or stimuli evoked lightening attacks of pain.
4. *Phantom limb pain* occurs after limb amputation. There is a very severe pain felt in the ghost limb.
5. *Post herpetic neuralgia* is caused by herpes zoster virus. It is associated with an intense burning pain and hyperalgesia along affected dermatomes of the peripheral nerve involved.
6. *Sciatica* is a shooting pain in the leg along the line of distribution of sciatic nerve caused by inflammation or compression of its spinal nerve roots.
7. *Carpal tunnel syndrome* is due to compression of median nerve in the wrist leading to a pain in proximal area of wrist and fingers.
8. *Chronic pain* disorders include disk degeneration causing damage to the spinal nerves.
9. *Pudendal neuralgia* is due to a pressure over pudendal nerve leading to pain in pelvis.
10. *Central pain syndrome* caused by a damage to nervous system, e.g. post, stroke pain and neurological diseases.
11. *Complex regional pain syndrome* has sympathetic nervous system related pain after nerve injury, responding fully to sympathetic blocks.[2]
12. *Failed back surgery syndrome* after discectomy or spinal fusion may be due to pain generator produced because of recurrent spinal stenosis, degeneration of next level, inadequate decompression, nerve damage or epidural fibrosis.

MECHANISM OF NEUROPATHIC PAIN

Peripheral Mechanisms

Abnormal Sodium Channels and Ectopic Neural Activity

There is an ectopic and spontaneous discharge due to neuroma formation at injury site or in dorsal root ganglion (DRG).[2] Such ectopic activity may be caused by abnormal or dysfunctional sodium channels and explain the benefit of sodium-channel blockers, e.g. lignocaine, mexiletine, phenytoin, carbamazepine and tricyclic antidepressants.[5-7]

Sympathetic Dysfunction

The damaged primary afferent fibers developing adrenergic sensitivity and surviving afferents acquiring noradrenergic sensitivity has been shown in animal studies. Complex regional pain syndrome has sympathetic system related pain after nerve injury, responding fully to sympathetic blocks.[2]

Neurogenic Inflammation

Neuropeptides for example substance P and prostaglandins (PGE_2) having inflammatory action are released at the site of primary afferent nociceptors and sympathetic postganglionic neurons following a neural trauma. This explains the pain relief in response to NSAIDs, lignocaine and capsaicin.[3] The connective tissue sheath is supplied by primary afferents (nervi nervorum) which may enter the nerve trunk with endovascular bundle. The compression and inflammation of the sheath leads to pain and tenderness. There is a sprouting of afferents and sympathetic neurons in DRG.[2]

Central Mechanisms

Central Sensitization

This occurs with intense and long-term C fibers input, e.g. post-herpetic neuralgia (PHN), leading to pain. Further, with central sensitization large diameter and low threshold Aβ mechanoreceptors become capable of generating pain. At NMDA receptor sites, the substance P and glutamate activity leads to central sensitization.[4]

Deafferentation Hyperactivity in Dorsal Horn Cells

After peripheral nerve damage or dorsal rhizotomy there is a spontaneous firing in many dorsal horn cells, e.g. brachial plexus avulsion pain.[8,9]

Central Reorganization

A peripheral nerve damage leads to loss of central terminals of unmyelinated primary afferents; however large diameter Aβ afferents start responding intensely to mild stimulation and sprouts to innervate the deafferented nociceptive neurons of dorsal horn.[3,4]

Loss of Inhibitory Large Diameter Myelinated Fiber Afferents

Nerve injury can lead to pain as per Gate control hypothesis. Pain relief after transcutaneous electrical nerve stimulation (TENS) in mononeuropathies in trauma and dorsal column stimulation induced selective activation of the central branches of large afferents explains it.[3]

CHANGES AFTER SPINAL NERVE INJURY

After injury to a spinal nerve, various changes occur at different sites in the sensory neurons (Fig. 1). These sites are summarized as under:[5]

a. Spontaneous neural discharge ectopic sensitivity at nerve injury site.
b. The expression in DRG is re-regulated due to loss of trophic support and development of spontaneous neural activity.
c. The development of Wallerian degeneration distal to injury leads to release of cytokines and growth factors at uninjured portions of the nerve.
d. Partial denervation at peripheral tissues causes release of trophic factors leading to primary afferent's sensitization.
e. The molecular expression in DRG of uninjured nerve is re-regulated, due to increased trophic support.
f. Postsynaptic dorsal horn cell sensitization, leading to an increased cutaneous stimuli response.
g. Activation of microglial cells leads to sensitization of dorsal horn.
h. Descending modulation of DRG neurons leads to its enhanced response.

ASSESSMENT OF NEUROPATHIC PAIN

It involves assessing the pain and other associated symptoms for diagnosis and planning the treatment. A detailed history of neuropathic pain may reveal a delay in onset of pain following injury/disease, localization of pain and sensory loss, paroxysms of unprovoked spontaneous pain leading to disturbed sleep/or a change in character of pain. The pain may be constant/intermittent and stabbing, burning, sharp, shooting, electrical, numbness or tingling. Pain may be caused or relieved by applying pressure.[3]

Pain intensity can be rated and validated with verbal, numerical or visual analogue scales.[10] The assessment of unusual abnormal sensations is done by Neuropathic Pain Scale[11] and Neuropathic Pain Questionnaire.[12] However, the former is still not validated while the latter differentiates neuropathic from nociceptive pain. Chronic pain negatively affects quality of life. Therefore, measuring physical and emotional function is used in evaluating the response

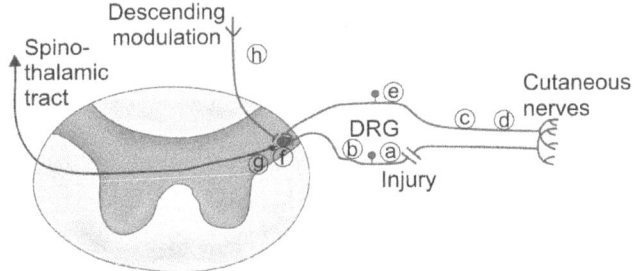

Fig. 1: Spinal nerve injury changes at different sites in sensory neurons.

to treatment.[5,13] The assessment of psychological co-morbidity (anxiety/depression), disturbed sleep, work related issues, treatment expectations, rehabilitation needs and family support is performed.[14]

On clinical examination, the somatosensory system should be evaluated for any positive sensory features without evidence of inflammation. One must look for *allodynia/hyperalgesia* when pain occurs in response to light touch or temperature. *Dynamic allodynia* may be present when evoked pain is worsened by light touch than with pressure, and/or the pain is relieved by pressure. *Hyperpathia* is the term to describe exaggerated response to normal painful stimuli stimulus, e.g. pinprick/temperature but with summation spread and / or prolonged pain after sensation.[3]

Quantitative sensory testing (QST) standardizes the sensory function measurement in controlled clinical trials to supplement neurological examination. The nerve conduction velocity test[5] and electromyography are useful to study large myelinated peripheral nerve function. Magnetic resonance imaging detects anatomical integrity of thermos-nociceptive sensory processing regions of brain, e.g. brainstem, thalamus, sensory cortex, etc., so as to assess their role in pain.[3]

TREATMENT OF NEUROPATHIC PAIN

Pharmacotherapy

Pharmacotherapy includes administration of specific drugs like anticonvulsants, antidepressants, antiarrhythmics, GABA receptor blockers and those acting on NMDA receptors. The *first line medications* include gabapentin, lignocaine patch, opioids, tramadol and tricyclic antidepressants (TCA) which are being used as initial treatment in neuropathic pain. Opioids and TCA require greater caution due to their side effects. Gabapentin has been used in phantom limb pain, herpes, spinal cord injury and Guillain-Barre syndrome.[3,15] The first line drugs with their doses is tabulated in Table 2.

Second line drugs are considered when first line medications are not effective.[4] Lamotrigine has been used in clinical trials for HIV sensory neuropathy,[16] diabetic neuropathy,[17] central post stroke pain[9] and spinal card injury.[18] Carbamazepine is most effective drug for trigeminal neuralgia pain. There are other anticonvulsants like oxcarbazepine, tiagabine, topiramate and zonisamide which are also awaiting result of controlled trials. Selective serotonin reuptake

Table 2: First line drugs used in neuropathic pain[3]		
Drug	Initial dose	Maximum dose
Gabapentin	100–300 mg at night or 3 times/day	3600 mg/day in 3 divided doses
5% Lignocaine patch	1–3 patches daily up to 12 h	Maximum of 3 patches daily in 12 hour
Opioid analgesics	5–15 mg every 4 h	120–180 mg/day
Tramadol hydrochloride	50 mg once/twice daily	400 mg/day (100 mg 4 times daily)
Tricyclic antidepressants (nortriptyline, desipramine)	10–25 mg at night	75–150 mg/day

inhibitors are tolerated better and have fewer side effects than TCA. Drugs like paroxetine, citalopram, fluoxetine, bupropion and venlafaxine are prescribed to patients not responding to nortriptyline.[4,19]

Beyond the second line medications, few drugs which have been often found effective in individual circumstances include capsaicin, clonidine, dextromethorphan and mexiletine.[4]

Stimulation Techniques

Transcutaneous electrical nerve stimulation (TENS), dorsal column stimulation and deep brain stimulation are being used to treat intractable neuropathic pain. The limitations of the invasive procedures include infection, bleeding or dislocation of electrodes.[2,3]

Chemical Neurolysis

This is being used successfully in gasserian gangliolysis, using glycerol. The patients with complex regional pain syndrome respond to sympathetic block using alcohol or local analgesics.[3]

Neurosurgical Procedures

Neurectomy, rhizotomy, dorsal root entry lesioning, cordotomy and thalamotomy are used for chronic intractable pain relief. These destructive pain procedures may lead to increased deafferentation and more severe pain. So, these procedures may not be used in neuropathic pain except for trigeminal neuralgia. Microvascular decompression of the trigeminal nerve by interposition or transposition is effective in treating trigeminal neuralgia.[3]

CONCLUSION

The diagnosis and management of neuropathic pain remains highly challenging because of complex pathophysiology and both peripheral and central mechanisms involvement. The pain is refractory to commonly used analgesics while available drugs in current use have limitations. Therefore, a proper clinical assessment, careful planning and monitoring is essential.

REFERENCES

1. Backonja M. Defining neuropathic pain. Anesth Analg. 2003;97:785-90.
2. Bennett GJ. Neuropathic pain. In: Wall PD, Melzack R. (Eds). Textbook of Pain. 3rd Ed. Edinburgh, Scotland: Churchill Livingstone; 1994. pp. 201-24.
3. Kumar P. Management of neuropathic pain. In: A Textbook of Pain. 2nd ed. New Delhi CBS publishers; 2008. pp. 254-7.
4. Dworkin RH, Backonja M, Rowbotham MC, et al. Advances in neuropathic pain. Diagnosis, mechanisms and treatment recommendations. Arch Neurol. 2003;60(11): 1524-34.
5. Campbell JN, Meyer RA. Mechanisms of neuropathic pain. Neuron. 2006;52(1):77-92.
6. Dellemijn PLI, Fields HL, Allen RR, et al. The interpretation of pain relief and sensory changes following sympathetic blockade. Brain. 1994;117:1475-87.
7. Devor M, Keller CH, Deerinck TJ, et al. Sodium channel accumulation on axolemma of afferent endings in nerve ending neuromas in Apteromotus. Neuro Sci Lett. 1989;102: 149-54.

8. Rowbotham MC, Petersen KL, Fields HL. Is postherpetic neuralgia more than one disorder? Pain Forum. 1998;7:231-7.
9. Fields HL, Rowbotham MC, Baron R. Post-herpetic neuralgia: irritable nociceptors and deafferentation. Neurobiol Dis. 1998;5:209-27.
10. Dworkin RH, Nagasako EM, Galer BS. Assessment of neuropathic pain. In: Turk DC, Melzack R (Eds). Handbook of Pain Assessment. 2nd ed. New York, NY: Guilford Press; 2001. pp. 519-48.
11. Galer BS, Jensen MP. Development and preliminary validation of a pain measure specific to neuropathic pain: the Neuropathic Pain Scale. Neurology. 1997;48:332-8.
12. Krause SJ, Backonja MM. Development of a neuropathic pain questionnaire. Clin J Pain. 2003 Sep-Oct;19(5):306-14.
13. Dworkin RH, Nagasako EM, Hetzel RD, et al. Assessment of pain and pain-related quality of life in clinical trials. In: Turk DC, Melzack R (Eds). Handbook of Pain Assessment. 2nd Ed. New York, NY: Guilford Press; 2001. pp. 659-92.
14. Haythornthwaite JA, Benrud-Larsen LM. Psychological aspects of neuropathic pain. Clin J Pain. 2000;16:S101-S105.
15. Backonja M, Beydoun A, Edwards KR, et al. For the Gabapentin Diabetic Neuropathy Study Group. Gabapentin for the symptomatic treatment of painful neuropathy in patients with diabetes mellitus: a randomized controlled trial. JAMA. 1998;280:1831-6.
16. Simpson DM, Olney R, McArthur JC, et al. For the Lamotrigine HIV Neuropathy Study Group. A placebo-controlled trial of lamotrigine for painful HIV-associated neuropathy. Neurology. 2000;54:2115-9.
17. Eisenberg E, Luria Y, Braker C, et al. Lamotrigine reduces painful diabetic neuropathy: a randomized, controlled study. Neurology. 2001;57:505-9.
18. Finnerup NB, Sindrup SH, Bach FW, et al. Lamotrigine in spinal cord injury pain: a randomized controlled trial. Pain. 2002;96:375-83.
19. McQuay HJ, Carroll D, Jadad AR, et al. Anticonvulsant drugs for management of pain: a systematic review. BMJ. 1995;311:1047-52.

CHAPTER 11

Management of Chronic Low Back Pain: An Overview

Babita Ghai, Dipika Bansal

KEY POINTS

- Chronic low back pain (LBP) is a highly prevalent and debilitating condition.
- Globally, LBP causes more disability than any other condition.
- Majority of the episodes are self-limiting and improve with time with a return to normal activity.
- Persistent pain can impact person's physical, mental and psychosocial ability to undertake normal activities of daily living.
- Emphasis must be given to communication and education of patient, family and caregiver regarding disease process, body mechanism, posture, exercise, early mobility and self-management practices.
- Personalized advice and information, tailored to the needs and capabilities, help patients self-manage their LBP.
- Prolonged bed rest is not advised as it causes deconditioning of body and weakens the muscles.
- Continuing with normal activities of daily living and return to work should be encouraged.
- A pragmatic multimodal treatment approach is required for management which may consider a group exercise program.
- Interventions are reserved for those who do not respond to conservative management.

INTRODUCTION

Low back pain (LBP) is a highly prevalent and debilitating condition. The emphasis on its management is of crying need nowadays. This chapter focuses on chronic low back pain (CLBP) with or without radicular pain and does not include the serious specific spinal pathologies (infections, malignancy, fracture, inflammatory causes, etc.) and potentially serious neurological sequelae (cauda equina syndrome).

EPIDEMIOLOGY

LBP stands among the top 10 diseases and injuries accounting for the highest number of disability associated living years (DALYs) globally as per 2010 Global Burden of Disease Study.[1] The data on prevalence and associated factors for CLBP are highly scattered in the literature due to variable definitions and heterogeneity of the condition. A global review reported the LBP point prevalence, one-month prevalence, one-year prevalence and lifetime prevalence to the extent of 12%, 23%, 38%, and 40%, respectively.[2] Considerable variation is reported in the lifetime prevalence ranging from 50% to 80%.[2,3] World health organization in a large back pain prevalence study conducted in adults aged more than 50 years spread over six low and middle income countries reported that the prevalence was highest in the Russian Federation (56%) and lowest in China (22%).[4] The prevalence was found to be 39.1% in India.[4] Other Indian studies have reported one-year LBP prevalence in medical students to be 47.5% while 83% housewives reported LBP.[5,6] Nearly 60% people in India have significant LBP at some time in their lifespan.[7] The ergonomic exposure at work causing LBP accounts for approximately 21.7 million DALYs. There is a 22% reported rise in overall LBP DALYs arising from occupational exposures between 1990 and 2010 due to population growth.[8]

IMPACT OF CLBP

Low back pain is a significantly disabling condition, responsible for long periods of absence from work and affecting health related quality of life (HRQoL). It is rarely fatal but profoundly affects functioning and reduces persons HRQoL due to suffering, failed treatments, difficulties at work and emotional distress.[9] It may also be associated with symptoms like chronic anxiety, fear, depression, sleeplessness, and impairment of social interaction.[10] Hence CLBP affects all aspects of life that is social, economical, psychological and spiritual.

RISK FACTORS

In the course of progression from a developing nation to an industrialized society, adaptation to westernized life style has made Indian society vulnerable to suffer from LBP. The interplay of working conditions, such as heavy physical work, awkward static and dynamic working postures, such as incorrect way of lifting and other lifestyle factors contribute to 85–90% cases of LBP.[11] The risk factors for LBP are listed in Table 1.

DEFINITION

Low back pain has diverse and variable definitions in the literature. Most widely used definition is by Chou et al.[12] LBP is characterized by pain or discomfort in the lumbar region, below the costal margin and above the gluteal fold that may or may not radiate to leg.[12] The nonspecific cases account for 75–85% where the exact etiology remains unknown[13] or multiple factors may play a role.

Table 1: Risk factors for low back pain
- Poor ergonomics/poor posture
- Prolonged sitting/poor posture
- Physical inactivity/lack of exercises
- Smoking
- Obesity
- Vitamin D deficiency

PAIN GENERATORS

There are various anatomical sources and pain generators for LBP symptoms like nerve roots, fascial structures, muscle, bones, joints, intervertebral disks and organs within the abdominal cavity. The symptoms can also generate from aberrant neurological pain processing causing neuropathic LBP.[14,15] A combination of these pain generators is usually observed in clinical practice. A pain physician is required to identify all pain generators and manage accordingly.

CLASSIFICATION

Low back pain can be classified into broad categories like **nonspecific LBP** (where the pain generator cannot be exactly identified),[12] **back pain potentially associated with radicular pain** (usually due to mechanically or chemically irritated nerve root or dorsal root ganglion), **low axial pain** (usually due to internal disk degeneration, or other midline pathologies), **lumbar canal stenosis** (may be due to soft tissue, such as disk protrusion/extrusion or bony stenosis, such as degenerative changes) or back pain potentially associated with another specific spinal cause, i.e. **facet joint or sacroiliac joint arthropathy**.[16] One must remember that these terminologies are not synonymous and should not be used interchangeably especially while generating evidence in systematic reviews.

Based upon the duration, LBP is classified as **acute** (pain lasting less than 6 weeks), **subacute** (6 to 12 weeks), **chronic** (more than 12 weeks) or **recurrent**.[17] International association for study of pain (IASP) classified the **leg pain** either **radicular pain** due to spinal nerve root involvement, or **referred pain** (non-specific) due to back pain that spreads down the leg from structures, such as ligament, joint or disk but not involving a spinal nerve root.[18]

LBP can also be classified **as nociceptive pain** (pain arising from actual or threatening damage to non-neural tissue due to activation of nociceptors), **neuropathic pain (NeP)** (pain arising from a primary lesion or disease of somatosensory nervous system) or **central sensitization** (increased neuronal response to the stimuli in central nervous system due to neurophysiological mechanisms, such as central excitability) pain.[19] NeP is associated with greater intensity, severe disability and worse HRQoL than non-NeP. A recent pooled analysis of 20 studies reported high NeP prevalence 0.56 (0.48–0.63) in LBP patients.[20]

EVALUATION OF CHRONIC LOW BACK PAIN

Chronic low back pain requires multidimensional assessment.[21]

History

Though it may not be possible to define a precise etiology of LBP symptoms for majority of patients, it is crucial to elicit the evidence of specific etiologies of LBP. The detailed history including an acronym L-OPQRSTUV (Table 2) but not limited to it must be elicited.

History about sick leaves and effect on job/job change/job resignation should also be obtained. Details of any prior back pain and its comparison with the present back pain must be obtained. Any other associated relevant medical

Table 2: Acronym L-OPQRSTUV for LBP history
L: **L**ocation (primarily back, paraspinal or leg),
O: **O**nset and duration (constant/intermittent),
P: **P**recipitating event (trauma, heavy weight lifting) and **P**rogression,
Q: **Q**uality (pins, needles, numbness, paresthesia, hot/cold sensation, dull/pricking which may differentiate nociceptive versus neuropathic),
R: **R**adiation or referred pain and **R**elieving or aggravating factors,
S: **S**everity of the pain (numerical rating scale/verbal rating scale/visual analogue scale/rupee scale/hundred paisa scale, etc,), **S**leep pattern (effect of pain on sleep) effect on **S**ocial life,
T: **T**iming of pain (morning/evening) past **T**reatment and its effect,
U: **U**nderstanding of patient about his condition,
V: **V**iews and feeling about symptoms that are important to patient and family

Table 3: Red flag signs for LBP
- Systemic symptoms: Fever, chills, fatigue, night sweats, unintentional weight loss, decrease in appetite
- Neurological deficit (sensory/motor weakness, urinary/bowel incontinence)
- History of malignancy
- Non mechanical pain (pain that gets worse with rest): Night pain
- Recent or current bacterial infection, especially skin infection or urinary tract infection
- History of intravenous drug use
- Immunosuppression
- Failure of response to initial treatment/therapy
- Prolonged corticosteroid use or diagnosis of osteoporosis
- Trauma

history and other comorbidities should also be elicited. Table 3 lists the "Red flag" signs (only suggestive and not conclusive of presence of specific problem) are evaluated for prompt management, if required.[22]

Various screening tools can assess the presence of neuropathic pain component. These include Neuropathic Pain Questionnaire, ID Pain, Pain DETECT, The Leeds Assessment of Neuropathic Symptoms and Signs pain Scale, and Douleur Neuropathic 4.[23] The functional disability can be assessed using Modified Oswestry Low Back Pain Disability Questionnaires (MODQ) or WHO disability assessment schedule.[24]

Patients should also be evaluated for social, psychological and behavioral distress. Screening for depression is also useful. Quality of life assessment is done using various questionnaires according to institutional protocol.

PHYSICAL EXAMINATION

The patient with LBP should be examined in standing, sitting and in lying down positions. The visual examination can assess for the presence of any asymmetry (scoliosis or kyphosis or skin abnormalities) around the lumbosacral spine. Any abnormal gait is also observed. The palpation of bony elements of spine, posterior pelvis and paraspinal muscles help to localize the patient's complaints. The discernible deformities, such as significant scoliosis or a high-grade spondylolisthesis may be tangible in a nonobese patient.[21] Paraspinal tenderness at the site of facet joint suggests facet joint involvement. Tenderness may be present at sacroiliac joint (SIJ) area in case of SIJ involvement.

NEUROLOGIC EXAMINATION

For patients suspected of having radicular pain or radiculopathy, neurologic testing should focus on the dermatomes involved. Testing sensation, muscle strength, and deep tendon reflexes can help identify the nerve roots are involved. Some rapid motor examination and reflexes are listed in Table 4 and these can help in screening the dermatome involved in a busy clinic.

Straight Leg Raise (SLR) and Cross-SLR tests are helpful in patients with radiating leg pain in an attempt to differentiate radicular from other causes of leg pain.[21,25,26]

The **Patrick or FABER test** (Flexion, Abduction, and External Rotation) is conducted to evaluate the SIJ pathology.[21]

To summarize, history and examination are crucial in the evaluation process to narrow down the differential diagnosis and for elucidating the pain generators. For instance, (1) **Discogenic LBP:** pain due to internal disk degeneration or lesion in the annulus. Pain usually increases on prolonged sitting or flexion while lumbar extension may relieve the pain. (2) **Disk herniation with sciatica:** pain radiates down the leg, SLR test is usually positive. (3) **Lumbar canal stenosis:** the hallmark is neurogenic claudication (increased pain while walking). The symptoms tend to get relieved with flexion while extension worsens them. (4) **SIJ dysfunctions:** localized tenderness, positive FABER and Patrick tests and diagnostic SIJ injection may help in diagnosis. (5) **Facet joint dysfunctions:** localized tenderness at the paraspinal area, pain usually increased on extension and lateral rotation and facet joint injections can help in the diagnosis. (6) **Ligaments and soft tissue:** usually musculoligamentous pain is a diagnosis of exclusion.[27]

IMAGING

Diagnostic imaging is required, if the patient suffers severe progressive neurological deficits or presents with the signs and symptoms suggestive of a serious or specific underlying disease. However, evidence indicates that routine imaging is

Table 4: Motor examination for LBP	

• Stand on toes: dorsiflexion with
  – L4,5
  – Extensor hallucis longus (EHL)
  – Big toe dorsiflexion: L5
• Stand on heal: plantar flexion
  – S1
• Hip flexor strength testing
  – L1,2,3
• Knee extension
  – L2-4
  – Buttock should rise from table
• Squat and rise
  – L4
	Reflexes
	• Patella reflex
	  – L4
	• Medial hamstring reflex
	  – L5
	• Pinprick sensation testing
	  – L2
	• Knee reflex
	  – L3-L4

not associated with clinically meaningful benefits in other patient population.[28] Guidelines do not advice the use of radiographs or laboratory tests in the initial evaluation process. The initial evaluation of possible vertebral compression fracture in selected higher risk patients (history of steroid use or osteoporosis) may require the use of plain radiography.[29] The exposure of unnecessary ionization radiation should be avoided as the gonadal radiation obtained from a single plain radiograph (2 views) of the lumbar spine is equivalent to being exposed to a chest radiograph for more than one year, which is of great concern.[30]

The American College of Physicians and the American Pain Society have suggested that clinicians should evaluate patients with persistent LBP and signs or symptoms of radiculopathy or spinal stenosis with magnetic resonance imaging (preferred) or computed tomography only if they are potential candidates for surgery or epidural steroid injection for suspected radiculopathy (strong recommendation, moderate-quality evidence).[12]

MANAGEMENT

Management of CLBP is challenging because of its heterogeneous etiologies, symptoms and underlying mechanisms. CLBP incurs substantial treatment and loss of productivity costs. Hence, it is of utmost concern to provide cost-effective and safe treatments. The initial intention to cure gradually shifts to improving pain, mood, functional ability and HRQoL. Clinicians help the patients by providing evidence-based information of the expected course of disease as well as various available therapeutic strategies.[31] The management modalities include nonpharmacological, pharmacological, minimally invasive interventions and surgery.

Nonpharmacologic Treatment Options

One of the important nonpharmacological options includes patient education and self-management. Other options include (but not limited to) acupuncture, behavior therapy, physiotherapy, massage, spinal manipulation, etc. The effectiveness of nonpharmacological treatment is not always sustainable.

1. *Patient education and self-management:* Patient education is simple and inexpensive option readily used by primary care practitioners. The patients are educated about the disease course, role of physical activity and exercises and management tailored to their need and capabilities to help them self-manage the appropriate body postures and ergonomics.[32] Evidence suggests that pain education changes pain-related attitudes and beliefs of patient.[33] It reduces catastrophization in people with chronic or subacute pain.[34]

   The patients are instructed about proper posture and life style modifications. They are also counseled regarding weight reduction so that burden on the spine can be reduced, regular exercises, maintaining correct posture during sitting and standing, use of firm mattresses while sleeping, lifting of things correctly and various stress management techniques as stress directly increases muscle tension and provoke more pain.[35] Bed rest is advised only for short duration (3-4 days) in case of severe acute on chronic LBP. Patients are encouraged to continue normal activities.[32]

2. *Physical activities and exercise therapy:* Patients with LBP are encouraged to continue with normal activities of daily living and return to work. Prolonged

bed rest is not advised as it causes deconditioning of body and may weaken the muscles. Muscle strength can decrease around 20-30% after only a week of complete bed rest and it takes much longer to regain that lost strength.

Exercise therapy is the most extensively used conservative form of treatment. It is reported to be effective at reducing pain and improving function in CLBP. The exercise should be delayed after waking up in the morning for 1-2 hours as the disks get swollen during night and make spine three times stiffer.[35] Systematic reviews have reported that exercise therapy is effective for chronic but not for acute LBP.[36] One may also consider a group exercise program in the form of biomechanical, aerobic, mind-body or a combination of approaches.[32]

3. *Acupuncture:* Acupuncture incorporates treatment with needles, which are either manipulated to produce a particular "needle sensation", or stimulated electrically for up to 20 minutes. The course consists of six or more sessions. Pain relief gradually accumulates, if the patient responds. It has been reported to be effective in providing symptomatic pain relief in CLBP patients.[37]

4. *Behavior therapy:* Cognitive behavioral therapy (CBT) is a form of psychotherapy effective in treating insomnia, anxiety, depression, addictions, and other mental disorders. It is also used in the treatment of CLBP.[38] The early and widespread adoption of CBT in treating and preventing CLBP is recommended.[39] It is employed for short-term relief of CLBP and shows similar effectiveness as exercise therapy.

Pharmacologic Treatment Options

Pharmacotherapy using oral analgesics remains the mainstay of the treatment in majority of the patients. Only safe and cost-effective drugs should be prescribed in conjunction with self-back care information. Baseline assessment of pain, functional deficits, and depression and potential risks of the prescribed drugs is crucial before initiating the therapy.

1. *Nonsteroidal anti-Inflammatory drugs (NSAIDs):* NSAIDs act by inhibiting both Cyclooxygenase enzyme (Cox) 1 and 2 that catalyzes the conversion of arachidonic acid to prostaglandin precursors. The anti-inflammatory and analgesic effects are selectively due to inhibition of Cox 2. The favored economical and safety profile makes them the first-line treatment for acute, chronic or acute on chronic LBP. All NSAIDs are reported to be equally effective. The major adverse events relate to renovascular and gastrointestinal systems.[12,40] The factors that are considered while prescribing NSAIDS to manage CLBP are potential differences in gastrointestinal, liver and cardiorenal toxicity and age of the patient. It is suggested that oral NSAIDs prescribed for LBP should be started at lowest effective dose and for the shortest period of time as per NICE guidelines 2016.[32]

2. *Acetaminophen (Paracetamol):* Acetaminophen possess similar spectrum as weak NSAIDS as it is a weak, reversible, nonspecific Cox inhibitor. The main effects are exerted by interaction with neurotransmitters in central nervous system. It should not be used alone for the management of LBP.[32]

3. *Opioid analgesics:* The NICE guidelines 2016 suggest that opioids are considered for managing acute LBP only if NSAIDS are contraindicated, not tolerated or found ineffective. These should not be used in the management of

CLBP. Tramadol, a nonopioid shares the mechanism of action of opioid analgesics by binding to mu receptors as well as by blocking the reuptake of norepinephrine. Various studies signal that it exhibits short-term improvements in pain and functional ability.[41,42] However, it should be used carefully in patients who are recovering from narcotic addiction. The main adverse effects are nausea, drowsiness and constipation.[41]

4. *Muscle relaxants:* Muscle relaxant may be used for short-term for severe muscle spasm in case of acute relapse on chronic LBP. They provide short-term relief in CLBP and causes sedation as side effect. The evidence regarding the long-term efficacy data is lacking.[43] Benzodiazepines carry the risk of dependency and are not advised.[32]

5. *Adjunctive analgesics:*
   - *Antidepressants:* Tricyclic antidepressants (TCAs) are commonly prescribed for the treatment of LBP with NeP component. TCAs like amitriptyline have demonstrated significant pain relief, improvement in sleep, reduce depression and can be a useful adjunct to analgesic therapy.[44] Duloxetine is another drug showing promising results in CLBP. However, NICE guidelines 2016 recommend against the use of selective serotonin reuptake inhibitors, serotonin-norepinephrine reuptake inhibitors, or TCAs for the management LBP.[32]
   - *Anticonvulsants:* Anticonvulsants are used for treating chronic and NeP. The results from the meta-analysis report that α-2-delta calcium-channel antagonists provide effective NeP relief for assessment periods ranging from 5 to 12 weeks. Pregabalin is found to be most effective and is associated with side effects like dizziness, somnolence, sedation, and peripheral edema.[45] The anticonvulsants licensed for the treatment of NeP include Gabapentin and Pregabalin.[46]
   - *Vitamin D supplementation:* Vitamin D is a steroidal fat-soluble vitamin. Various studies suggest that its low levels are associated with LBP.[47] The patients with persistent musculoskeletal pain are at high risk of the consequences of vitamin D deficiency. CLBP patients must be assessed for their vitamin D status and vitamin D supplementation should be advised, if found deficient.[48,49]

Minimally Invasive Interventions

Nowadays, minimally invasive interventions are preferred in the wake of unsatisfactory surgical outcomes.[50] These are usually employed when patients fail to respond to conservative pharmacological and nonpharmacological interventions. These interventions include but are not limited to trigger point injections, epidural injections, facet or SIJ injections, medial branch block, intradiscal procedures and other advanced procedures.[51]

1. *Trigger point injections (TPIs):* TPIs are the most basic and least invasive intervention for myofascial LBP.[52] Various pharmacological agents like local anesthetic (LA) and/or steroid, botulinum toxin, etc. are injected into the trigger points.[53] Another technique employed is "dry needling" which is reported to be equieffective as LA when combined with physical therapy.[54] However, TPIs may not provide long-term relief and have to be combined with other modalities.

2. *Epidural injections (EIs):* EIs are the most commonly performed minimally invasive intervention in managing CLBP with radicular pain with a reported rise from 2000 to 2013 of 165% per 100,000 Medicare beneficiaries.[55] EIs can be performed through interlaminar (either midline or parasagittal), transforaminal and caudal approaches. The approaches (parasagittal and transforaminal), which allow a high concentration of drug to be delivered precisely at the targeted site of disk herniation, i.e. ventral aspect of epidural space, are reported to be more effective than midline interlaminar approach.[56,57]

   There are conflicting results and ample amount of evidence in favor[58,59] or against EIs in general.[60] Despite these debates effectiveness of EIs for short to intermediate term has been observed in selected patients, i.e. lumbosacral radicular pain associated with disk herniation and radiculitis. However, there is insufficient data for role of EIs for central lumbar canal stenosis.

   EI of lignocaine alone has been reported to be equieffective with some superiority of adding steroid to it.[61] Recent systematic reviews have suggested that clinician may use nonparticulate steroid as first line drug for EI.[62] This evidence is particularly important with recent concerns and warning issued by US FDA regarding particulate steroids.[63] Though this warning has been highly criticized by other researchers.[64,65]

3. *Facet joint interventions and medial branch block:* Facet joints are one of the common pain generators accounting for 15–45% of LBP. There is strong evidence (Level I or II) for the diagnostic accuracy of lumbar facet joint blocks. These are recommended for patients with suspected facet joint pain.[66] Once the diagnostic block is successful, therapeutic intra-articular injection with lignocaine and steroid or radiofrequency ablation of medial branch block can be performed.[67]

4. *Sacroiliac joint (SIJ) injections:* The prevalence of SIJ pain is likely to be 20–30% among patients that have suspected SIJ pain based on history and physical examination. There is moderate evidence for the diagnostic accuracy of SIJ intra-articular injection and thus is recommended for patients with suspected SIJ pain.[68] Radiofrequency denervation of SIJ innervation can be performed after successful diagnostic SIJ injection.

5. *Other interventions:* Various intradiscal procedures (diagnostic discography, disk decompression, thermal annular procedures, etc.) and further advanced procedures (spinal cord stimulations, intrathecal infusion pumps, peripheral nerve field stimulation, etc.) may be required for selected patients or extremely refractory patients and are beyond the scope of this chapter.

CONCLUSION

Low back pain is a highly prevalent debilitating condition. It adversely affects the economic, social and HRQoL. In real clinical scenario multiple pain generators may be responsible for CLBP. As far as possible all the pain generators must be identified and managed accordingly. The wide spectrum of therapeutic options is available. A pragmatic multidisciplinary approach including self-management should be deployed for proper care and rehabilitation of the patient with emphasis on cost effectiveness. The emphasis on patient education, self-care, active life style and exercises should also be laid upon.

ACKNOWLEDGMENT

Authors would like to acknowledge the substantial and valuable contribution of Mr Mir Mahmood Asrar (PhD Scholar, NIPER, Mohali) in data acquisition of updated resource material and chapter preparation throughout the entire process of composition of the chapter.

REFERENCES

1. Al Mazroa, Mohammad A. Years lived with disability (YLDs) for 1160 sequelae of 289 diseases and injuries 1990-2010: a systematic analysis for the Global Burden of Disease Study 2010. Lancet. 2012;380:2163-96.
2. Hoy D, Bain C, Williams G, et al. A systematic review of the global prevalence of low back pain. Arthritis Rheum. 2012;64:2028-37.
3. Badley EM, Rasooly I, Webster GK. Relative importance of musculoskeletal disorders as a cause of chronic health problems, disability, and health care utilization: Findings from the 1990 Ontario Health Survey. J Rheumatol. 2010;2:505-14.
4. Stewart J, Peltzer K, Yawson A, et al. Risk factors and disability associated with low back pain in older adults in low- and middle-income countries. Results from the WHO Study on Global Ageing and Adult Health (SAGE). PLoS One. 2015;10:0127880.
5. Aggarwal N, Anand T, Kishore J, et al. Low back pain and associated risk factors among undergraduate students of a medical college in Delhi. Educ Health (Abingdon). 2013;26:103-8.
6. Gupta G, Nandini N. Prevalence of low back pain in nonworking rural housewives of Kanpur, India. Int J Occup Med Environ Health. 2015;28:12-25.
7. Bindra S, Sinha AGK, Benjamin AI. Epidemiology of low back pain in Indian population: a review. Int J Basic Appl Med Sciences. 2015;5:166-79.
8. Driscoll T, Jacklyn G, Orchard J, et al. The global burden of occupationally related low back pain: estimates from the Global Burden of Disease 2010 study. Ann Rheum Dis. 2014;73:975-81.
9. Nickel R, Egle UT, Eysel P, et al. Health-related quality of life and somatization in patients with long-term low back pain. Spine. 2001;26:2271-7.
10. Mathew J, Singh SB, Garis S, et al. Backing up the stories: the psychological and social costs of chronic low-back pain. Int J Spine Surgery. 2013;7:e29-e38.
11. Lionel KA. Risk factors for chronic low back pain. J Community Med Health Educ. 2014;4:71-5.
12. Chou R, Qaseem A, Snow V, et al. Diagnosis and treatment of low back pain: a joint clinical practice Guideline from the American College of Physicians and the American Pain Society. Ann Intern Med. 2007;147:478-91.
13. Posadzki P, Lizis P, Hagner-Derengowska M. Pilates for low back pain: a systematic review. Complementary Ther Clin Pract. 2011;17:85-9.
14. Smart KM, Blake C, Staines A. Mechanisms-based classifications of musculoskeletal pain: part 1 of 3: symptoms and signs of central sensitization in patients with low back (+/- leg) pain. Man Ther. 2012;17:336-44.
15. Garland EL. Pain processing in the human nervous system: a selective review of nociceptive and biobehavioral pathways. Prim Care. 2012;39:561-71.
16. Allegri M, Montella S, Salici F, et al. Mechanisms of low back pain: a guide for diagnosis and therapy. F1000 Research 2016, 5 (F1000 Faculty Rev): 1530. doi: 10.12688/f1000research.8105.2
17. Koes BW, van Tulder M, Lin CW, et al. An updated overview of clinical guidelines for the management of non-specific low back pain in primary care. Eur Spine J. 2010;19:2075-94.

18. Merskey H, Bogduk N. Classification of Chronic Pain. Seattle: IASP Press; 1994.
19. Nijs J, Apeldoorn A, Hallegraeff B, et al. Low back pain: guidelines for the clinical classification of predominant neuropathic, nociceptive, or central sensitization pain. Pain Physician. 2015;18:333-46.
20. Gudala K, Bansal D, Vatte R, et al. High prevalence of neuropathic pain component in patients with low back pain: evidence from meta-analysis. Pain Physician. 2017. Accepted for publication (In press).
21. Patrick N, Emanski E, Knaub MA. Acute and chronic low back pain. Med Clin North Am. 2014;98:777-89.
22. Williams CM, Henschke N, Maher CG, et al. Red flags to screen for vertebral fracture in patients presenting with low-back pain. Cochrane Database Syst Rev. 2013;1:CD008643.
23. Gudala K, Ghai B, Bansal D. Usefulness of four commonly used neuropathic pain screening questionnaires in patients with chronic low back pain: a cross-sectional study. Korean J Pain. 2017;30:51-8.
24. Fairbank JC, Couper J, Davies JB, et al. The Oswestry low back pain disability questionnaire. Physiotherapy. 1980;66:271-3.
25. Deville' WL, van der Windt DA, Dzaferagic A. The test of Lasègue: systematic review of the accuracy in diagnosing herniated discs. Spine. 2000;25:1140-7.
26. Tabesh H, Tabesh H, Fakharian E, et al. The effect of age on result of straight leg raising test in patients suffering lumbar disc herniation and sciatica. J Res Med Sci. 2015;20:150-3.
27. Nasser MJ. How to approach the problem of low back pain: an overview. J Family Community Med. 2005;12:3-9.
28. Chou R, Qaseem A, Owens DK, et al. Clinical Guidelines Committee of the American College of Physicians. Diagnostic imaging for low back pain: advice for high-value health care from the American College of Physicians. Ann Intern Med. 2011;154:181-9.
29. Jarvik JG, Deyo RA. Diagnostic evaluation of low back pain with emphasis on imaging. Ann Intern Med. 2002;137:586-97.
30. Jarvik JG. Imaging of adults with low back pain in the primary care setting. Neuroimaging Clin N Am. 2003;13:293-305.
31. Gourlay DL, Heit HA, Almahrezi A. Universal precautions in pain medicine: a rational approach to the treatment of chronic pain. Pain Med. 2005;6:107-12.
32. National Institute for Health and Care Excellence. Low back pain and sciatica in over 16s: assessment and management (NICE guideline NG59). 2016. https://www.nice.org.uk/guidance/ng59.
33. Traeger AC, Moseley GL. Evidence for a direct relationship between cognitive and physical change during an education intervention in people with chronic low back pain. Eur J Pain. 2004;8:39-45.
34. Traeger AC, Moseley GL. Pain education to prevent chronic low back pain: a study protocol for a randomized controlled trial. BMJ Open. 2014;4:e005505.
35. Londhey VA (2013). Approach to Low Back Pain. In Medicine Update, pp. 719-23. www.apiindia.org/medicine_update_2013/chap165.pdf.
36. van Middelkoop M, Rubinstein SM, Verhagen AP, et al. Exercise therapy for chronic nonspecific low-back pain. Best Pract Res Clin Rheumatol. 2010;24:193-204.
37. Xu M, Yan S, Yin X, et al. Acupuncture for chronic low back pain in long-term follow-up: a meta-analysis of 13 randomized controlled trials. Am J Chin Med. 2013;41:1-19.
38. Ehde DM, Dillworth TM, Turner JA. Cognitive-behavioral therapy for individuals with chronic pain: efficacy, innovations, and directions for research. Am Psychol. 2014;69:153-66.
39. Hanscom DA, Brox JI, Bunnage R. Defining the role of cognitive behavioral therapy in treating chronic low back pain: an overview. Global Spine J. 2015;5:496-504.

40. Roelofs PD, Deyo RA, Koes BW, et al. Nonsteroidal anti-inflammatory drugs for low back pain. Cochrane Database Syst Rev. 2008;1:CD000396.
41. Schnitzer TJ, Gray WL, Paster RZ, et al. Efficacy of tramadol in treatment of chronic low back pain. J Rheumatol. 2000;27:772-8.
42. Ruoff GE, Rosenthal N, Jordan D, et al. For the Protocol CAPSS-112 Study Group. Tramadol/acetaminophen combination tablets for the treatment of chronic lower back pain: a multicenter, randomized, double-blind, placebo-controlled outpatient study. Clin Ther. 2003;25:1123-41.
43. Malanga G, Wolff E. Evidence-informed management of chronic low back pain with nonsteroidal anti-inflammatory drugs, muscle relaxants, and simple analgesics. Spine J. 2008;8:173-84.
44. Staiger TO, Gaster B, Sullivan MD, et al. Systematic review of antidepressants in the treatment of chronic low back pain. Spine. 2003;28:2540-5.
45. Baidya DK, Agarwal A, Khanna P, et al. Pregabalin in acute and chronic pain. J Anaesthesiol Clin Pharmacol. 2011;27:307-14.
46. Sakai Y, Ito K, Hida T, et al. Pharmacological management of chronic low back pain in older patients: a randomized controlled trial of the effect of pregabalin and opioid administration. Pain. 2016;157:1499-507.
47. Ghai B, Bansal D, Kapil G, et al. High prevalence of hypovitaminosis D in Indian chronic low back patients. Pain Physician. 2015;18:E853-62.
48. Lewis PJ. Vitamin D deficiency may have role in chronic low back pain. BMJ. 2005;331:109.
49. Ghai B, Bansal D, Kanukula R, et al. Vitamin D supplementation in patients with chronic low back pain: an open label, single arm clinical trial. Pain Physician. 2017;20:E99-E105.
50. Chou R, Atlas SJ, Stanos SP, et al. Nonsurgical interventional therapies for low back pain: a review of the evidence for an American Pain Society Clinical Practice Guideline. Spine. 2009;34:1078-93.
51. Patel VB, Wasserman R, Imani R. Interventional therapies for chronic low back pain: a focused review (efficacy and outcomes). Anesth Pain Med. 2015;5:e29716.
52. Saeidian SR, Pipelzadeh MR, Rasras S, et al. Effect of trigger point injection on lumbosacral radiculopathy. Anesth Pain Med. 2014;4:e15500.
53. Jabbari B. Treatment of chronic low back pain with botulinum neurotoxin. Curr Pain Headache Rep. 2007;11:352-8.
54. Cotchett MP, Landorf KB, Munteanu SE. Effectiveness of dry needling and injections of myofascial trigger points associated with plantar heel pain: a systematic review. J Foot Ankle Res. 2010;3:1-9
55. Manchikanti L, Pampati V, Falco FJ, et al. An updated assessment of utilization of interventional pain management techniques in the medicare population: 2000-13. Pain Physician. 2015;18:115-27.
56. Ghai B, Bansal D, Kay JP, et al. Transforaminal versus parasagittal interlaminar epidural steroid injection in low back pain with radicular pain: a randomized, double-blind, active-control trial. Pain Physician. 2014;17:277-90.
57. Ghai B, Vadaje KS, Wig J, et al. Lateral parasagittal versus midline interlaminar lumbar epidural steroid injection for management of low back pain with lumbosacral radicular pain: a double-blind, randomized study. Anesth Analg. 2013;117:219-27.
58. Kaye AD, Manchikanti L, Abdi S, et al. Efficacy of epidural injections in managing chronic spinal pain: a best evidence synthesis. Pain Physician. 2015;18:939-1004.
59. Manchikanti L, Knezevic NN, Boswell MV, et al. Epidural injections for lumbar radiculopathy and spinal stenosis: a comparative systematic review and meta-analysis. Pain Physician. 2016;19:365-410.

60. Chou R, Hashimoto R, Friedly J, et al. Epidural corticosteroid injections for radiculopathy and spinal stenosis: a systematic review and meta-analysis. Ann Intern Med. 2015;163:373-81.
61. Ghai B, Kumar K, Bansal D, et al. Effectiveness of parasagittal interlaminar epidural local anesthetic with or without steroid in chronic lumbosacral pain: a randomized, double-blind clinical trial. Pain Physician. 2015;18:237-48.
62. Feeley IH, Healy EF, Noel J, et al. Particulate and non-particulate steroids in spinal epidurals: a systematic review and meta-analysis. Eur Spine J. 2017;26:336-44.
63. US Food and Drug Administration (2014, April 23). FDA Drug Safety Communication: FDA requires label changes to warn of rare but serious neurologic problems after epidural corticosteroid injections for pain. https://www.fda.gov/Drugs/DrugSafety/ucm394280.html.
64. Manchikanti L, Candido KD, Singh V, et al. Epidural steroid warning controversy still dogging FDA. Pain Physician. 2014;17:E451-E74.
65. Manchikanti L, Falco FJ, Benyamin RM, et al. Epidural steroid injections safety recommendations by the Multi-Society Pain Workgroup (MPW): more regulations without evidence or clarification. Pain Physician. 2014;17:E575-88.
66. Bernstein IA, Malik Q, Carville S, et al. Low back pain and sciatica: summary of NICE guidance. BMJ. 2017;356:i6748.
67. Manchikanti L, Hirsch JA, Falco FJ, et al. Management of lumbar zygapophyseal (facet) joint pain. World J Orthop. 2016;7:315-37.
68. Kennedy DJ, Engel A, Kreiner DS, et al. Fluoroscopically guided diagnostic and therapeutic intra-articular sacroiliac joint injections: a systematic review. Pain Med. 2015;16:1500-18.

CHAPTER 12

Intracranial Pressure versus Brain Relaxation

Dilip Kumar Kulkarni

KEY POINTS

- Intracranial pressure is defined as the force exerted by the intracranial contents against the wall of closed cranium vault. This definition is not valid, once the cranium is opened.
- Intracranial pressure is dynamically maintained by the intracranial components namely: brain, arterial and venous blood flow, extracellular fluid and CSF.
- When the cranium is opened, the concept of brain relaxation is considered. Brain relaxation is the relationship between the volume of the intracranial components and the capacity of the intracranial space when the cranium and dura are opened.
- Both ICP and BR are inter-related but the concepts are different. Most of management strategies are same for both ICP and BR.
- Brain relaxation can be achieved by hyperosmolar therapy with mannitol and hypertonic saline.
- Current consensus is to maintain normocapnia and reserve hyperventilation as a temporary measure for BR when brain is resistant to other measures.
- Head up tilt and CSF drainage help in BR but the latter has the risk of infection and cerebral herniation.
- Glucocorticoids are not recommended by Brain Trauma Foundation for management of traumatic brain injury.

INTRODUCTION

Intracranial pressure (ICP) and brain relaxation (BR) are inter-related terms but if we closely observe, the definition of ICP is applied when cranium is closed and dura is not opened. The brain relaxation is usually described when cranium and dura are opened. ICP can be measured by different methods using transducers, but the brain relaxation is usually observed subjectively either by surgeon or by anesthesiologist. The details of these two concepts will be discussed.

INTRACRANIAL PRESSURE

Intracranial Pressure is usually defined as the force exerted by the intracranial contents against the wall of closed cranium vault. The contents of the cranium are brain, cerebrospinal fluid (CSF), extracellular fluid (ECF) arterial and venous system. In an adult, the volumes of each compartment is distributed as follows, brain parenchyma 1200–1600 mL, CSF 100–150 mL, ECF 100–150 mL and blood volume (BV) 100–150 mL. The normal range of ICP is 3 and 4 mm Hg before the age of one year, and between 10 and 15 mm Hg in adults.

The Monro-Kellie hypothesis states that the cranial compartments are incompressible and that the volume inside the cranium is fixed. The cranium and its constituents (blood, CSF, ECF and brain tissue) create a state of volume equilibrium, such that any increase in volume of one of the cranial constituents must be compensated by a decrease in volume of another, once the compensatory mechanism reaches to the maximum, the ICP rises drastically (Fig. 1).[1]

Dynamic Components of Intracranial Pressure

In Monro-Kellie hypothesis an equal importance is given to blood and CSF. The CSF is secreted slowly at the rate of 0.3 to 0.4 mL/min, on the other hand the blood flow is 700 mL/min in and out of the brain.[2] If CSF is removed the ICP usually is reduced but accumulation of CSF will be slow to increase ICP compared to blood accumulation which can occur in case of trauma, where the ICP increases rapidly. The real dynamicity of components has not been highlighted in the original Monro-Kellie hypothesis.[3]

Arterial and Venous Influence on ICP

Cerebral blood flow is dependent on cerebral perfusion pressure (CPP), which usually its calculation from mean arterial pressure (MAP) with a formula CPP = MAP − ICP, when the ICP is higher than jugular venous pressure (JVP), it means that there is little involvement of venous pressure. This CPP equation has resulted in diverse guidelines that advocate MAP and CPP targets in the management of brain injury. For example, The Brain Trauma Foundation recommendation is to avoid systolic pressure below 90 mm Hg to maintain CPP. It is well recognized that gentle pressure to the neck over the jugular veins causes an ICP rise and the formula in fact to be written as CPP = MAP − JVP. Thus, venous obstruction also plays an important role in maintaining CPP.

The internal jugular veins are fed from three main intracerebral venous drainage systems:[4,5]
1. Cortical veins draining via bridging veins
2. Deeper (anterior) veins and
3. A series of small veins draining into the internal cerebral veins superiorly and the basal veins of Rosenthal inferiorly.

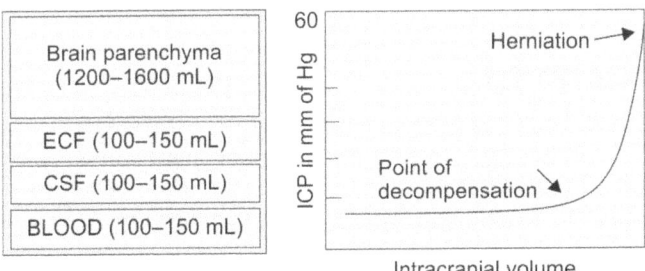

Fig. 1. Components of cranium and volume-pressure curve.

Unlike the strong muscular arterial walls, those of the venous sinuses are susceptible to dilatation and compression. Interpreting the value of and regulating ICP, without interrogating increasing central venous pressure (CVP) results in increasing ICP when compliance is lost, and this in turn results in the formation of brain edema and swelling.[6,7]

Causes of Raised Cerebral Venous Pressure

Intracranial venous hypertension can be caused by increased venous resistance/pressures within the cranium or outside it. Within the cranium this can be focal (from outside the sinus, within the sinus wall or within the sinus lumen) or it can be diffuse compression. Further, venous hypertension can originate in the neck, thorax or abdomen.

Poor head position is often overlooked but is an incredibly important cause of raised ICP. Mavrocordatos et al.[8] in a study of elective neurosurgery patients without raised ICP demonstrated that ICP was lowest with the head in a neutral position. Flexion and flexion with rotation caused significant increases in ICP.[9]

Cervical collars can increase ICP from about 4.5 mm Hg to as much as 14.5 mm Hg, the rise being greater in those with baseline ICP >15 mm Hg.[10-12] This probably reflects the degree of intracranial compliance: a patient who can accommodate less cerebral venous engorgement will have a more immediate rise in ICP. These mean pressure increases may be small, but they can have profound effects if sustained[11-13] or if the patient is at the limit of their compliance.[12]

Intrathoracic positive pressure ventilation in the treatment of chest infection and adult respiratory distress syndrome (ARDS) can severely raise intrathoracic pressure as can the application of positive end expiratory pressure (PEEP) with interindividual variation in ICP possibly reflecting deference in venous compliance.

Abdominal compartment syndrome (raised intra-abdominal pressure causing organ dysfunction) raises ICP in brain-injured patients which can be reduced by decompressive laparotomy (DL).[14] It has also been suggested that the raised intra-abdominal pressures in pre-eclampsia cause raised cerebral venous and ICP and contribute to the intracerebral hemorrhage that is sometimes seen.[15]

Thus, the ICP is dynamically maintained by the compartments namely, compressible brain to some extent, CSF secretion and drainage, arterial blood flow and equally important venous outflow. The definition and concept of ICP may not apply when the dura mater is opened during craniotomy. However, the surgeons will be complaining that brain is tense and not relaxed despite dura being open and CSF drained. Here the concept completely changes and the content-space relationship is important.

BRAIN RELAXATION

Brain relaxation describes the relationship between the volume of the intracranial contents and the capacity of the intracranial space when the cranium and dura are opened by the neurosurgeon. If brain relaxation is adequate the volume of the intracranial components will be either equal to or less than intracranial space available.

Thus, concept of brain relaxation can be defined as an ideal volume of the intracranial contents in relationship to the capacity of the intracranial space.

At the same time, the brain relaxation should also provide optimal conditions to perform neurosurgical operations. There is subtle difference in the concept of brain relaxation and ICP. But most of the extent the etiology and management of both the conditions are same.[16] These two entities are also intrinsically related. This relationship is corroborated by studies demonstrating that an elevated ICP correlates with a higher incidence of clinical brain swelling after dural opening.[17,18]

Assessment of Brain Relaxation

Subjective Assessment

Once the cranium and dura are opened, the status of brain relaxation can be evaluated by direct inspection and palpation. Different grading methods were used in different studies. Some use a five-point scale assessing brain relaxation from excellent to poor, including ideal, less ideal, tense, bulging, and the worst conditions for surgery. Others categorized brain relaxation as satisfactory or not.[16,19] Other studies classified the brain as tight, adequate, or soft.[20,21] A four-point scale, grading the brain as completely relaxed, satisfactorily relaxed, firm, and bulging, has also been used.[22-26] In general, it is best to avoid scales that have an easily defined midpoint (e.g. a three-point scale), as there is a tendency to select the midpoint level. However, direct visual and tactile assessment by the surgeon and the anesthetist is subjective, which may be influenced by factors such as the firmness of the tumor and the size of the surgical opening. A previous study demonstrated that the neurosurgeon's tactile estimation of dural tension in posterior fossa surgery was poorly predictive of subsequent brain swelling or herniation.[27]

Till date subjective assessment remains the most convenient and accessible method of grading brain relaxation during craniotomy.

Objective Measurement

The subdural pressure measured when the cranium is opened while the dura is closed has been used as an objective indicator of brain relaxation. This method is relatively easy, reliable, and minimally invasive, as long as the dura is not torn during the craniotomy.[27,28]

In patients with supratentorial tumors, Cold and colleagues[28] showed that the subdural pressure is correlated with the tactile estimation of dural tension and the risk of brain herniation. These authors found that brain herniation rarely occurs when the subdural pressure is <6 mm Hg, whereas pronounced brain herniation is much more likely at a subdural pressure that is =11 mm Hg.[28]

Another study conducted during posterior fossa surgery showed that brain swelling or herniation occurs rarely if the subdural pressure <10 mm Hg, and some degree of brain swelling and herniation is always present if subdural pressure is =10 mm Hg. These studies suggest that the subdural pressure is an objective and valuable supplement to the surgeon's subjective estimation of brain relaxation.[24]

Comparison between Brain Relaxation and Intracranial Pressure

It is important to differentiate the concept of brain relaxation from the practice of measuring ICP. Intracranial pressure is the pressure in a closed cranium, and objectively can be measured with a transducer. Brain relaxation, in contrast, is a more subjective assessment by the surgeon primarily based on the intracranial content–space relationship when the cranium and dura are opened. Intracranial pressure decreases to the atmospheric level (referred to as zero) when both the cranium and dura are opened, yet the degree of brain relaxation may not change or may worsen if the brain tissue suddenly expands. However, these two entities are also intrinsically related. This relationship is corroborated by studies demonstrating that an elevated ICP correlates with a higher incidence of clinical brain swelling after dural opening.[17,18]

In summary, brain relaxation and ICP are distinct concepts and are applied in different clinical scenarios. However, they overlap in some aspects of etiology and management related to poor brain relaxation and intracranial hypertension.

Incidence of Inadequate Brain Relaxation

The incidence of poor intraoperative brain relaxation, as manifested by brain swelling through the craniotomy site, is variably reported, ranging from 0.7% to 30% depending on the definition used and population studied.[29]

Etiology of Unsatisfactory Brain Relaxation

Any alteration of the balance between intracranial contents and available space leads to unsatisfactory brain relaxation and cause tight brain. The causes can be space occupying lesions of the brain like tumors, cysts, hemotomas etc.

Other causes are excessive CSF, excessive blood volume, hypoxia, hypercapnia, any factor increasing the JVP like neck compression, vasodilators, anesthetic agents like inhalational anesthetics with high MAC values.

MANAGEMENT OF ICP AND BRAIN RELAXATION

Most of the methods used to reduce ICP are also applicable for treating tight brain except decompressive craniotomy.

Hyperosmolar Therapy

Mannitol and hypertonic saline are commonly used hypertonic agents to reduce ICP as well as for brain relaxation. Both the agents extract free water from the brain and extracellular water into intravascular space by osmosis across the blood-brain barrier. There is initially increase in cerebral blood flow followed by vasoconstriction and lead to brain shrinkage.[30-32]

Mannitol is commonly used in the intraoperative period to produce brain relaxation in elective surgeries. However, in case of acute stroke patients undergoing decompressive craniotomy, the sudden shrinkage of brain can worsen the situation and cause midline shift and may cause herniation. The characteristics and adverse effects of mannitol and hypertonic saline (HS) shown in Tables 1 and 2.

Previous studies have shown that hypertonic saline and mannitol both are effective in reducing intracranial hypertension.[33] However, the current evidence does not support choosing one agent over the other.[34]

Furosemide is frequently used alone or in combination with a hyperosmolar agent to treat a tight brain. However, present studies does not support that furosemide acts synergistically with mannitol to reduce brain water content.[35]

Table 1: Characteristics of mannitol and hypertonic saline (HS)

Characteristics	Mannitol	Hypertonic saline
Dosing (Neurotrauma guidelines)	2 mL/kg 20% mannitol infused over 20 min	30–60 mL 23.4% saline infused over 20 min
Rheologic effect	Yes	Yes
Diuretic effect	Osmotic diuretic	Diuretic action via ANP (atrial natriuretic peptide.)
Hemodynamic effect	Diuresis may compromise intravascular volume causing hypotension, hypovolemia.	Augments intravascular volume, maintains MAP, CVP, CO
Proposed cellular effects	Antioxidant via free radical scavenging	Restores resting membrane potential and cell volume Modulates inflammation.
Potential for rebound edema	Yes	Yes
Half-life	2–4 h	Not known

Table 2: Adverse effects of mannitol and hypertonic saline (HS)

Mannitol	Hypertonic saline
- Rebound elevation in ICP - Hyperkalemia - Hemolysis - Hypotension - Diuresis - Hypovolemia - Congestive heart failure - Renal failure	- Rebound elevation in ICP - Hypokalemia – cardiac arrhythmias, hypernatremia - Hemolysis - Congestive heart failure - Coagulopathy - Central pontine myelinolysis

Hyperventilation

Hyperventilation has been used to reduce ICP for 50 years. Hyperventilation acts by constriction of cerebral blood vessels and lowering of CBF. Decreasing the $PaCO_2$ to the range of 30–35 mm of Hg, is an effective and rapid means to reduce ICP.[36]

This vasoconstrictive effect on cerebral arterioles lasts only 11 to 20 h because the pH of the CSF rapidly equilibrates to the new $PaCO_2$. However, $PaCO_2$ level below 20 may cause severe vasoconstriction and can lead to cerebral ischemia.[36] Prophylactic prolonged hyperventilation correlates with poorer 3 and 6 months outcomes in head-injured patients and should be avoided.[37]

The current consensus is to maintain normocapnia during intracranial surgery and to reserve hyperventilation as a temporary measure for brain relaxation when the tight brain is resistant to other means of treatment.[38]

Cerebrospinal Fluid Drainage

Cerebrospinal fluid draining procedures will reduce ICP and cause brain relaxation, however it is an invasive method with inherent risk of infection, hematoma

| Table 3: Effect of different anesthetic agents ||||||
Agent	CBF	CSF Production	CSF Absorption	CBV	ICP
Isoflurane	+	±	+	++	+
Sevoflurane	+	?	?	?	++
Desflurane	+	+	-	?	++
Enflurane	++	+	-	++	++
Nitrous oxide	+	±	±	±	+
Barbiturates	- - -	±	+	- -	- - -
Etomidate	- -	±	+	- -	- -
Propofol	- - - -	?	?	- - -	- - -
Benzodiazepines	?	±	+	-	- -
Ketamine	++	±	-	++	++
Opioids	±	±	+	±	±
Lignocaine	- -	?	?	- -	- -

Note: + means Increase, – means Decrease, ± means No Change

formation and nerve injury. Cerebral herniation is also a potential risk of CSF drainage, especially if lumbar drainage is used.[39]

Head-up Tilt

Head-up tilt usually reduces ICP by relocation of CSF from intracranial space to extracranial intrathecal space and by reducing CBV by the gravitational facilitation of cerebral venous blood drainage, and possibly, by the gravitational traction on the brain. Elevation of head by 30 degrees reduces ICP in head injured patients.[40] While undergoing surgery 10 degree elevation reduces ICP without reducing cerebral perfusion.[41]

Intravenous and Inhalation Anesthesia

It is very difficult to decide which technique is better between inhalational or intravenous anesthesia with present available scientific evidence. The inhalational agents do not significantly increase ICP and brain bulk if <0.5 MAC is used.[42] The effect of different anesthetic agents is given in Table 3.

Steroids

Glucocorticoids are not recommended by Brain Trauma Foundation for the management of traumatic brain injury.[43] The glucocorticoids have not been shown to reduce edema (both vasogenic and cytotoxic) effectively in the setting of intracerebral hemorrhage or ischemic stroke. But glucocorticoids such as dexamethasone are often administered in the perioperative period to reduce tumor-associated edema, although the precise mechanisms behind these effects are not clear.[44]

CONCLUSION

Intracranial pressure by definition is valid only when the cranium is closed, whereas in anesthesia practice during surgery once the dura is opened, the definition of ICP does not apply and a content-space relationship between the volume of the intracranial contents and the capacity of the intracranial space come into play. Although brain relaxation is correlated with intracranial pressure, the concept differs. The outcomes of patients depend on defining, evaluating, and managing not only ICP but also brain relaxation.

REFERENCES

1. Mokri B. The Monro-Kellie hypothesis: applications in CSF volume depletion. Neurology. 2001;56(12):1746-8.
2. Milhorat TH. The third circulation revisited. J Neurosurg. 1975;42:628-645.
3. Wilson MH. Monro-Kellie 2.0: The dynamic vascular and venous pathophysiological components of intracranial pressure. J Cereb Blood Flow Metab [Internet]. 2016;36(8): 1338-50. Available at: http://journals.sagepub.com/doi/10.1177/ 0271678X16648711.
4. Wilson MH, Imray CHE, Hargens AR. The headache of high altitude and microgravity-similarities with clinical syndromes of cerebral venous hypertension. High Alt Med Biol. 2011;12:379-86.
5. Beards SCS, Yule SS, Kassner AA, et al. Anatomical variation of cerebral venous drainage: the theoretical effect on jugular bulb blood samples. Anaesthesia. 1998;53: 627-33.
6. Boushel R, Durgun BB, Ilglt ETE, et al. Evaluation by angiography of the lateral dominance of the drainage of the dural venous sinuses. Surg Radiol Anat. 1993; 15:125-30.
7. Lavoie P, Metellus P, Velly L, et al. Functional cerebral venous outflow in swine and baboon: feasibility of an intracranial venous hypertension model. J Invest Surg. 2008; 21:323-9.
8. Mavrocordatos P, Bissonnette B, Ravussin P. Effects of neck position and head elevation on intracranial pressure in anaesthetized neurosurgical patients: preliminary results. J Neurosurg Anesthesiol. 2000;12:10-14.
9. Goldberg RN, Joshi A, Moscoso P, et al. The effect of head position on intracranial pressure in the neonate. Crit Care Med. 1983;11:428-30.
10. Mobbs RJ, Vuyk J, Van Den Bos J, et al. Effect of cervical hard collar on intracranial pressure after head injury. ANZ J Surg. 2002;72:389-91.
11. Davies G, Deakin C, Wilson A. The effect of a rigid collar on intracranial pressure. Injury. 1996;27:647-9.
12. Hunt K, Hallworth S, Smith M. The effects of rigid collar placement on intracranial and cerebral perfusion pressures. Anaesthesia. 2001;56:511-3.
13. Craig GR and Nielsen MS. Rigid cervical collars and intracranial pressure. Intensive Care Med. 1991;17:504-5.
14. Scalea TM, Bochicchio GV, Habashi N, et al. Increased intra-abdominal, intrathoracic, and intracranial pressure after severe brain injury: multiple compartment syndrome. J Trauma. 2007;62:647-56.
15. Sugerman HJ. Hypothesis: preeclampsia is a venous disease secondary to an increased intra-abdominal pressure. Med Hypotheses. 2011;77:841-9.
16. Li J, Gelb AW, Flexman AM, et al. Definition, evaluation, and management of brain relaxation during craniotomy. Br J Anaesth. 2016;116(6):759-69.
17. Iversen BN, Rasmussen M, Cold GE. The relationship between intracranial pressure and the degree of brain swelling in patients subjected to infratentorial surgery. Acta Neurochirurgica. 2008;150:337-44.

18. Turner CR, Losasso TJ, Muzzi DA, et al. Brain relaxation and cerebrospinal fluid pressure during craniotomy for resection of supratentorial mass lesions. J Neurosurg Anesthesiol. 1996;8:126-32.
19. Gemma M, Cozzi S, Tommasino C, et al. 7.5% hypertonic saline versus 20% mannitol during elective neurosurgical supratentorial procedures. J Neurosurg Anesthesiol. 1997;9:329-34.
20. Sneyd JR, Andrews CJ, Tsubokawa T. Comparison of propofol/remifentanil and sevoflurane/remifentanil for maintenance of anaesthesia for elective intracranial surgery. Br J Anaesth. 2005;94:778-83.
21. Wu C-T, Chen L-C, Kuo C-P, et al. A comparison of 3% hypertonic saline and mannitol for brain relaxation during elective supratentorial brain tumor surgery. Anesth Analg. 2010;110:903-7.
22. Dostal P, Dostalova V, Schreiberova J, et al. A comparison of equivolume, equiosmolar solutions of hypertonic saline and mannitol for brain relaxation in patients undergoing elective intracranial tumor surgery: a randomized clinical trial. J Neurosurg Anesthesiol. 2015;27:51-6.
23. Todd MM, Warner DS, Sokoll MD, et al. A prospective, comparative trial of three anesthetics for elective supratentorial craniotomy. Propofol/fentanyl, isoflurane/nitrous oxide, and fentanyl/nitrous oxide. Anesthesiology. 1993;78:1005-20.
24. Gelb AW, Craen RA, Rao GSU, et al. Does hyperventilation improve operating condition during supratentorial craniotomy? A multicenter randomized crossover trial. Anesth Analg. 2008;106:585-94.
25. Citerio G, Pesenti A, Latini R, et al. A multicentre, randomised, open-label, controlled trial evaluating equivalence of inhalational and intravenous anaesthesia during elective craniotomy. Eur J Anaesthesiol. 2012;29:371-9.
26. Quentin C, Charbonneau S, Moumdjian R, et al. A comparison of two doses of mannitol on brain relaxation during supratentorial brain tumor craniotomy. Anesth Analg. 2013; 116:862-8.
27. Jorgensen HA, Bundgaard H, Cold GE. Subdural pressure measurement during posterior fossa surgery. Correlation studies of brain swelling/herniation after dural incision with measurement of subdural pressure and tactile estimation of dural tension. Br J Neurosurg. 1999;13:449-53.
28. Cold GE, Tange M, Jensen TM, et al. 'Subdural' pressure measurement during craniotomy. Correlation with tactile estimation of dural tension and brain herniation after opening of dura. Br J Neurosurg. 1996;10:69-75.
29. Rasmussen M, Bundgaard H, Cold GE. Craniotomy for supratentorial brain tumors: risk factors for brain swelling after opening the dura mater. J Neurosurg. 2004;101: 621-6.
30. Muizelaar JP, Wei EP, Kontos HA, et al. Mannitol causes compensatory cerebral vasoconstriction and vasodilation in response to blood viscosity changes. J Neurosurg. 1983;59:822-8.
31. Prough DS, Whitley JM, Taylor CL, et al. Regional cerebral blood flow following resuscitation from hemorrhagic shock with hypertonic saline. Influence of a subdural mass. Anesthesiology. 1991;75:319-27.
32. Muizelaar JP, Lutz HA III, Becker DP. Effect of mannitol on ICP and CBF and correlation with pressure autoregulation in severely head-injured patients. J Neurosurg. 1984;61: 700-6.
33. Kamel H, Navi BB, Nakagawa K, et al. Hypertonic saline versus mannitol for the treatment of elevated intracranial pressure: a meta-analysis of randomized clinical trials. Crit Care Med. 2011;39:554-9.

34. Prabhakar H, Singh GP, Anand V, et al. Mannitol versus hypertonic saline for brain relaxation in patients undergoing craniotomy. Cochrane Database Syst Rev. 2014; 7:CD010026.
35. Wang LC, Papangelou A, Lin C, et al. Comparison of equivolume, equiosmolar solutions of mannitol and hypertonic saline with or without furosemide on brain water content in normal rats. Anesthesiology. 2013;118:903-13.
36. Sankhyan N, Raju KNV, Sharma S, et al. Management of raised intracranial pressure. Indian J Pediatr. 2010;77(12):1409-16.
37. Muizelaar JP, Marmarou A, Ward JD, et al. Adverse effects of prolonged hyperventilation in patients with severe head injury: a randomized clinical trial. J Neurosurg. 1991;75:731-9.
38. Talke PO, Sharma D, Heyer EJ, et al. Society for Neuroscience in Anesthesiology and Critical Care Expert consensus statement: anesthetic management of endovascular treatment for acute ischemic stroke: endorsed by the Society of NeuroInterventional Surgery and the Neurocritical Care Society. J Neurosurg Anesthesiol. 2014;26:95-108.
39. Grady MS. Editorial. Lumbar drainage for increased intracranial pressure. J Neurosurg. 2009;110:1198-9.
40. Feldman Z, Kanter MJ, Robertson CS, et al. Effect of head elevation on intracranial pressure, cerebral perfusion pressure, and cerebral blood flow in head-injured patients. J Neurosurg. 1992;76:207-11.
41. Tankisi A, Rolighed Larsen J, Rasmussen M, et al. The effects of 10° reverse Trendelenburg position on ICP and CPP in prone positioned patients subjected to craniotomy for occipital or cerebellar tumours. Acta Neurochir (Wien). 2002;144:665-70.
42. Chui J, Mariappan R, Mehta J, et al. Comparison of propofol and volatile agents for maintenance of anesthesia during elective craniotomy procedures: systematic review and meta-analysis. Can J Anaesth. 2014;61:347-56.
43. Brain Trauma Foundation, American Association of Neurological Surgeons, Congress of Neurological Surgeons. Guidelines for the management of severe traumatic brain injury. J Neurotrauma. 2007;24(Suppl 1):S1-106.
44. Ryken TC, McDermott M, Robinson PD, et al. The role of steroids in the management of brain metastases: a systematic review and evidence-based clinical practice guideline. J Neurooncol. 2010;96:103-14.

CHAPTER 13

Sepsis and the Anesthesiologist

Krishna HM, Basavaraj Herekar

KEY POINTS

- Only emergency surgeries are done in septic patients. Bundled care for sepsis management is continued all along the perioperative period.
- Hypotension and hypoxemia are the common problems encountered during anesthetic management of septic patients. One has to be prepared to manage these.
- General anesthesia or locoregional anesthesia are the commonly used techniques.
- Goal directed fluid therapy, use of norepinephrine as vasopressor, use of relatively hemodynamically stable drugs like ketamine, etomidate, short acting opioids and benzodiazepines, invasive monitoring, protective lung ventilation form the core principles in the anesthetic management of septic patients.

INTRODUCTION

The syndrome of sepsis accounts for high incidence of death and intensive care unit (ICU) admissions worldwide and the incidence is increasing. Sepsis is different from infection because the host response, in sepsis, is uncontrolled and lacks the regulatory mechanism. It is also characterized by organ dysfunction.[1] Research into the pathophysiology of sepsis has enabled us to define and identify patients in sepsis better. Initially sepsis was viewed as a spectrum encompassing systemic inflammatory response syndrome (SIRS), severe sepsis and septic shock. The focus was solely on inflammatory excess. But now it is being understood that along with the proinflammatory response the anti-inflammatory response is also activated.

The existing definitions, since the 1991 consensus conference, were re-examined by The European Society of Intensive Care Medicine (ESICM) and the Society of Critical Care Medicine (SCCM) in January 2014. They put out the third international consensus definitions for sepsis and septic shock (Sepsis-3) in 2015 which is summarized in Table 1.[1] The mortality rate is found to be more than 10% even in the presence of mild degree of organ dysfunction secondary to an infection.[2] In view of this the term "severe sepsis" included in the previous definitions has been removed.

SURGERY IN A PATIENT WITH SEPSIS

The commonest indication for surgery in a patient with sepsis is for source control of the infection. Source control measures should be initiated within 12 h

Table 1: New terms and definitions of sepsis

Sepsis: Life-threatening organ dysfunction caused by a dysregulated host response to infection.

Organ dysfunction: An acute change in total sequential organ failure assessment (SOFA) score ≥ 2 points consequent to the infection. Baseline SOFA score is taken as zero in patients without pre-existing organ dysfunction.

Septic shock: Subset of sepsis in which underlying circulatory and cellular/metabolic abnormalities are profound enough to substantially increase mortality. It is identified by persistent hypotension requiring vasopressors to maintain mean arterial pressure (MAP) ≥ 65 mm Hg and having a serum lactate level >2 mmol/L (18 mg/dL) despite adequate volume resuscitation.

Table 2: Etiology of sepsis

Infective causes	Primarily noninfective causes with super-added infections
• Central nervous system (meningitis, encephalitis)	• Severe trauma and hemorrhage
• Cardiovascular system (infective endocarditis)	• Myocardial infarction
• Respiratory system (pneumonia)	• Pulmonary embolism
• Urinary tract infection	• Burns
• Gastrointestinal tract (peritonitis)	• Cardiac tamponade
• Infection of skin and soft tissues	• Drug overdose
• Infections of bone and joints	• Diabetic ketoacidosis
	• Acute pancreatitis
	• Adrenal insufficiency
	• Anaphylaxis

after arriving at the diagnosis. Infected peripancreatic necrosis is an exception. The invasive intervention in this case is delayed till demarcation of viable and nonviable tissues occurs. Though infection is the predominant cause of sepsis there are other noninfective causes as well (Table 2).

Blood cultures need not be positive in all the cases. They are positive in only one third of the cases. Respiratory and cardiovascular systems are most commonly affected organ systems. Classical involvement of the respiratory system is in the form of acute respiratory distress syndrome (ARDS). The diagnostic criteria for sepsis is given in Table 3.[2]

ANESTHETIC CONCERNS IN A SEPTIC PATIENT

Almost all the surgeries in a septic patient are emergent surgeries. There may be inadequate information about the diagnosis and physiologic status of the patient. Mobilizing the resources for safe conduct of anesthesia for these patients can be challenging. The time available for preoperative optimization of these patients can also be limited. It is difficult to maintain adequate tissue perfusion pressure (due to hypotension) and oxygenation (due to dysfunctional oxygen delivery and uptake).[4,5]

Table 3: Diagnostic criteria for sepsis

General variables

Fever (core temperature >38.3°C), hypothermia (core temperature <36°C), tachycardia (> 90 beats/min or >2 SD above the upper limit of normal range for age), tachypnea, substantial edema or positive fluid balance (>20 mL/kg body weight over a 24-hr period), altered mental status, hyperglycemia (>120 mg/dL) without diabetes

Inflammatory variables

Leukocytosis (>12,000/mm^3), leukopenia (<4000/mm^3), normal white-cell count with >10% immature forms, elevated plasma C-reactive protein (>2 SD above the upper limit of the normal range), elevated plasma procalcitonin (>2 SD above the upper limit of the normal range)

Hemodynamic variables

Arterial hypotension (SBP <90 mm Hg; MAP <70 mm Hg; or SBP fall >40 mm Hg or to > 2 SD below the lower limit of the normal range for age), elevated mixed venous oxygen saturation (>70%), elevated cardiac index (>3.5 L/min/m^2 body surface area)

Organ-dysfunction variables

Arterial hypoxemia (PaO$_2$/FiO$_2$ < 300), acute oliguria (urine output < 0.5 mL/kg/h or 45 mL/h for at least 2 h), increase in creatinine level of > 0.5 mg/dL), coagulation abnormalities (INR >1.5; or aPTT >60 sec), paralytic ileus (absence of bowel sounds), thrombocytopenia (<1 lakh/mm^3), hyperbilirubinemia (plasma total bilirubin >4 mg/dL)

Tissue-perfusion variables

Hyperlactatemia (lactate >18 mg/dL), decreased capillary refill or mottling

PREOPERATIVE ASSESSMENT, PREPARATION AND OPTIMIZATION

Optimizing the patient's condition preoperatively improves the surgical outcome especially in high risk patients. Surgery may have to be delayed for a short period of time for resuscitating the patient to ensure adequate oxygen delivery, cardiac output and blood pressure. However, surgery should not be delayed unnecessarily in the name of preoperative optimization. There has to be a continuum of care from the emergency department/intensive care unit to the operation theatre. Resuscitation is continued throughout the perioperative period. Initial resuscitation and measures to control the infection are summarized in Table 4.[3]

As the major problems encountered in these patients are hypovolemia, hypotension, anemia, coagulation abnormalities, dyselectrolytemia and acidosis they require thorough assessment and detailed investigations. Preoperative investigations as indicated for the patient are listed in Table 5.[4]

CHOICE OF ANESTHESIA AND MONITORING

The interplay between anesthesia, sepsis, blood loss and the stress of the surgery accounts for greater hemodynamic instability seen in these patients during the perioperative period. General anesthesia or locoregional anesthesia are preferred due to hemodynamic instability.[5,6] Central neuraxial blockade (spinal and epidural anesthesia) is usually avoided because the ensuing hypotension is difficult to treat and reverse. Epidural hematoma and abscess formation are

Table 4: Resuscitation and infection control in sepsis

Initial Resuscitation

Goals during first 6 hour

Mean arterial pressure (MAP) ≥ 65 mm Hg
Central venous pressure 8–12 mm Hg
Urine output ≥ 0.5 mL/kg/h
Central venous oxygen saturation 70%
Mixed venous oxygen saturation 65%
Target resuscitation to normalize elevated lactate levels

Complete within 3 hour

Obtain blood cultures prior to administration of antibiotics
Administer broad spectrum antibiotics
Measure lactate level
Administer 30 mL/kg crystalloid for hypotension or lactate > 4 mmol/L

Complete within 6 hour

Administer vasopressors when hypotension is unresponsive to initial fluid resuscitation to maintain hemodynamic goals listed above

Antimicrobial therapy

Empiric IV antimicrobials have to be administered within 1 hour
Reassess antimicrobial regimen for de-escalation periodically
Procalcitonin level or other similar biomarkers can be used to assist in de-escalation
Antiviral treatment is started as early as possible in patients with septic shock of viral etiology
Antimicrobial agents have no role in severe inflammatory states of noninfectious cause

Table 5: Preoperative investigations

Hematological	Hemoglobin, total and differential count, coagulation screen
Biochemistry	Renal function test, serum electrolytes, liver function tests, blood sugar, serum amylase
Arterial blood gas (ABG) analysis	To assess the respiratory functions and acid base status
Electrocardiogram/ echocardiography	To rule out the cardiac causes for hypotension
Chest X-ray	To exclude lung pathology, confirmation of central line or endotracheal tube, if present
Ultrasound/CT scan	To confirm deep seated infection, if any
Microbiology (if not sent already)	Blood cultures (2 or 3 sets) Sputum, if indicated Wound swabs from suspected sites

the other concerns. If central neuraxial blocks are contemplated in patients with mild sepsis then normal coagulation profile has to be confirmed. Regional infiltration with local anesthetics or blockade of the peripheral nerves may be used. Analgesia and anesthesia must not be withheld because of hypotension. Rather the anesthetic agents should be chosen judiciously anticipating the hemodynamic disturbances.

Meticulous monitoring is required because of the rapidity in hemodynamic changes. In addition to standard monitoring, an invasive arterial pressure monitoring should also be established. Wide bore intravenous access and central venous access with central venous pressure monitoring should also be established. Dynamic variables like pulse pressure variations are useful to estimate fluid responsiveness.

INDUCTION, INTUBATION AND MAINTENANCE OF ANESTHESIA

Having a second anesthetist or trained assistant during the course of anesthesia or at least during induction of anesthesia is desirable. A hypoxic patient should never be left unattended. Oxygen (100%) at the flow rate of 15 L/min should be administered whilst preparing equipment for airway management.[7,8] A widebore IV access (14G or 16G cannula) should be obtained and an attempt should be made to improve the volume status of the patient preinduction. Vital signs such as BP, heart rate and capillary refill time may not be reliable to guide fluid therapy.

Since the respiratory reserve of these patients is likely to be poor, they should be preoxygenated for at least 3 minutes before induction of anesthesia. Dyspneic patients may require assisted ventilation. Severe hypotension during anesthetic induction should be anticipated. Slow induction with titrated, small doses of IV anesthetic agents minimizes hypotension. Ketamine, etomidate or benzodiazepines like midazolam with fentanyl provide better hemodynamic stability during induction of anesthesia compared to propofol or thiopentone. Etomidate, though known for hemodynamic stability, can inhibit adrenal mitochondrial 11-beta hydroxylase and induce adrenal suppression. Vasopressors should be prepared and kept ready before induction of anesthesia. Rapid sequence induction or its modification might have to be considered. Avoid suxamethonium, if hyperkalemia is likely and rocuronium is a better alternative for rapid sequence induction. Choice of neuromuscular blocking agent does not matter, if postoperative mechanical ventilation is considered. Atracurium and cisatracurium may be preferred nondepolarizing muscle relaxants due to their organ-independent metabolism.

Maintenance of anesthesia can be either with inhalation or intravenous agents. Inhalational volatile anesthetics cause vasodilation. Some of them (halothane) are cardiac depressants. Hence, caution needs to be exercised. Minimum alveolar concentration of inhalational agents is reduced. Ketamine is a good anesthetic for analgesia and anesthesia in unstable patient. Short acting opioids like remifentanil 0.25–0.5 µg/kg/min provide good hemodynamics. Fentanyl is a good alternative as well. It is prudent to use short acting opioids while avoiding agents which tend to have active metabolites like morphine unless the patient is intubated. It is better to avoid nonsteroidal anti-inflammatory drugs (NSAIDs) as they may cause renal dysfunction and gastrointestinal bleed. In this regard IV paracetamol may have favorable profile when used judiciously. The anesthesia technique is best chosen by the anesthetist depending on what is best for the individual patient and their own experience and expertise.

Volume resuscitation should continue as indicated. Crystalloids are preferred over colloids for resuscitation in sepsis and septic shock and are used as maintenance fluids as well. Hydroxyethyl starch should be avoided for fluid resuscitation.

Albumin can be used for resuscitation, if substantial amounts of crystalloids are required. Additional vasopressor therapy may be required to maintain the MAP of 65 mm Hg. The first choice of vasopressor is norepinephrine but epinephrine can also be used. Additional infusion of vasopressin 0.03 units/min may be considered to increase the MAP or decrease the dose of norepinephrine. Dopamine may be used in selected patients with low risk of tachycardia or in those with bradycardia. Phenylephrine infusion is generally not recommended. However, it may be considered when arrhythmias are seen with norepinephrine and when blood pressure is low despite a known high cardiac output. Dobutamine infusion may be considered in the presence of myocardial dysfunction.

Depending on the blood loss during the surgery, transfusion of blood products may have to be considered. Hemoglobin of 7 to 9 g/dL is an acceptable target after transfusion. If there is no bleeding or plan for an invasive procedure, then fresh frozen plasma should not be merely transfused to correct the abnormal values of coagulation profile. Prophylactic platelet transfusion is considered when platelet counts are <10,000/mm^3 in the absence of bleeding, or when counts are < 20,000/mm^3 with significant risk of bleeding, or ≥50,000/mm^3, if active bleeding is present or the patient is undergoing surgery/invasive procedures.

Patients in sepsis have poor lung compliance. Protective lung strategies need to be implemented for ventilation. Low tidal volume strategy (6–8 mL/Kg of predicted body weight), limiting plateau pressures to ≤30 cm H$_2$O and application of PEEP to prevent alveolar collapse is recommended. In refractory hypoxemia recruitment maneuvers may be used.

Stress dose of hydrocortisone is administered, if the patient is already on corticosteroid therapy. Blood glucose levels are monitored every 1–2 h and is maintained at <180 mg/dL using glucose insulin infusion, if necessary. Intraoperative hypothermia is avoided by using warm blankets and fluid warmers as it can cause coagulation dysfunction.

Most patients being critically ill are not reversed from neuromuscular blockade and are shifted with the endotracheal tube in-situ to the ICU. Supportive measures like deep vein thrombosis prophylaxis, stress ulcer prophylaxis, renal replacement therapy (if required) and nutritional therapy have to be continued in the perioperative period.

POSTOPERATIVE MANAGEMENT

The patients in sepsis are managed according to the protocolized bundled care guidelines and this care is continued in the postoperative period. Adequate analgesia should be ensured and frequent re-assessment of the patient in the ICU is important.

CONCLUSION

Anesthetic management in patients with sepsis is extremely challenging. Optimization, resuscitation and the perioperative management go hand-in-hand. Tailoring the anesthesia to maintain the organ perfusion and oxygenation is important.

REFERENCES

1. Singer M, Deutschman CS, Seymour CW, et al. The third international consensus definitions for sepsis and septic shock (Sepsis-3). JAMA. 2016;315(8):801-10.
2. Angus DC, van der Poll T. Severe sepsis and septic shock. N Eng J Med. 2013;369(9): 840-51.
3. Dellinger KP, Levy MM, Carlet JM, et al. Surviving sepsis campaign: international guidelines for management of severe sepsis and septic shock. Crit Care Med. 2008; 36(1):296-327.
4. Eissa D, Carton EG, Bugg DJ. Anaesthetic management of patients with severe sepsis. Br J Anaesth. 2010;105:734-43.
5. Yoon SH. Concerns of the anesthesiologist: anesthetic induction in severe sepsis or septic shock patients. Korean J Anesthesiol. 2012;63(1):3-10.
6. McCormick B. Management of sepsis: overview. World anaesthesia tutorial of the week. www.AnaesthesiaUK/WorldAnaesthesia.
7. Khanna AK, Laudanski K. Septic shock and anesthesia: much ado about nothing? J Anaesthesiol Clin Pharmacol. 2014;30(4):481-3.
8. Battaglin FS, de Oliveira Filho GR. SBA Recommendations for anesthetic management of septic patient. Rev Bras Anestesiol. 2013;63(5):377-84.

CHAPTER 14

Congenital Tracheoesophageal Fistula: Anesthetic Considerations and Management

Sharmila Ahuja, Medha Mohta

KEY POINTS

- Congenital tracheoesophageal fistula (TEF) has an incidence of 1 in 2500–3000 live births. It manifests within few hours to days after birth.
- There are five types of TEF, esophageal atresia with distal tracheoesophageal fistula being the commonest (86%).
- Common congenital anomalies associated with TEF include vertebral, anorectal, cardiac, renal and limb (VACTERL) malformations.
- TEF typically presents with symptoms of excessive salivation and repeated episodes of coughing, gagging, choking, regurgitation and cyanosis while feeding. Diagnosis is confirmed by inability to pass a 10–12 French gauge catheter beyond 9–10 cm from the lower alveolar ridge, and coiling of catheter on X-ray chest.
- Surgical repair of this anomaly is commonly performed within 24–72 hours, primary treatment being a right thoracotomy using extrapleural approach, division of fistula and end to end anastomosis of esophageal ends. Thoracoscopic approach is a newer method with less morbidity.
- Accurate diagnosis, identification of associated congenital anomalies and optimizing the general condition of the neonate are cornerstones of anesthesia management that influences outcome. This requires correction of fluid-electrolyte and acid-base abnormalities and optimization of chest condition by antibiotics and regular suction of upper esophageal pouch and oropharynx.
- The challenges specific to TEF repair are placement of tracheal tube below the level of fistula but above the carina to avoid gastric insufflation; poor lung condition due to aspiration of gastric contents and/or respiratory distress syndrome of prematurity; and associated cardiac or other congenital anomalies.
- Awake intubation or inhalation induction with spontaneous ventilation is most commonly used to secure airway. Positive pressure ventilation with administration of muscle relaxants can be safely started once the airway has been secured.
- Causes of intraoperative hypoxemia include compression of the lung by the surgeons; endobronchial intubation; tracheal tube obstruction due to kinking, secretions or bleeding; kinking of bronchus or trachea; and atelectasis.
- Postoperative care should be provided in an intensive care unit. Postoperative ventilation may be required in cases with poor preoperative lung condition or low birth weight.
- Complications include anastomotic leak, esophageal stricture, tracheomalacia, repeated chest infections and gastroesophageal reflux. Other long-term sequelae include chronic pain, obstructive and restrictive ventilatory defects and hyper-reactive airway.

INTRODUCTION

Congenital tracheoesophageal fistula (TEF) is a fistulous communication between esophagus and trachea or a main bronchus. It has an incidence of 1 in 2500 to 3000 live births.[1] Some patients may have isolated esophageal atresia (EA) without any fistula. Congenital TEF manifests within few hours to days of neonatal life. It requires surgical correction which presents a major challenge to the pediatric anesthesiologist. Survival following TEF repair has improved over the years due to advances in pediatric anesthesia. However, prematurity and associated cardiac anomalies significantly contribute to mortality in these neonates.[2]

EMBRYOLOGY

The trachea and esophagus develop from primitive foregut during third week of embryonic life. The exact mechanism for formation of TEF is not known; however, various theories have been suggested. According to the simplest theory, a ventral diverticulum develops from the foregut. There is growth of endodermal cells on its lateral aspect, the fusion of which divides the foregut into tracheal and esophageal tubes. Any defect or failure of this process results in fistulous connections between the trachea and the esophagus.[3]

CLASSIFICATION

The TEF has been classified in different manners; however, it is most important to understand the anatomical defect present in each type (Table 1 and Figs. 1A to E). The commonest variety is esophageal atresia with distal tracheoesophageal fistula, which occurs in about 86% of patients.

Vogt type I refers to esophageal agenesis, whereas Gross type F is for esophageal stenosis.

Besides classifications based on anatomical variations, prognostic classifications have also been described.[1,4,5] Spitz prognosticated these anomalies based on the birth weight and the presence of cardiac defects (Table 2).

Major cardiac anomaly has been defined as cyanotic congenital heart disease requiring palliative or corrective surgery or noncyanotic heart disease requiring medical or surgical treatment for cardiac failure.

Table 1: Classification of tracheoesophageal fistula (TEF)[1]			
Anatomical defect	Incidence	Gross classification	Vogt classification
Pure esophageal atresia (no fistula)	7%	A	II
Esophageal atresia with proximal TEF	2%	B	III
Esophageal atresia with distal TEF	86%	C	IIIb
Esophageal atresia with both proximal and distal TEF	<1%	D	IIIa
H-type TEF (no atresia)	4%	E	

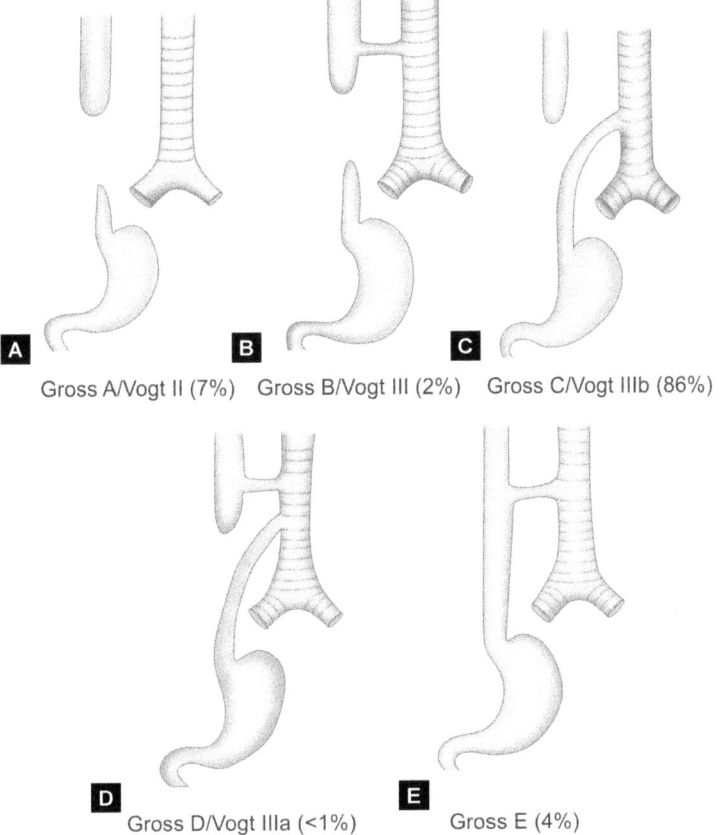

Figs. 1A to E: Classification of tracheoesophageal fistula.

Table 2: Spitz classification[1]		
Group	Features	Survival rate (%)
I	Birth weight ≥ 1.5 kg **with no** major cardiac anomaly	98
II	Birth weight < 1.5 kg **or** major cardiac anomaly	82
III	Birth weight < 1.5 kg **and** major cardiac anomaly	50

ASSOCIATED ANOMALIES

In about 50% cases, EA/TEF is associated with congenital malformations in other organ systems.[6,7] Cardiovascular system is the most commonly involved. Of several malformation associations involving EA/TEF, the best described is the VACTERL association which includes vertebral (17%), anorectal (12%), cardiac (20%), tracheoesophageal, renal (16%), and limb malformations (10%).[8] In addition, there may be other abnormalities in gastrointestinal and genitourinary

Table 3: Congenital anomalies associated with tracheoesophageal fistula[6-8]	
Anomaly	Examples of malformations
Cardiac	Ventricular septal defect, patent ductus arteriosus, atrial septal defect, tetralogy of Fallot, coarctation of aorta
Vertebral	Vertebral defects, scoliosis
Gastrointestinal	Imperforate anus, duodenal atresia, malrotation, pyloric stenosis, omphalocele
Genitourinary	Renal agenesis, hypospadias, polycystic kidney, ureteric or urethral abnormalities
Limb	Radial anomalies, polydactyly, lower limb defects

systems. The common anomalies associated with TEF are listed in Table 3. It is, therefore necessary to perform a thorough clinical examination and relevant radiological investigations to rule out these anomalies in any neonate suspected to have EA/TEF.

DIAGNOSIS

There is no definite sign for prenatal diagnosis of TEF with EA. The presence of EA may be suspected by an ultrasound examination after 18th week of gestation which may demonstrate a small or absent fetal stomach bubble. As the fetus is unable to swallow amniotic fluid due to EA, polyhydramnios may be present.[9] These ultrasound signs are nonspecific and have a positive predictive value of only 44%.[6] However, they enable the parents and the caregivers to be prepared for prompt management of the neonate and earlier identification of associated anomalies.[10]

After birth, neonates with EA/TEF present with excessive salivation, repeated episodes of coughing, gagging, choking, regurgitation and cyanosis while feeding.[1] This condition may also manifest as sudden onset respiratory distress following feeding attempts. As these infants are unable to swallow saliva due to esophageal atresia, excessive salivation requiring repeated suctioning is a typical diagnostic feature of this anomaly. A stiff 10–12 French gauge catheter should be passed through the mouth into the esophagus in such babies before the first feed. In esophageal atresia, the catheter is seen to be arrested at about 9–10 cm from the lower alveolar ridge.[6] A plain X-ray of chest and abdomen will show the tip of the catheter curled up in the upper chest or neck while gas in the stomach and intestine signifies the presence of a distal tracheoesophageal fistula (Fig. 2).[11] The absence of gastrointestinal gas is indicative of an isolated esophageal atresia (Fig. 3).

TREATMENT

The definitive treatment for EA and TEF is surgical repair of the defect. Surgery is generally performed within 24 to 72 hours in otherwise healthy neonates. Any delay in surgical repair predisposes the child to pneumonitis due to aspiration of saliva accumulated in upper pouch or reflux of gastric acid through the tracheo-esophageal fistula.[8]

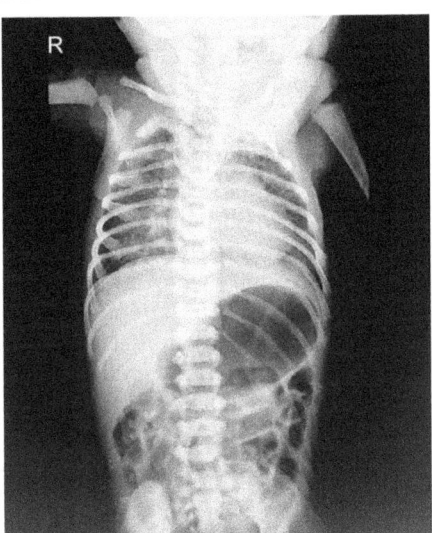

Fig. 2: X-ray showing coiled catheter in distal tracheoesophageal fistula.

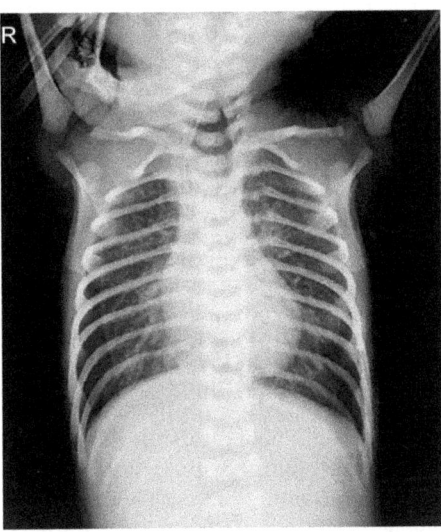

Fig. 3: X-ray showing coiled catheter in isolated esophageal atresia.

In the commonest variety, after stabilization, primary treatment includes right thoracotomy using extrapleural approach, division of tracheoesophageal fistula, and end-to-end anastomosis of two esophageal ends. This procedure can also be performed by thoracoscopic approach where surgical expertise and facilities exist.[12] In pure atresia and wide gap esophageal atresia, cervical esophagostomy with gastrostomy may be performed as the primary procedure. Esophageal continuity can then be restored by different surgical methods available after the child grows.[13]

ANESTHETIC MANAGEMENT

Preoperative Preparation

The goal of an effective preoperative preparation is to stabilize the general condition of the neonate before surgery. Important considerations include prevention of dehydration and hypoglycemia by intravenous fluid infusions, and administration of prophylactic antibiotics to reduce the risk of respiratory infections.[7] The neonate should be nursed in supine position with head raised or in the lateral position. Continuous suction using Replogle tube or repeated suction of the upper esophageal pouch and oropharynx is required to clear the secretions and thus reduce the risk of aspiration. Fluid-electrolyte and acid-base abnormalities should be corrected and chest condition should be optimized.

Echocardiography is required to diagnose any cardiac or vascular abnormality which could affect anesthetic and surgical management and outcome.[7] Hematological and biochemical profiles should be obtained and blood sample should be sent for grouping and cross matching.

Intraoperative Management

The anesthetic management of a neonate undergoing TEF repair is very challenging. There are basic concerns related to neonatal anesthesia due to their anatomic and physiologic differences from adults, such as greater difficulty in securing airway, vulnerability to have flip-flop circulation, less compliant ventricles, immature renal and hepatic function, susceptibility to develop hypothermia, need for very careful and strict fluid balance, risk of postoperative apnea in preterm infants and risk of anesthetic overdose.[14]

The concerns specific to anesthetic management of TEF include: the need to avoid tracheal tube placement above or in the fistula to prevent gas insufflation into fistula and stomach; poor lung condition due to aspiration of gastric contents and/or respiratory distress syndrome of prematurity; and associated cardiac or other congenital anomalies.[8] Inadvertent tracheal tube placement in the fistula can lead to ineffective ventilation and massive gastric dilation, which can further result in gastric reflux, hypotension and hypoxemia.

A very important requirement while anesthetizing TEF patients is the ability to ventilate lungs without ventilation of the fistula.[8] To achieve this, it is preferable to avoid giving muscle relaxants before appropriately securing the airway. Either awake intubation or inhalation induction with spontaneous ventilation may be used to secure airway, as positive pressure ventilation with bag and mask may cause gastric inflation. The tip of the tracheal tube should be placed below the fistula and above the carina. For proper placement, the tube is inserted as far as possible and then is slowly withdrawn until bilateral air entry is present on auscultation. Auscultation over stomach also helps to identify the correct location. It is very important to reconfirm the correct position of tracheal tube after positioning the patient as the tube can migrate into the fistula during this time.[15]

If the fistula is large and just above the carina, various techniques have been suggested to prevent entry of tip of the tracheal tube into it. The simplest is to adjust the tube position very gradually, while auscultating over lungs as well as stomach. Alternatively, the fistula may be occluded by using a cuffed tracheal tube, directing the bevel of the tube anteriorly or using a Fogarty catheter until ligation of the fistula.[6,9]

In occasional cases with the fistula being at the carina or more distally, bronchial intubation and one lung ventilation is required until the fistula is ligated.[7] If facilities and expertise are available, a preoperative rigid bronchoscopy is helpful to define the location of the fistula and assess for other airway abnormalities.[6,8] Tracheoscopy using flexible fibreoptic bronchoscope has been described to facilitate delineation of the airway anatomy, rapid surgical control by transillumination of fistula and assessment of postoperative bleeding, secretions and tracheomalacia.[16] Once airway has been secured with adequate ventilation without gastric inflation, muscle relaxants can be administered and positive pressure ventilation started.

The patient is positioned for right thoracotomy in left lateral position with right arm raised across the head. This requires use of padding, tapes, and gel blocks. During the procedure, the surgeon usually compresses the lung to mobilize distal segment of esophagus. This can result in desaturation which requires intermittent expansion of the lung. Other causes of intraoperative hypoxemia include endobronchial intubation; endotracheal tube obstruction due to kinking, secretions or bleeding; kinking of bronchus or trachea; and atelectasis.[8]

To aid the surgeon in identification of the upper esophageal pouch, the anesthesiologist is required to insert a nasogastric tube which is then pushed whenever asked by the surgeon, to make the proximal pouch prominent. The nasogastric tube is guided into the stomach by the surgeon before completing the esophageal anastomosis and is used to feed the baby in postoperative period.

Once the procedure is complete, the thoracic cavity is filled with saline. Absence of any bubbles on application of positive airway pressure confirms secure closure of the tracheal end of the fistula.

Intraoperatively, the mandatory monitoring standards for a neonate are followed. Of these, monitoring of oxygen saturation, heart rate, ventilation and body temperature are of paramount importance. Standard noninvasive monitors often suffice, including use of a precordial stethoscope. However, invasive arterial monitoring is indicated in patients with associated comorbid conditions, e.g. complex congenital heart disease or pulmonary disease, and during thoracoscopic surgery.[6]

Postoperative Care

All these neonates require intensive monitoring in neonatal intensive care unit. Care should be taken to not extend the neck of the neonate at any time during extubation or while nursing otherwise the anastomosis can give way. Routine care includes use of appropriate analgesics, intravenous fluids and antibiotics. Feeding through nasogastric tube is usually started 48 hours after surgery. Postoperative ventilation may be indicated in cases with low birth weight, significant associated anomalies or poor preoperative lung condition. The decision to electively ventilate should be taken carefully as prolonged ventilation can cause abrasion at the site of tracheal fistula repair. On the other hand, laryngoscopy and reintubation, if required, can cause trauma to the fistula site and traction to the esophageal repair.[17]

Pain Management

Intraoperatively, narcotics can be safely administered after isolating the fistula and securing the airway.[11] Regional techniques in the form of caudal, epidural or paravertebral blocks are also helpful.[18] A catheter inserted through caudal needle and advanced to T6-T7 level gives good intraoperative as well as postoperative analgesia.[8] Non-narcotic analgesics should be added to provide multimodal analgesia.[18]

COMPLICATIONS

Patients operated for TEF can have many complications and long-term sequelae.[7-9] The common complications include anastomotic leak, esophageal stricture, tracheomalacia and repeated chest infections.[7] The most common gastrointestinal sequelae of TEF repair is gastroesophageal reflux, with an incidence as high as 50%.[19] This is secondary to abnormal peristalsis and decreased lower esophageal sphincter tone due to abnormal development of mesenteric plexus in these patients. In some cases, repeated episodes of aspiration, recurrence of TEF and scoliosis can occur. Wound infection, gastric perforation, missed fistulae, lung collapse, phrenic nerve palsy, vocal cord palsy, chylothorax and pleural fistula formation also have been reported.[11,20]

Chronic pain may develop, if acute pain is not managed adequately.[11] Long term respiratory sequelae also include obstructive and restrictive ventilatory defects and hyper-reactive airway.[8]

CONCLUSION

Anesthetic management of a neonate undergoing TEF repair is a challenging task. It may become more complex due to coexisting anomalies in other organ systems, especially cardiac anomalies. Good preoperative assessment and preparation are required to identify problems and optimize the patient's condition. Neonates require stabilization and correction of fluid-electrolyte imbalance, hypothermia, hypoglycemia, and poor chest condition. Airway management during TEF repair may present great challenges. Postoperatively, these patients need vigilant postoperative monitoring and care in neonatal intensive care unit.

REFERENCES

1. Spitz L. Oesophageal atresia. Orphanet J Rare Dis. 2007;2:24.
2. Diaz LK, Akpek EA, Dinavahi R, et al. Tracheoesophageal fistula and associated congenital heart disease: implications for anesthetic management and survival. Pediatr Anesth. 2005;15:862-9.
3. Merei J, Hutson J. Embryogenesis of tracheoesophageal anomalies. Saudi Med J. 2003;24(5 Suppl):39-40.
4. Niramis R, Tangkhabuanbut P, Anuntkosol M, et al. Clinical outcomes of esophageal atresia: comparison between the Waterston and the Spitz classifications. Ann Acad Med Singapore. 2013;42:297-300.
5. Okamoto T, Takamizawa S, Arai H, et al. Esophageal atresia: prognostic classification revisited. Surgery. 2009;145:675-81.
6. Broemling N, Campbell F. Anesthetic management of congenital tracheoesophageal fistula. Pediatr Anesth. 2011;21:1092-9.

7. Al-Rawi O, Booker PD. Oesophageal atresia and tracheoesophageal fistula. Contin Educ Anaesth Crit Care Pain. 2007;7:15-9.
8. Gayle JA, Gómez SL, Baluch A, et al. Anesthetic considerations for the neonate with tracheoesophageal fistula. MEJ Anesth. 2008;19:1241-54.
9. Gupta A. Tracheoesophageal fistula oesophageal atresia and anaesthetic management. Indian J Anaesth. 2002;46:353-5.
10. Krishan S, Solanki R, Sethi SK. Radiological case of the month. Applied Radiology. 2005;34:31-4.
11. Motshabi P. Anaesthesia for oesophageal atresia with or without tracheo-oesophageal atresia. S Afr J Anaesth Analg. 2014;20:202-8.
12. Rothenberg SS. Thoracoscopic repair of esophageal atresia and trachea-esophageal fistula in neonates: evolution of a technique. J Laparoendosc Adv Surg Tech A. 2012;22:195-9.
13. Ron O, De Coppi P, Pierro A. The surgical approach to esophageal atresia repair and the management of long-gap atresia: results of a survey. Semin Pediatr Surg. 2009;18:44-9.
14. Cote CJ. Pediatric anesthesia. In: Miller RD (Ed). Miller's Anesthesia, 8th edn. Philadelphia. Elsevier Saunders; 2015. pp. 2757-98.
15. Alabbad SI, Shaw K, Puligandla PS, et al. The pitfalls of endotracheal intubation beyond the fistula in babies with type C esophageal atresia. Sem Pediatr Surg. 2009;18:116-8.
16. Deanovic D, Gerber AC, Dodge-Khatami A, et al. Tracheoscopy assisted repair of tracheoesophageal fistula (TARTEF): a 10-year experience. Pediatr Anesth. 2007;17:557-62.
17. Maxwell LG. Anesthetic management for newborns undergoing emergency surgery. ASA Refresher Courses Anesthesiol. 2007;35:107-26.
18. Hammer GB. Pediatric thoracic anesthesia. Anesthesiol Clin N Am. 2002;20:153-80.
19. Rintala RJ, Sistone S, Pakarinen MP. Outcome of esophageal atresia beyond childhood. Semin Pediatr Surg. 2009;18:50-6.
20. Knottenbelt G, Costi D, Stephens P, et al. An audit of anesthetic management and complications of tracheoesophageal fistula and esophageal atresia repair. Pediatr Anesth. 2012;22:268-74.

CHAPTER 15

Extremely Premature Infants and Anesthesia

Elsa Varghese

KEY POINTS

- Survival of extremely premature infants (<28 weeks GA), low or extremely low birth weight (<1500 g and <1000 g respectively) is on the increase.
- They are susceptible to developing respiratory distress syndrome (RDS), retinopathy of prematurity (ROP), patent ductus arteriosus (PDA), intraventricular hemorrhage (IVH), periventricular leukomalacia and necrotizing enterocolitis (NEC).
- Safe anesthesia includes adjustment of inspired oxygen concentration (SpO_2 85–95%), hemodynamic stability and aggressive prevention of hypothermia and hypoglycemia. The lower MAC of inhalation agents and lower dosage of opiates and sedatives require careful titration yet providing adequate anaesthesia and analgesia.
- Regional analgesia in competent hands can provide adequate analgesia for procedures in the extremities and inguinal hernia repair with minimal incidence of apnea.

INTRODUCTION

The World Health Organization published its premature birth fact sheet in 2010, stating that "more than 1 in 10 of the world's infants (>15 million children) were born prematurely".[1] In India along with other countries in South East Asia, the premature birth rate is 18% of live births. Extremely premature infants are very vulnerable and anesthesiologists are faced with the challenge of caring for them perioperatively. Anesthesiologists need to be familiar with respiratory consequences of therapies and neurological outcomes of the extremely premature babies especially since management of these infants pose a multitude of challenges.[2,3]

Current terminology of prematurity includes: *Gestational age* (GA) which is defined as the age of the fetus in terms of pregnancy duration in weeks, from the first day of last menstrual period; *Postmenstrual age* (PMA) is the duration in weeks between the first day of the last menstrual period of the mother and the current day. *Viability* is defined as the gestational age at which there is a 50% chance of survival regardless of the medical care provided; in high income countries, this ranges between 22 and 24 weeks GA and around 34 weeks GA in low-middle income countries.[2] Table 1 shows some of the current terminology of prematurity.

Table 1: Prematurity terminology	
Term	Gestational age (GA) in weeks
Extremely preterm	<28
Very preterm	28–<32
Moderate preterm	32–<34
Late preterm	34–<37
Early preterm	37–39
Term	38–41
Very low birth weight (VLBW)	<1500 g
Extremely low birth weight (ELBW)	<1000 g

PHYSIOLOGICAL CONSEQUENCES AND OUTCOMES OF THE EXTREMELY PREMATURE INFANTS

Survival and Morbidity

Infants born less than 34 weeks GA comprise almost 60% of infant deaths.[2] Improvement in clinical outcomes of extremely premature babies is due to marked improvements in medical care. Continuous positive airway pressure (CPAP), improved modes of mechanical ventilation, exogenous surfactant treatment and administration of antenatal steroids have all contributed to better outcomes. Improved design of artificial airways and breathing circuits and reduction in ventilator airway distending pressures have also helped reduce complications. Oxygen therapy has also contributed to complications of chronic lung disease and retinopathy of prematurity especially in extremely premature infants. With increased survival, there are an increasing number of these infants who subsequently face severe problems such as; bronchopulmonary dysplasia (BPD), necrotizing enterocolitis (NEC) and intraventricular hemorrhage (IVH). Chronic lung disease, cerebral palsy (CP), severe visual and hearing impairment and cognitive developmental delay are problems that persist as the child develops. Extremely premature infants have 30-50% mortality and 20-50% risk of disability, despite all the above technological advances in management.[3]

Respiratory System

Fetal alveoli form at 17-28 weeks GA and pulmonary capillaries at 28-36 weeks GA. Prior to 32-34 weeks GA, production of surfactant is inadequate, therefore the infant born prior to this period is predisposed to respiratory distress syndrome. Physiological development of the lung in the postnatal period, can be disrupted by inflammation, infection, volutrauma and barotrauma, mechanical ventilation and hyperoxia. Pathological lung changes secondary to the above-mentioned effects include; larger but fewer alveoli, abnormal vascular growth and smooth muscle hypertrophy, inflammation and fibroproliferation. Ultimately these changes result in a reduced alveolar surface area and impaired gas exchange. Pulmonary hypertension (incidence ranging from 17-43%) which occurs secondary to disrupted pulmonary vascular development, contributes quite significantly to morbidity and mortality.[3,4] The requirement for oxygen increases in these infants and in addition, diminished lung compliance and reversible airway obstruction may persist for an extended period of time into childhood.[5,6]

Bronchopulmonary dysplasia (BPD) is a sequela in infants born between 24 and 28 weeks GA and is due to factors mentioned above. Infants born <32 weeks GA who require a FiO_2 >0.3 after the age of 36 weeks PMA, are considered to have *severe* BPD. BPD is associated with diminished pulmonary residual capacity, impaired oxygen diffusion capacity, markedly increased metabolic demands to cope with the increased oxygen consumption, along with a reduction in cardiovascular reserve. Symptoms of cough and wheeze, may be responsive to bronchodilators and anti-inflammatory drugs. Newer ventilatory modes of high frequency ventilation and nasal CPAP may reduce the incidence of BPD. Infants who require prolonged intubation can in addition develop complications like subglottic stenosis or tracheomalacia.[6-8]

Control of respiration and apnea. Chemoreceptor responses are blunted in preterm infants. Apnea replaces the normal biphasic response to hypoxemia (hyperventilation and hypoventilation). Apnea is pathological when the duration is more than 20 s and is associated with bradycardia, cyanosis, pallor or hypotonia. Fewer type I fibers in the preterm diaphragm also contribute to apnea during stressful situations of hypoglycemia, hypoxia, anemia, hypothermia and sepsis. The incidence of apnea in extremely premature infants can be as high as 84%.[9,10]

Cardiovascular System

The risk of cardiovascular compromise during anesthesia and surgery is considerable in these infants. They often have poor diastolic function, poor left ventricular compliance, heart rate dependent cardiac output and very small blood volumes. Minimal blood loss can rapidly cause hypovolemia, hypotension and shock. The neonatal immature myocardium is less compliant with limited ability to improve cardiac output. The autonomic system is underdeveloped with a predominant parasympathetic system, the heart rate may not increase when the infant is hypovolemic.[11]

Cardiac malformations are more common, e.g. pulmonary atresia with ventricular septal defect, complete atrioventricular septal defect, coarctation of aorta, tetralogy of Fallot and pulmonary valve stenosis.[12]

The presence of a patent ductus arteriosus, atrial and ventricular defects can result in a left to right shunt, along with an increase in pulmonary blood flow and resultant congestive cardiac failure. Increased pulmonary vascular resistance secondary to hypoxia along with increased airway pressures, can lead to right to left shunting, with resultant worsening hypoxia and acidosis.[3]

Persistent raised pulmonary vascular resistance eventually leads to impaired right ventricular function and a low cardiac output state, pulmonary edema and sudden death.[13] Prevention of pulmonary hypertension is the key to successful management and involves strategies to decrease pulmonary vascular resistance and provide inotropic support for the right ventricle.[14]

Surgery and anesthesia may be required for palliative or curative interventions for these defects. Patent ductus arteriosus (PDA), may require fluid restriction and diuretic therapy. About 50% of extremely premature or extremely low birth weight (ELBW) babies receive indomethacin for closure of a PDA, with 12% having to undergo surgical ligation through a left thoracotomy or video-assisted thoracoscopic clipping.[15,16]

Neurological Outcomes

The incidence of neurodevelopmental (mental and psychomotor) abnormalities is high. Autoregulation of cerebral blood vessels is disturbed. The ELBW infant has very variable blood pressure and the lower limit of blood pressure at which cerebral blood flow autoregulation is intact is unknown in this age group.[2] *Intraventricular hemorrhage* (IVH) occurs in 25% of these babies, often within a few days after birth. Perinatal injuries disrupt the coordinated brain growth with resultant global deficits in higher cognitive function.[3] Ventricular dilatation may progress to hydrocephalus, parenchymal infarctions and cystic periventricular injury. Risk factors include; respiratory distress syndrome, hypotension, fluctuating blood pressure and aggressive fluid resuscitation. Imaging with ultrasound, MRI and CT along with focused cerebral protection, have become the standard of care to diagnose congenital and acquired conditions and predict prognosis.[17] Periventricular leukomalacia changes in the white matter are a strong predictor for development of cerebral palsy, cognitive disabilities and epilepsy.[18]

Supportive care to minimize neurological complications includes:

Oxygenation at the same time avoiding hyperoxia and oxygen toxicity especially during reperfusion which can occur with tissue damage.

Ventilation aimed at avoiding hypocapnea, which can disrupt cerebral autoregulation and blood flow.

Cardiovascular support which can be achieved by avoiding rapid changes and ensuring a stable blood pressure, thereby avoiding a low perfusion state and intraventricular hemorrhage.

Temperature control with normothermia to be maintained as far as practically possible avoiding hypothermia as well as hyperthermia, which can exacerbate brain injury.

Glucose management is done by maintaining blood glucose at physiological levels as hypoglycemia can cause brain injury.[3]

Hematology

Extremely premature infants at birth have lower hemoglobin levels (13–15 g/dL) compared to a term baby (18–20 g/dL). Of this, 70–80% of hemoglobin may be fetal hemoglobin (HbF). The total blood volume is 95–100 mL. The ability to compensate by increasing cardiac output is markedly reduced and therefore, early preoperative blood transfusion is required with the aim of achieving a target hematocrit of 40–45%. Deficiency in vitamin K and vitamin K-dependent coagulation factors may result in a lower platelet count.[4]

Renal Function

The renal tubules have a limited capacity to reabsorb bicarbonate in a state of "normal" acidosis seen in newborns. Retention of sodium by renal tubules does not develop till 32 weeks GA. This results in a limited response to aldosterone (till 34 weeks GA) and high levels of antidiuretic hormone with a tendency for hyponatremia. The total body water in these babies is higher than in the term neonate, i.e. 90% of total body weight.[1]

Gastrointestinal Disorders

These infants have limited glycogen stores and immature hepatic function and are therefore prone to *hypoglycemia*. Drug metabolism is immature.

Short bowel syndrome is more common and may require enteral feeding. They are at high-risk of developing electrolyte abnormalities, dehydration and necrotizing enterocolitis (NEC), an inflammatory condition that affects the gut. NEC usually presents with abdominal distension, blood stained stool and gut perforation with signs of systemic sepsis. *Gastroesophageal reflux* is common, especially in preterm infants because of an incompetent lower esophageal sphincter and neurological immaturity. Reflux can lead to laryngospasm, laryngitis, tracheitis, apnea, chronic cough, otitis media and asthma. The degree of reflux may influence decisions during induction (IV versus inhalation) and airway management.[4,9]

Temperature Regulation, Skin and Body Surface

In infants <32 weeks GA, the epidermis is thinner and more susceptible to fluid and temperature loss. The large surface area, increased thermal conductance along with increased permeability of the epidermis, results is more evaporative water loss (15-fold increase), therefore predisposing to dehydration.[7] Thermoregulation is limited with a significant potential for heat loss. In addition, these is limited heat production from brown fat metabolism. The importance of maintaining a warm neutral thermal environment is critical. The immature, thin skin can be easily damaged with trivial trauma.[19]

Retinopathy of Prematurity

There is incomplete retinal vascularization as part of a vasculoproliferative disorder of the retina of premature infants. This problem can be detected as early as 30–32 weeks GA.

TIMING AND INDICATIONS FOR SURGERY

The optimal timing of surgery for the extremely premature infant depends on the risks of delaying the procedure. The availability of appropriate resources and personnel for perioperative care and postoperative monitoring, also determines the appropriateness of surgery. Anesthesia is requested for the extremely premature infant for the following procedures which do require special considerations as mentioned briefly below.[19,20]

- *PDA ligation:* Surgery is performed in the left lateral position. Immediately following ligation of the duct, a rise in blood pressure may be observed, which increases the risk of intraventricular hemorrhage. To avoid this situation, the concentration of the inhalational agent can be transiently increased, in addition the duct should be clamped gently.
- *Laparotomy:* Performed for NEC, spontaneous perforation, reanastomosis or release of adhesions. These are generally in sick babies with acid-base abnormalities and coagulopathy often requiring vitamin K injections, fresh frozen plasma and platelets.
- *Inguinal hernia repair:* Incidence of inguinal hernia is 38% of ELBW babies. This surgery is usually performed once the baby has been weaned from mechanical ventilation.
- *Fundoplication:* This is performed for symptomatic esophageal reflux.
- *Vascular access:* For difficult IV access and central line insertion under radiological guidance.

- *Vitrectomy or laser surgery:* These are performed for retinopathy of prematurity and can be performed with combination of sedation and local anesthesia.
- *CSF drainage:* Drainage or insertion of ventriculoperitoneal shunt is done for treatment of obstructive hydrocephalus.
- *CT and MRI:* These are done for diagnosis of intraventricular hemorrhage and other abnormalities.
- *Other coexisting diseases:* Which may require urgent surgery, e.g. esophageal or intestinal atresia, congenital diaphragmatic hernia, tracheoesophageal fistula.

ANESTHETIC MANAGEMENT

These infants require meticulous attention in all aspects of their care. The following are a brief summary of details of the care of these fragile infants.[7,8,19]

Preoperative Evaluation

A detailed history and physical evaluation, a clear perioperative management plan and communication between the neonatologist, pediatric surgeon and pediatric anesthesiologist go a long way in providing optimal management of anesthesia and postoperative care. Explaining to the parents the risks involved is necessary. Routine investigations of hematocrit, coagulation profile, serum electrolytes and blood glucose levels should ideally be within acceptable limits. Arterial blood gases, chest X-ray and echocardiogram should preferably be done. Packed red blood cells should be cross matched and available. Information on duration of fasting helps calculate fluid deficits. Breastmilk and formula feed are considered as solids. Infants < 32–34 weeks gestation are unable to nipple feed and are fed via a nasogastric tube. Intravenous fluids must be supplemented if the baby is kept fasting.[4]

Premedication: These babies should receive their usual medications, e.g. anticonvulsants, bronchodilators. Sedative premedication is avoided. All babies should receive vitamin K prior to surgery.

Operating Room Preparation

Personnel: Extra nursing and technical personnel and preferably two anesthesiologists working together make a difference in providing smooth conduct of the procedure.

Equipment: Prechecking of anesthetic equipment, availability of a ventilator with the capability of delivering low tidal volumes, pressure-controlled ventilation and PEEP is essential. Infusion pumps should be available and connected. Generally, these infants have an endotracheal tube in place and mechanically ventilated. However, appropriate sized intubation equipment should be ready at hand including; "000" size face mask, "0" Miller blade, "0" size laryngeal mask airway and endotracheal tube of 2.5 mm outer diameter with an appropriate size stylet, along with appropriate sized suction catheters.

Operating room temperature: The ambient temperature should be kept at 27°C. A warming mattress and/or a warm air blanket, pediatric heat and moisture exchanger, equipment for warming IV fluids, irrigation fluid, blood and blood products should be available. Application of waterproof surgical drapes on nonoperating areas also help keep the infant dry and warm.

Positioning: Transfer of the baby from the incubator to the operating table must be achieved carefully, avoiding accidental disconnections and decannulations. To have better access to the baby, the foot and head end of the operating table can be removed.

Other important strategies include gentle, minimal handling of these infants, using finger tips and not ones' whole hand. Avoiding pressure complications on the occiput, heels and caused by the nasogastric tube on the nose, blood pressure cuffs and saturation probes. In addition, one has to be cautious and meticulous with drug administration, dilutions and fluid flushes. Providing the minimum FiO_2 to maintain oxygen saturation between 88% and 95%. Being patient with obtaining IV access and ensuring adequate analgesia.[19]

Monitoring

Two pulse oximeter probes (neonatal probes) should preferably be used; on the right hand (preductal) and the other on a lower limb (postductal). An appropriate sized blood pressure cuff and its appropriate application is important (repeated measurement can fracture poorly ossified bones). Removal of electrocardiogram adhesive stickers or adhesive tape can cause skin damage, similar to a partial thickness burn injury. End-tidal carbon dioxide readings may be less accurate (because of the very small tidal volume), but needs to be monitored. Transcutaneous CO_2 monitoring can be used if available. Obtaining an arterial line is technically challenging and potentially dangerous, with the risk of an ischemic compromised limb. If an umbilical arterial line is in place, rapid sampling or flushing of the line is to be avoided. Temperature monitoring with an esophageal or rectal probe or a combined esophageal stethoscope and temperature probe is useful. These probes should be inserted with great care to avoid perforation.

General Anesthesia

Premature infants are vulnerable to developing metabolic and respiratory abnormalities precipitated by stress, triggered by anesthetic techniques, anesthetic agents and surgery. The current controversy over the neurodevelopmental effects of anesthetic medications gives us cause for concern for administering general anesthesia.

Induction of Anesthesia

The majority of infants who present for surgery, are already intubated and mechanically ventilated and may be on inotropic support. Induction can be achieved with moderate concentrations of sevoflurane or narcotic-based (fentanyl or sufentanyl) with additional drugs, e.g. midazolam, ketamine or thiopentone. Clearance of propofol is slower in the preterm baby. Drugs that depend on hepatic clearance have a prolonged duration of action. These include sedatives, opioids and neuromuscular blocking agents which should be titrated to effect. Fentanyl administration reduces hormonal response and protein breakdown after surgery in premature infants.[21]

Airway and Intubation

Ill-fitting face masks and difficult mask ventilation, especially when a nasogastric tube is in place may require it to be removed prior to induction (after gentle aspiration). Securing the airway can be a challenge in these tiny infants. Awake intubation should generally be avoided as this may result in raised blood pressure and intraventricular pressure, apnea, desaturation and airway trauma. Gentle intubation can be performed with analgesia, local anesthesia and sedation or general anesthesia. During intubation, providing a stable head and good positioning, improves visibility of the larynx. The tracheal length may be as short as 4 cm and accurate tube position should be carefully confirmed. Securing the endotracheal tube may be difficult. Use of adhesive tape which causes minimal damage to the fragile skin of the face should be used.[14] The possibility of subglottic stenosis contributing to a difficult intubation should be kept in mind.[20] Avoiding exposure to high oxygen levels helps reduce morbidity and mortality with oxygen saturations not exceeding 95%.[19]

Maintenance of Anesthesia

Sevoflurane or desflurane help towards rapid recovery. The importance of adequate analgesia and anesthesia in the premature newborn needs to be emphasized and can be provided with fentanyl or sufentanyl, given as boluses or infusion. Higher doses of fentanyl 30 μg/kg or sufentanyl are associated with better arterial oxygenation.[15,21,22] A marked metabolic response increases mortality and morbidity. General anesthesia, controlled ventilation combined with local infiltration, regional or caudal block is a popular technique in high-risk premature neonates. The appropriate levels of anesthesia for various procedures are unclear.

Normal blood pressure in the extremely low birth weight infants has not been clearly defined. The guideline to follow is, if the mean arterial pressure is less than the gestational age + 5 mm Hg, it should be treated as hypotension. Tachycardia and hypertension can be deleterious in view of an underdeveloped cerebral autoregulation. Careful titration of anesthetic agents and narcotic agents is required therefore. If extubation is planned, analgesia should be provided with non-narcotic analgesia, combined with local anesthetic (infiltration or blocks). On the other hand, a high dose narcotic-based anesthetic technique should be used if postoperative ventilation is planned.[14]

Intraoperative Ventilation

Mechanical ventilation should be provided with a PEEP of 3-5 cm H_2O, an I:E ratio of 1:1, at 40-60 breaths per minute with a ventilatory mode allowing a degree of permissive hypercapnea.

Regional Anesthesia

Performing spinal and caudal blocks can be technically difficult. They have a high failure rate and when they do work, have a short duration. Regional blocks may need to be converted to or combined with general anesthesia. Levobupivacaine 1 mg/kg can be used for spinal anesthesia, and for caudal block, 2 mg/kg bupivacaine with 0.25% adrenaline can be used.[13]

Dose Modification of Anesthetic Agents in Neonates

- *Inhalation agents:* In neonates, the MAC for sevoflurane is 3.3. The MAC of isoflurane decreases steadily in neonates as gestational age decreases.
- *Propofol:* It has a low clearance at birth with a longer duration of action.
- *Opioids:* The tolerance to synthetic opioids develops in 3-5 days, faster than with morphine. Fentanyl may cause muscular rigidity and laryngospasm in doses of 2 µg/kg IV. Respiratory depression persists longer than its analgesic effect. Remifentanil may cause concentration dependent respiratory depression and muscle rigidity in doses greater than 3 µg/kg. The loading dose of remifentanil infusion may cause hypotension and bradycardia.
- *Other analgesics:* Ibuprofen causes a reduction in GFR in preterm neonates, indirectly prolonging aminoglycoside clearance. Ibuprofen has not been found to increase the incidence of intraventricular hemorrhage.[23]

Intravenous Fluid Replacement

Administration of 10% dextrose at 110-120 mL/kg/day maintains normoglycemia. Ongoing fluid loss should be replaced based on clinical judgment with isotonic 0.9% saline or lactated Ringer's as slow boluses of 10-20 mL/kg. Prompt but slow replacement of warmed blood products, prevents hypovolemia and avoids volume overload. Hypotension is common in this group of patients. Dopamine infusion 5 µg/kg/min. starting dose, is an effective therapy. Blood glucose levels should be checked with a glucometer and a blood glucose level ≥45 mg/dL is acceptable. Some ELBW infants may become hyperglycemic and require lower glucose intake and/or insulin. In the older ex-premature baby, alternatively, 25 mL 50% dextrose can be added to 500 mL of Ringer's lactate solution to make a 2.5% solution at 4 mL/kg/h infusion rate.[24]

Postoperative Management

If these infants require surgery soon after birth, postoperative management continues in the neonatal ICU. Postoperative complications of apnea, atelectasis and aspiration has been reported to be 33% in preterm babies.[25]

The decision to extubate, depends of the preoperative state of the baby and the type of surgery performed and should be performed once the baby is normothermic, fully awake with adequate tidal volume and maintaining adequate oxygenation. CPAP can be delivered by a flow device or via a ventilator and nasal prongs. Nasal prongs may increase the risk of nasal trauma.

Apnea is the main postoperative risk. Early apnea detection depends on the level of monitoring. Clinical observation, pulse oximetry and ECG monitoring helps with detecting bradycardia and hypoxemia. In the older infant close monitoring during the first 12-24 hours postoperatively is required as it is during this period that apnea is likely to occur. Infants with comorbidities of anemia, intraventricular hemorrhage, seizures, bronchopulmonary dysplasia requiring CPAP and oxygen, are at higher risk for postoperative apnea. Caffeine in a dose of 10 mg/kg can prevent apnea.

Multimodal approach is used for postoperative pain management. Paracetamol 7.5 mg/kg IV is used for babies 28-32 weeks. The oral and per rectal dose of paracetamol is 20 mg/kg followed by 10-15 mg/kg 8-12 hourly. Ketorolac in a dose of 1 mg/kg and tramadol 1 mg/kg or infusion of 0.18 mg/kg/h can be administered after the age of 40 weeks PMA.[26]

CONCLUSION

The anesthesiologist who provides care for the extremely premature infant is faced with a plethora of physiological, pathological, ethical and equipment challenges. The balancing act of avoiding hypoxemia, hemodynamic instability, respiratory and neurological complications remains a daunting task. These infants are best managed in the tertiary hospital setting. Despite advances in technology and specialized care, extremely premature and extremely low birth weight infants are at high-risk of death and disability.

REFERENCES

1. World Health Organization. Premature birth fact sheet No 363. Available at: http://www.who.int/mediacentre/factsheets/fs363/en/.
2. World Health Organization; March of Dimes; The partnership for maternal, newborn and child health; save the children. Born too soon: the global action report on preterm birth. Geneva: World Health Organization, 2012.
3. Glass HC, Costarino AT, Stayer SA, et al. Outcomes for extremely premature infants. Anesth Analg. 2015;120(6):1337-51.
4. Taneja B, Srivastava V, Saxena KN. Physiological and anaesthetic considerations for the preterm neonate undergoing surgery. J Neonat Surg. 2012;1(1):14-9.
5. Mourani PM, Abman SH. Pulmonary vascular disease in bronchopulmonary dysplasia: pulmonary hypertension and beyond. Curr Opin Pediatric. 2013;25:329-37.
6. Carraro S. Filippone M, Da Dalt L, et al. Bronchopulmonary dysplasia, the earliest and perhaps the longest lasting obstructive pulmonary disease in humans. Early Hum Dev 2013;89(Suppl 3):S3-5.
7. Frawley G. Special considerations in the premature and ex- premature infant. Anesth & Intensive Care Medicine. 2017;18:79-83.
8. Gurria J, Kuo P, Kao A, et al. General endotracheal vs. nonendotracheal regional anesthesia for elective inguinal hernia surgery in very preterm neonates: a single institution experience. J Pediatr Surg. 2017;52:56-9.
9. Peiris K, Fell D. The prematurely born infant and anaesthesia. Continuing Education in Anaesthesia, Critical Care & Pain. 2009;9:73-7.
10. Santin RL, Porat R. Apnea of prematurity. Available from http://www.emedicine.com/ped/topic1157 htm (2005).
11. Brett C, Robinowitz D. Physiology and development of the term and preterm neonate. In: Lerman J, editor. Neonatal Anesthesia. New York: Springer; 2015. pp. 17-66.
12. Tanner K, Sabrine N, Wren C. Cardiovascular malformations among preterm infants. Pediatrics. 2005;116:e833.
13. Raiesdana Department of Medicine, Brigham and Women's Hospital, Harvard Medical School, Boston, MA, USA, Loscalzo Department of Medicine, Brigham and Women's Hospital, Harvard Medical School, Boston, MA, USA J. Pulmonary arterial hypertension. Ann. of Med. 2006;38(2):95-110.
14. Thomas J. Reducing the risk in neonatal anesthesia. Pediatr Anesth. 2013;24:106-13.
15. Janvier A, Martinez JL, Barrington K, et al. Anesthetic technique and postoperative outcome in preterm infants undergoing PDA closure. J Perinatol. 2010;30:677-82.
16. Wyllie J. Treatment of Patent Ductus Arteriosus. Semin Neonatol. 2003;8:425-35.
17. Volpe J. Neurology of the Newborn. 4th ed. Philadelphia: WB Saunders; 2008. pp. 154-202.

18. McCann ME, Schouten AN, Dobija N, et al. Infantile postoperative encephalopathy: perioperative factors as a cause for concern. Pediatrics. 2014;133:e751-7.
19. Bayley G. Special considerations in the premature and ex-premature infants. Anesth Int Care. 2010;12(3):91-4.
20. Pang LM. Anesthesia for ex-premature infants and children. UpToDate 2017. wwwuptodate.com.
21. Hiller SC, Krishna G, Brasoveanu E. Neonatal anesthesia. Semin Pediatr Surg. 2004;13(3):142-51.
22. Shew SB, Keshen TH, Glass NI, et al. Ligation of a patent ductus arteriosus under fentanyl anesthesia improves protein metabolism in premature neonates. J Pediatr Surg. 2000;35(9):1277-81.
23. Anderson BJ, Larsson P, Lerman J. Anesthesia and ancillary drugs and the neonate, In: Lerman J, editor. Neonatal Anesthesia. New York: Springer; 2015. pp. 67-130.
24. Lai M, Inglis GDT, Hose K, et al. Methods for securing endotracheal tubes in newborn infants. Cochrane Database of Systematic Reviews. 2014, Issue 7. Art. No.: CD007805.
25. Collins C, Koren G, Crean P, et al. Fentanyl pharmacokinetics and hemodynamic effects in preterm infants during ligation of patent ductus arteriosus. Anesth Analg. 1985;64:1078-108.
26. Pribul V. Anesthesia for preterm infant. WFSA Tutorial for the week 259. 2012 www.totw.anaesthesiologists.org.

CHAPTER 16

ECMO: Need of the Hour

Poonam Malhotra Kapoor, Shivani Aggarwal

KEY POINTS

- Extracorporeal membrane oxygenation or ECMO is used for cardiac and/or respiratory failure when all other treatment modalities fail. It is increasingly being used today in all ICUs because of its sleek design and portability.
- Two types of ECMO are known, the veno-venous (V-V) and veno-arterial (V-A) and indications for both are different.
- Though the basic mechanism is the same, cannulation sites and ECMO flows are different in V-V and V-A types.
- Complications like bleeding, thrombosis and emboli are known which decrease the ECMO flows.
- Echocardiography, NIRS, central/mixed venous oxygenation with precept/pulmonary artery catheter, serum lactate and coagulation monitoring parameters like prothrombin time and fibrinogen level are essential parameters for monitoring in smooth ECMO run.
- ECMO requires a teamwork, involving intensivists, pulmonologists, perfusionists and nurses.

INTRODUCTION

In case of a failing heart and lungs, several mechanical assist devices like extra corporeal membrane oxygenation (ECMO), intra aortic balloon pump (IABP) and ventricular assist devices (VAD) are now available. ECMO is a form of partial cardiopulmonary bypass where venous blood from the patient is carried by an artificial circulation to a membrane oxygenator made of specialized material for gas exchange. The blood is oxygenated and carbon dioxide removal takes place and this oxygenated blood is then sent back to the patient through different cannula. Patients with acute cardiac failure/dysfunction, acute respiratory failure/dysfunction or both not responding to conventional therapy are usually candidates for ECMO support. ECMO provides the time required for recovery from the underlying pathology. Therefore, it is vital that the patient's disease/condition should be reversible.

Initially, ECMO was used only for oxygenating the blood, but later more emphasis was laid on removing carbon dioxide and the term extracorporeal carbon dioxide removal was coined.[1] Today the new paradigm shift is more to do with carbon dioxide removal then oxygenation. Recently a new term - Extracorporeal life support (ECLS), has come into vogue. This term also includes other methods for circulatory support, such as ventricular assist devices and extracorporeal circuits. Extracorporeal support was used for providing postoperative support in post-cardiotomy patients when there was failure to wean from cardiopulmonary bypass.[2] Developments in its design and careful selection of patients have enabled its use in variety of conditions making it a necessity in cases of cardiac and/or respiratory failure in the ICU where facilities for ECLS exists. It provides a bridge while awaiting definitive treatment such as heart or lung transplant (Fig. 1).

HISTORY OF ECMO

The developments for the safe conduct of cardiopulmonary bypass for complex congenital heart diseases laid the stepping stone for the present day ECMO. It all started when artificial oxygenation was first used by Gibbon for the first successful open heart surgery in 1953. The first successful open heart operation was possible with perfusion support in 1954.[3] As live cardiopulmonary bypass apparatuses Lillehei developed the cross-circulation technique by using slightly anesthetized adult volunteers during the repair of definitive congenital cardiac disorders.[4] In 1955, at the Mayo Clinic, Kirklin et al. improved on Gibbon's device and successfully repaired an atrial septal defect in a baby who was suffering from meconium aspiration.[5]

In 1965, a neonate was dying of respiratory failure, Rashkind and coworkers were the first to use a bubble oxygenator as support to save the neonate.[6] The membrane oxygenator in infants was used by Dorson and colleagues in 1969.[7] Prior to 1970s, attempts at long-term extracorporeal support were limited by

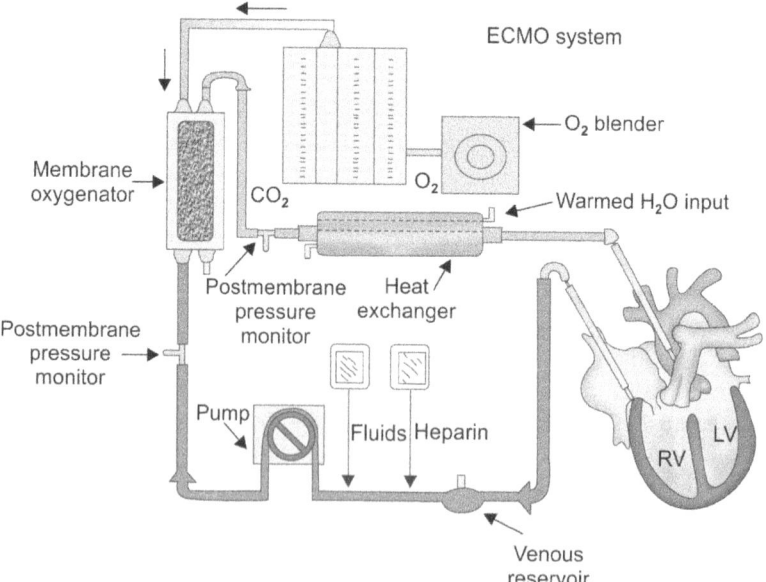

Fig. 1: A diagram of extracorporeal membrane oxygenation is shown with a membrane oxygenator pump and heat exchange as essential component of ECMO circuit.

gas-exchange devices ("oxygenators") which did not separate the gas from the blood and this led to hemolysis, thrombocytopenia and coagulopathy if used for hours at a time. With development of silicone membrane oxygenators, the whole scenario changed. From 1971 onwards first reports of bedside CPB being used for long-term cardiopulmonary support emerged.

In 1970, Baffes et al. reported the successful use of extracorporeal membrane oxygenation as support in infants with congenital heart defects who were undergoing cardiac surgery.[8] In 1972, the ECMO was used for the first times by Hill et al. in an adult with respiratory failure following trauma.[9] In 1976, first successfully use of V-A ECMO in neonates with severe respiratory distress was by Bartlett et al.[10] Haiduc et al. started the era of ECMO in critical care by using bedside CPB for treating a newborn with meconium aspiration.[11] With formation of ICU units and better understanding of positive pressure ventilation, increased survival of infants, children, and adults following cardiac/pulmonary insults was observed. Acute respiratory distress syndrome (ARDS) emerged as the major problem in ailing ICUs. Several clinical trials published demonstrating clear survival benefit of ECMO in infants suffering from severe respiratory failure, meconium aspiration, persistent fetal circulation and so on.[12] Randomized controlled studies in adults with ARDS demonstrated no such benefit.[13] Though several smaller studies and case reports emerged with reports of >50% survival in those treated with ECMO in addition to maximal ventilatory management, ECMO fell out of favor for use in adults. The interest in ECMO revived with reports of Bartlett et al. and O'Rourke et al. demonstrating favorable outcome in infants and children in early 1980s.[14,15]

ECMO AND THE ELSO REGISTRY

In an attempt to formulate guidelines for development of a common consensus, ELSO or Extracorporeal Life Support Organization was established in 1989.[16] ELSO registry database was formed in 1984. It provided platform for 1991 NIH conference on diffusion of ECMO technology. Till date, about 141 centers worldwide report to this registry providing valuable information regarding ECMO. These have been divided into 9 chapters across the globe. For example, the 39 centers of ECMO in India called under the banner of The South and West Asia Chapter of Extracorporeal Life Support Organization (SWACELSO) which includes south west Asian and African countries besides India.

TYPES OF ECMO

There are two types of ECMO: the venovenous (V-V) ECMO and the veno-arterial (V-A) ECMO. While V-V ECMO is used primarily in patients of respiratory failure with good cardiac functions, the V-A ECMO is used exclusively for patients with cardiac failure or combined cardiorespiratory failure. The ECMO is different from cardiopulmonary bypass (CPB) in that:
- ECMO can be frequently instituted using only cervical cannulation under local anesthesia; standard CPB requires transthoracic cannulation under general anesthesia.
- Standard CPB is used for short-term support measured in hours while ECMO is used for longer-term support ranging from 3 to 10 days.

- The purpose of ECMO is to allow time for intrinsic recovery of the lungs and heart; a standard CPB provides support during various types of cardiac surgical procedures.

Veno-Venous (V-V) ECMO

In veno-venous ECMO, venous blood is removed from the patient via large central veins "access line" and then returned to the right atrium "return line" after it has been oxygenated by the oxygenator. It is used to provide support in cases of severe respiratory failure without any cardiac dysfunction.

Very often the ECMO flow rate may be very high as in cases of severe respiratory failure. This may require a second venous cannula over and above a single access cannula. This decreases the suction and speed of the venous flow line, thus improving the hemodynamic disturbances. V-V ECMO enhances the oxygenation of a diseased lung by reducing the amount of blood that passes through it. This allows reduction in the level of ventilatory support which in turn decreases the ongoing ventilator induced lung injury (Fig. 2).

It is the patients cardiac output that derives the pump flow of the ECMO circuit and thus determines the oxygenation of the patient on ECMO. Increased ECMO flow rates should increase the patient's oxygenation, or/else, recirculation of blood between the inflow and outflow cannula will occur and hamper the ECMO flow.

Veno-Arterial (V-A) ECMO

In veno-arterial ECMO blood from the patient's central vein flows into an oxygenator and return into a major arterial vessel. In cases of severe heart failure and in postcardiotomy patients along with associated pulmonary failure VA ECMO is useful (Fig. 2).

Low Flow V-A ECMO

Low flow V-A ECMO is invoked today as smaller percutaneous cannula can be inserted faster percutaneously during emergency resuscitative measures as in viral myocarditis and cardiogenic shock. This form of ECMO used for resuscitation is known as extracorporeal CPR of E-CPR.[17]

FACTOR AFFECTING GASEOUS EXCHANGE

The efficiency of oxygenation by the ECMO circuit depends on the pump flow relative to the patient's cardiac output. The patient's oxygenation should increase with increasing ECMO flow rate. However, if this does not occur, recirculation of blood between the inflow and outflow cannula should be suspected.

The factors which affect the gas exchange from the ECMO are:
- Native cardiac output
- Native pulmonary function
- Ventilator setting and FIO_2
- ECMO sweep and FIO_2
- ECMO flow
- Hemoglobin
- Site of mixing of ECMO circulation and native circulation.

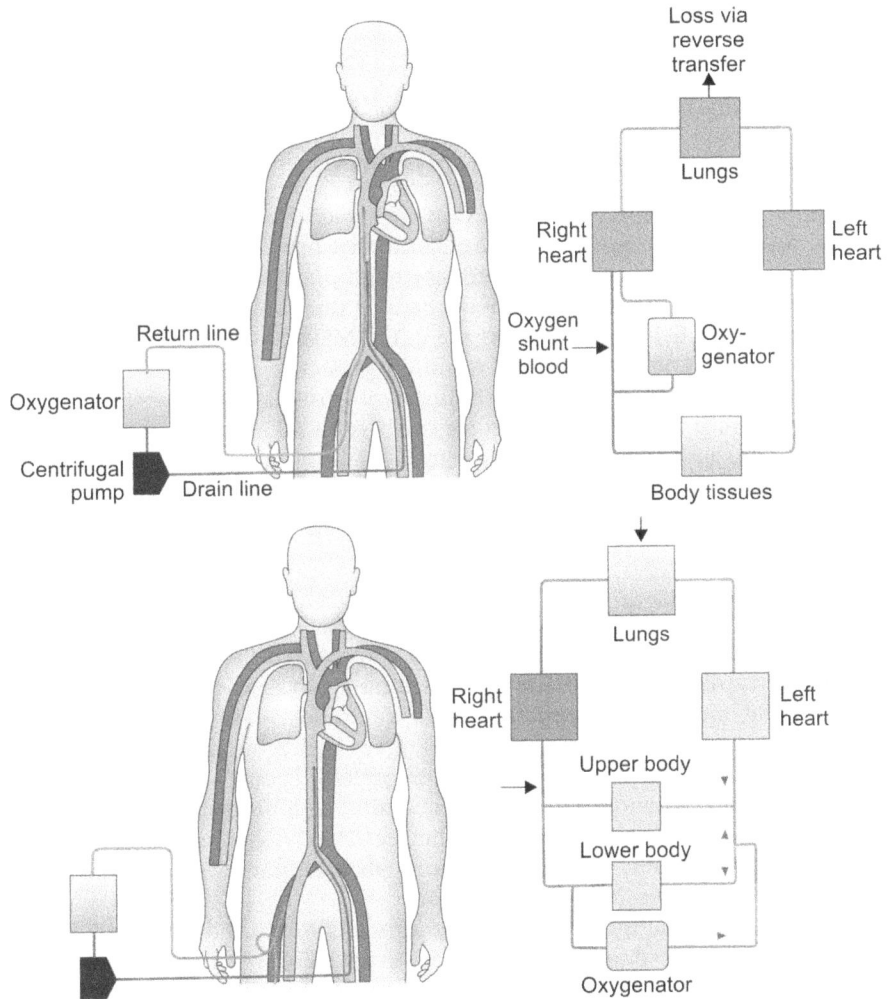

Fig. 2: Veno-venous ECMO and veno-arterial ECMO circuits.

Between the V-V and V-A ECMO, it is the former that is more efficient in removing carbon dioxide of the patient. V-A ECMO is better for oxygenation of the patient. The ECMO flow determines the carbon dioxide removal and thus these two determines the cardiac output. Increased ECMO flow rates will decrease the carbon dioxide of the blood. The oxygen flow rate should be double the ECMO flow rate. All of patient's carbon dioxide production can be removed by the ECMO oxygenator if the flow through the oxygenator is double the ECMO pumps flow rate, maintaining an ECMO flow rate with two-thirds the patient's cardiac output and an oxygen flow rate of twice the pump flow, nearly all of the patient's CO_2 production can be removed by the oxygenator.

The low flow V-V ECMO which enables carbon dioxide removal but not oxygenation of blood is more aptly referred to as extracorporeal carbon dioxide removal. It has emerged as a potential therapy for ventilatory management in diseases apart from ARDS like exacerbations after chronic obstructive pulmonary disease, severe asthma and bridge to transplant and is a burning need in every medicine, pediatric and pulmonary intensive care unit.

WHICH TO CHOOSE: VENO-VENOUS OR VENO-ARTERIAL ECMO?

Though V-V ECMO scores over V-A ECMO in avoiding any major arterial vessel tear or any air or clot embolism, we must remember that V-V ECMO is a low pressure circuit and therefore easier to insert and can remain for long. The latter also produces less hemodynamic perturbations than V-A ECMO. For example, the RA pressure will fall on increasing the V-A ECMO flows, but no change will be seen in V-V ECMO. The features of V-A and V-V ECMO are enumerated in Table 1.

V-V ECMO is better for managing pulmonary sepsis as it preserves pulmonary blood flow. However, V-A ECMO scores over V-V ECMO in providing complete hemodynamic and respiratory support to the failing heart. Thus, V-A ECMO is ideal as a bridge to recovery or bridge to transplant. Other indications for V-A ECMO in an adult are cardiogenic shock associated with myocarditis, poisoning or hypothermia.

PRESENT DAY ECMO

The present-day applications of ECMO have surpassed the traditional use for support of cardiac and respiratory failure long ago. Cardiac ECMO is used in the neonatal and pediatric populations for a number of indications, including postoperative support following cardiac surgery and acute myocarditis. In the adult population, it is rapidly becoming the preferred acute short-term therapy for postcardiotomy syndrome, acute myocarditis, as a bridge to recovery or as a bridge to decision. Ventricular assist devices (VADs) are not being reserved for bridge to transplant or destination, although some patients recover function during support to have their VAD explanted.

Support of respiratory failure remains the most common indication for ECMO. Historically it was used for patients with acute reversible respiratory failure with expected recovery, and this still remains the most common application. With recent improvements in technology, in particular with dual-lumen single cannulation of the internal jugular vein (Figs. 3A and B), patients are being supported till lung transplant is done. With development of portable ECMO, patients can participate

Table 1. Comparative features of V-A and V-V ECMO	
Veno-Arterial (V-A) ECMO	**Veno-Venous (V-V) ECMO**
Provides support for severe cardiac and respiratory failure, most commonly after cardiac surgery	Provides support for severe respiratory failure when reasonable heart function is assessed
Induces high hemodynamic disturbances depending on the chosen return access sites	Induces low hemodynamic disturbances
Can be used as a bridge to cardiac recovery or to another destination therapy	1 or 2 access cannulae can be used depending on the bypassed blood flow

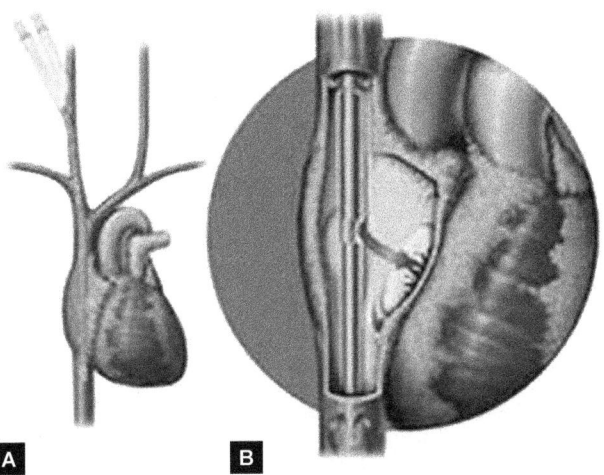

Figs. 3A and B: (A) Different types of ECMO cannulas: Arterial and venous; (B) Dual-lumen single cannulation of the internal jugular vein.
Source: With permission from Goyal and Oza (2013).[23]

in physical rehabilitation, including ambulation, thereby improving their ability to successfully undergo transplantation. The newest and most rapidly growing indication is for the support during cardiopulmonary arrest. Extracorporeal cardiopulmonary resuscitation (ECPR) entails the rapid deployment of femoral veno-arterial ECMO in patients not responding to conventional CPR. Survival rates of 30% and more without any neurological sequelae are being reported, higher than the historically reported rates of 12–15% with conventional CPR.

Rapid deployment is facilitated by recent technological improvements, including hollow fiber oxygenators with centrifugal pumps, which can be rapidly primed with crystalloid solutions. Results following in-hospital cardiac arrest are encouraging, while its use in out-of-hospital arrest is still associated with poor outcomes.[18,19] The challenge in the latter may be in selection of patients, since in-hospital arrest is usually witnessed, while out-of-hospital often is not.

Our knowledge regarding outcome of the two therapies is still in initial phases. Some randomized control trials such as Cochrane review have yielded inconclusive results in adults while some such as CESAR trial have shown promising results.[20,21] Given the lack of studies with appropriate control groups, future studies on the use of ECMO are needed to clarify its role,[22] i.e. when to use and its effects on various organ systems in all age groups.

MONITORING OF ECMO

The success of critical care lies with the vigilant monitoring which helps in early recognition and diagnosis of the problem and the timely, and accurate action. Right action at right times saves the life. Monitoring can be done by observing the clinical parameters, the biochemical and laboratory parameters, radiological monitoring and last but not the least is circuit monitoring. While the patient is on ECMO, monitoring of the patient's parameter becomes more vital as he/she is critically ill. In addition, it is equally important to monitor ECMO system so as to prevent the life-threatening complications, and if it does occurs, manage it appropriately. The practical aspects of all these parameters are discussed in length in ECMO volume I, practical manual.[23] Echocardiography, NIRS, central/mixed venous oxygenation with precept/pulmonary artery catheter, serum lactate and coagulation monitoring parameters like prothrombin time and fibrinogen level are today essential parameters for monitoring in smooth ECMO run.

Echocardiographic monitoring on ECMO helps in patient selection, monitoring during support, for insertion and correct placement of cannulas, in detecting complications and in decision-making for cardiac recovery, weaning and bridge to transplant (Figs. 4 and 5).

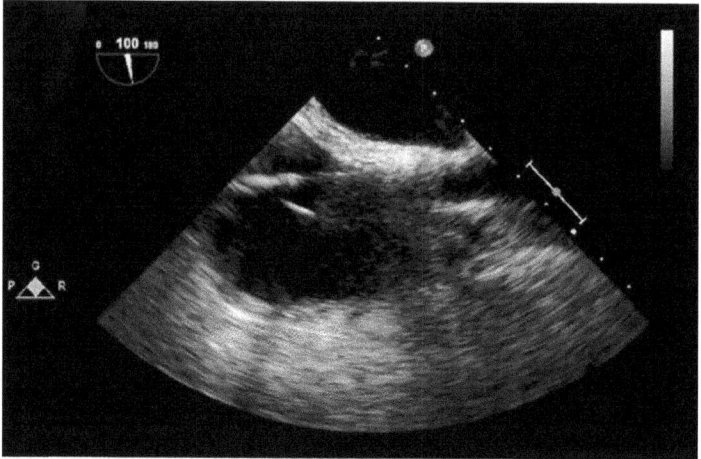

Fig. 4: Echocardiography can visualize the correct position of both wires and cannula.

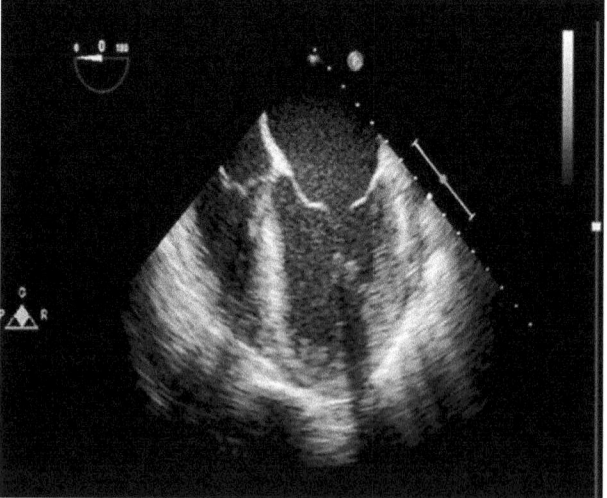

Fig. 5: Monitoring of the patient on VA-ECMO adequate LV unloading.

FUTURE OF ECMO

As we recruit more and more new patient population and increase the horizons of ECMO, simultaneous improvements in technology are must for maintaining this trend in future. Miniaturization and automation of support systems will help ECMO to move towards the current status enjoyed by CRRT, with nurse-driven bedside management. Development of Maquet Cardiohelp® system has bought a revolution in the ECMO era (Figs. 6 and 7). It enhances the mobility of patients and even permits excursion outside the hospital. Future systems may even allow the use of ECMO as a replacement for mechanical ventilation. Some ECMO centers are already actively pursuing extubation of patients on ECMO, removing a source of further injury and infection. It is not inconceivable that ECMO could emerge as a first line therapy in selected patients, avoiding intubation altogether. This is particularly true for hypercapnic respiratory failure, such as COPD exacerbation, for which dedicated CO_2 removal systems are currently hitting the market.

The greatest hurdle still is perhaps anticoagulation. Use of antithrombotic coatings can reduce heparin requirements but not eliminate its use, requiring complex monitoring and management. Advanced coatings have the potential to eliminate this restriction altogether. Nitric oxide releasing coatings are currently under development and shown promising results in preclinical studies.

Another exciting extension of ECMO is the artificial implantable lung for destination therapy of chronic heart failure. In this capacity, blood would be pumped by the right ventricle, eliminating the need and problems of a blood pump. Animal experiments had clearly demonstrated the feasibility, yet work remains on optimal hemodynamic configuration, oxygenator design and antithrombotic coatings. With continued development, these advances should be realizable in the not-too-distant future.

CONCLUSION

To conclude, extracorporeal membrane oxygenation or ECMO is a useful modality for patients with cardiac and/or respiratory failure when all other

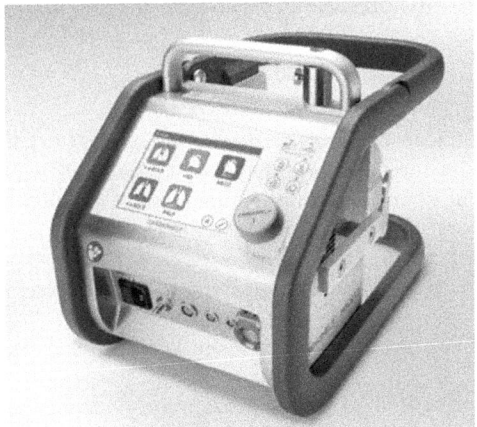
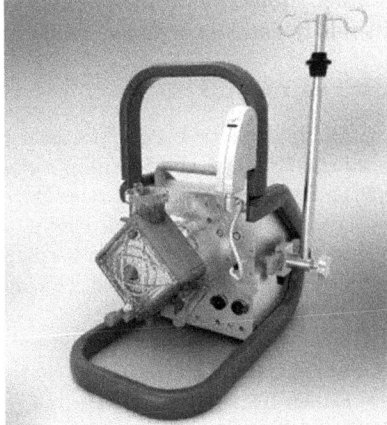

Fig. 6: The future of ECMO—Cardio help, the mobile ECMO.

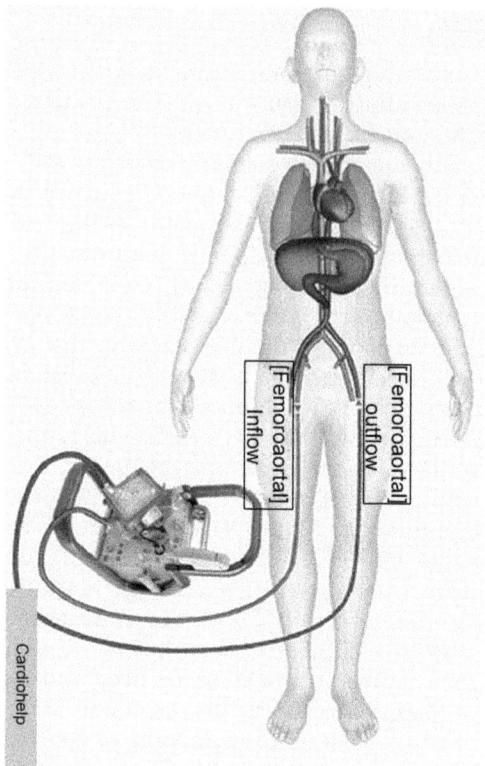

Fig. 7: Cardiohelp: Femoroaortal inflow and outflow.

treatment modalities have failed. ECMO therapy requires teamwork between the intensivists, pulmonologists, cardiologists, perfusionists and the nurses. It is increasingly being used in all ICUs because of the sleek design and portability but there are conflicting results regarding its usefulness from various studies. Future studies should focus on the effect of ECMO on various organ systems and clarify its role in patients in all age groups.

REFERENCES

1. Morelli A, Sorbo L, Pesenti A, et al. Extracorporeal carbon dioxide removal ($ECCO_2R$) in patients with acute respiratory failure. Intensive Care Medicine. 2017;43(4):519-30.
2. Lowry AW, Morales DL, Graves DE, et al. Characterization of extracorporeal membrane oxygenation for pediatric cardiac arrest in the United States: Analysis of the kids' Inpatient Database. Pediatr Cardiol. 2013;34(6):1422-30.
3. Gibbon JH Jr. Application of a mechanical heart and lung apparatus to cardiac surgery. Minn Med. 1954;37:180-5.
4. Lillehei CW. A personalized history of extracorporeal circulation. Trans Am Soc Artif Intern Organs. 1982;28:5-16.
5. Kirklin JW, Donald DE, Harshbarger HG, et al. Studies in extracorporeal circulation. I. Applicability of Gibbon-type pump-oxygenator to human intracardiac surgery: 40 cases. Ann Surg. 1956;144(1):2-8.

6. Rashkind WJ, Freeman A, Klein D, et al. Evaluation of a disposable plastic, low volume, pumpless oxygenator as a lung substitute. J Pediatr. 1965;66:94-102.
7. Dorson W Jr, Baker E, Cohen ML, et al. A perfusion system for infants. Trans Am Soc Artif Intern Organs. 1969;15:155-60.
8. Baffes TG, Fridman JL, Bicoff JP, et al. Extracorporeal circulation for support of palliative cardiac surgery in infants. Ann Thorac Surg. 1970;10(4):354-63.
9. Hill JD, O'Brien TG, Murray JJ, et al. Prolonged extracorporeal oxygenation for acute post-traumatic respiratory failure (shock-lung syndrome). Use of the Bramson membrane lung. N Engl J Med. 1972;286(12):629-34.
10. Bartlett RH, Gazzaniga AB, Jefferies MR, et al. Extracorporeal membrane oxygenation (ECMO) cardiopulmonary support in infancy. Trans Am Soc Artif Intern Organs. 1976;22:80-93.
11. Haiduc NJ, Wetmore N, Jefferies MR, et al. Prolonged extracorporeal circulation in a neonatal meconium aspiration: A case report. JECT 1977;9:183-6.
12. RH Bartlett, AB Gazzaniga, SW Fong, et al. Extracorporeal membrane oxygenator support for cardiopulmonary failure. Experience in 28 cases. J Thorac Cardiovasc Surg. 1977;73(3):375-86.
13. Zapol WM, Snider MT, Hill JD, et al. Extracorporeal membrane oxygenation in severe acute respiratory failure. A randomized prospective study. JAMA 1979; 242(20):2193-6.
14. Bartlett RH, Andrews AF, Toomasian JM, et al. Extracorporeal membrane oxygenation for newborn respiratory failure: forty-five cases. Surgery. 1982;9(2):425-33.
15. O'Rourke PP, Crone RK, Vacanti JP, et al. Extracorporeal membrane oxygenation and conventional medical therapy in neonates with persistent pulmonary hypertension of the newborn: a prospective randomized study. Pediatrics. 1989;84(6):957-63.
16. ECMO registry of Extracorporeal Life Support Organization. www.elso.org.
17. Chen YS, Yu HY, Huang SC, et al. Extracorporeal membrane oxygenation support can extend the duration of cardiopulmonary resuscitation. Crit Care Med. 2008;36:2529-35.
18. Maekawa K, Tanno K, Hase M, et al. Extracorporeal cardiopulmonary resuscitation for patients with out-of-hospital cardiac arrest of cardiac origin: a propensity-matched study and predictor analysis. Crit Care Med. 2013;41:1186-96.
19. Shin TG, Jo IJ, Sim MS, et al. Two-year survival and neurological outcome of in-hospital cardiac arrest patients rescued by extracorporeal cardiopulmonary resuscitation. Int J Cardiol. 2013;168:3424-30.
20. Tillmann BW, Klingel ML, Iansavichene AE, et al. Extracorporeal membrane oxygenation (ECMO) as a treatment strategy for severe acute respiratory distress syndrome (ARDS) in the low tidal volume era: A systematic review. J Crit Care. 2017; 41:64-71.
21. Tramm R, Ilic D, Davies AR, et al. Extracorporeal membrane oxygenation for critically ill adults. Cochrane Database of Systematic Reviews. 2015, Issue 1. Art. No.: CD010381. DOI: 10.1002/14651858.CD010381.pub2.
22. Hitt E. Efficacy and economic assessment of conventional ventilatory support versus extracorporeal membrane oxygenation for severe adult respiratory failure (CESAR): a multicentre randomised controlled trial. Lancet. 2009;374:1351.
23. Goyal V, Oza P. Monitoring on Extracorporeal Membrane Oxygenation. Manual of ECMO in ICU. New Delhi: Jaypee Brother Medical Publishers; 2013. pp. 76.

CHAPTER 17

Anesthesia for Laryngotracheal Stenosis

Amit Rai, Gunjan Singh

KEY POINTS

- Laryngotracheal stenosis (LTS) is a rare but a life-threatening condition and may be congenital but the most common cause is postintubation injury.
- The management of LTS varies from endoscopic tracheal dilatation to placement of tracheal stents to tracheal reconstruction and depends on the location, degree of airway lumen narrowing, etiology and impact on patient's functional status.
- Since the airway is "shared" close collaboration and communication between the anesthesiologists and surgeons is required. A well-structured, coordinated plan is the key to successful management of these patients.
- Depending on the severity and location of the stenosis and the type of surgical procedure, there may be a variety of choices for perioperative airway management and ventilation.
- Smooth extubation and emergence is the preferred goal since mechanical ventilation has the potential for disruption of the anastomosis.

INTRODUCTION

Laryngotracheal stenosis (LTS) is a broad-spectrum term commonly used for narrowing of the airway lumen involving the larynx, trachea or both. The narrowing can occur at the level of larynx, trachea, carina or main bronchi. Tracheal stenosis (TS) is the term used for narrowing of the airway lumen from the cricoid cartilage to the main carina. It is different than subglottic stenosis (SGS), which involves narrowing of the airway between vocal cord (glottis) and cricoid cartilage.[1] Subglottic stenosis is more common in the pediatric age group and is therefore used commonly to describe airway lumen narrowing in children and laryngotracheal stenosis is more often used in adults. The incidence of laryngotracheal stenosis varies from 1% to 8% in both the pediatric and adult population.[2] The normal diameter of an adult trachea is 1.8 to 2.5 cm. Stenosis of the trachea causes functional impairment, which can be objectively measured in terms of fall in peak expiratory flow. The management of LTS is a collaborative effort between the otolaryngologist, pulmonologist, anesthesiologist and at times the thoracic surgeon, and it depends on the location, extent and shape of the stenosis, degree of airway lumen narrowing, etiology and the impact on patient's functional status.

The involvement of multiple specialties in the management of this disease has resulted in the development of various classification systems with varied criteria, though none of them have included all parameters relevant to treatment decisions and none of them are universally accepted. The lack of uniformity has made it difficult to provide evidence-based recommendations for managing patients suffering from LTS. This chapter sums up the disease process along with treatment modalities and the role of the anesthesiologist.

ETIOLOGY

Laryngotracheal stenosis may be congenital or acquired. The cause of congenital LTS is in-utero malformation of the cricoid cartilage. The diagnosis is considered to be congenital if the patient has not had a history of endotracheal intubation and has an absence of other potential causes of stenosis. Congenital laryngeal webs are the commonest cause of congenital LTS, with almost 75% occurring at the glottis followed by subglottic level. Severe conditions typically present during childhood, while milder forms can present in adolescence or even in adult life.

Acquired forms of subglottic stenosis most commonly occur from trauma to airway tissue, with more than 90% of them following endotracheal intubation. Endotracheal intubations are the most common of all the causes of LTS.[3] The factors that are consistently cited as causative include the duration of intubation, the size of the endotracheal tube, frequent manipulation or movement of the endotracheal tube, and repeated intubations. Amongst these, the duration of intubation is most important. Usually a 7-10 days duration of intubation is acceptable, beyond which the chances of development of LTS are very likely. Other factors that contribute are systemic illness (relapsing polychondritis, sarcoidosis, Wegener's granulomaosis, inflammatory bowel disease), malnutrition, anemia, and hypoxia. Local bacterial infections like tuberculosis and diphtheria may play an important role in the development of LTS. Iatrogenic causes that are implicated in LTS include high tracheostomy (even percutaneous tracheostomy), radiotherapy (LTS after radiation therapy can occur up to 20 years later), external trauma (penetrating and blunt), inhalational injury (thermal and caustic) and neoplasms (benign and malignant). Gastroesophageal reflux (GER) may play an important role in the development of LTS because it causes the airway to be continually bathed in acid, which irritates and inflames the area and prevents it from healing correctly. Not only has it been implicated as a cause of acquired LTS, it also may be the cause of restenosis after laryngotracheal reconstruction or repair (LTR). It is important for the surgical team to know the etiology of tracheal stenosis as it helps in planning the management.

A thorough history from the patient or his relatives is of utmost importance as it may help in zeroing down the etiology since treatment options will shift from surgical to medical and vice versa in patients with LTS. Tracheal stenosis when diagnosed, needs urgent attention as it can cause respiratory disorders ranging from dyspnea to stridor and even respiratory failure.[4]

CLASSIFICATION

Since LTS affects all age groups, most experts differentiate the disease and its process based on a pediatric or adult presentation. The same is also true for classifying LTS. The Myer Cotton grading system is used for assessing the severity of pediatric laryngotracheal stenosis. This system uses endotracheal size as a measure of airway diameter. It consists of four grades (Table 1). This system is a

Table 1: Classification systems for laryngotracheal stenosis	
Meyer Cotton classification	
Grade 1	No obstruction to 50%
Grade 2	51% to 70% obstruction
Grade 3	71% to 99% obstruction
Grade 4	No detectable lumen
McCaffrey classification	
Stage I	Confined to the subglottis or trachea and length is less than 1 cm
Stage II	The lesions are subglottic, stenosis is longer than 1 cm within the cricoid ring and not extending to the glottis or trachea
Stage III	The lesions are subglottic, stenosis that extend into the upper trachea but do not involve the glottis
Stage IV	The lesions involve the glottis and cause fixation or paralysis of one or both of the vocal cords.

useful tool to assess the grade of subglottic severity and to predict the success rate of decannulation of pediatric tracheostomy patients. However, it has less value as a prognostic indicator in patients with multiple sites of airway disease, or with airway inflammation, or when there is trauma from multiple intubation attempts. However, in adults, just using cross sectional area as a guide to consistently determine successful decannulation may not be enough and therefore the McCaffrey system (Table 1) for adults was created. It is a four-stage system based on the vertical extent. It predicts decannulation in adult patients based on the anatomic location and extent of the stenosis. Generally, 90% of stage I and II, 70% of stage III, and 40% of stage IV patients are successfully decannulated. Other classifications mentioned are Lano's, Nouri's, and recently introduced FEMOS (functional status, extent and location, morphology, origin and severity of stenosis) classification.[5-9]

CLINICAL PRESENTATION

Clinical manifestation differs in children and adults. In children with LTS, there is airway obstruction, which may manifest in several different ways. Whenever a smaller than appropriate endotracheal tube for age and weight has to be used, narrowing of the airway may be present, and we must suspect LTS. In neonates and infants, it may manifest as stridor and obstructive breathing immediately after extubation that requires re-intubation. The stridor in LTS depends on the site of stenosis. Biphasic stridor is associated with glottic, subglottic, and upper tracheal lesions. Inspiratory stridor usually is associated with supraglottic lesions, whereas expiratory stridor usually is associated with tracheal lesions.

In mild LTS, only exercise-induced stridor or obstruction may be present. In severe LTS, complete airway obstruction may be present and may require immediate surgical intervention. Some children with LTE may present with a history of recurrent croup. Older children may present with either hoarse or a weak voice.

Most patients do not develop symptoms at rest until they have reached 70% stenosis. Adult patients with acquired stenosis may get diagnosed within days following an initial insult to the airway or may go undiagnosed for years, though most patients get diagnosed within a year. Symptoms include the following:
a. Stridor
   ➢ Dyspnea (on exertion or at rest, depending on severity of stenosis). Some patients of tracheal stenosis can be an asymptomatic with complaints of shortness of breath on exertion and may be falsely diagnosed to have asthma. It may be accompanied with noisy breathing or there may be complaints of cough and wheeze that does not respond to bronchodilators.
b. Hoarseness
c. Brassy cough
d. Recurrent pneumonitis
e. Cyanosis.

In patients with a history of intubation and onset of respiratory distress thereafter, there should be a very high index of suspicion of developing LTS.

PREOPERATIVE EVALUATION

History

Iatrogenic trauma is the commonest cause of LTS. A clear history of any antecedent airway management and intensive care admission needs to be taken. Detailed history should include progression of the disease and any other pertinent symptoms that the patient has experienced with emphasis on hoarseness after general anesthesia and recurrent respiratory tract infections. However, there are numerous causes of LTS, which must be ruled out specially if there is no history of any prior trauma. A detailed history of the patient should be taken, and a review of systems including difficulty clearing secretions, stridor, effort tolerance, gastroesophageal reflux and orthopnea, should be elicited. Patients with dyspnea on exertion have decreased severity of obstruction than the patients complaining of dyspnea at rest or minimal exertion.[10]

Physical Examination

Airway assessment, including neck mobility, palpation of the trachea, mouth opening and prediction of successful mask ventilation is necessary. However, a reassuring airway exam may not necessarily predict successful endotracheal intubation. Neck mobility of the patient is an important assessment as it is an important determinant of intraoperative visualization of the field as well as postoperative healing of the patient.[10]

The trachea and lungs should be auscultated. All patients that have a history of ventilation (postoperative or intensive care unit), need to be evaluated for the presence of other comorbidities, that have been associated with the development of LTS.

Investigations

A complete blood count (CBC) is usually enough and specific laboratory studies are not required unless indicated due to other comorbidities. Cardiac evaluation is required if the patient is incapable of physical activity due to the stenosis. In such cases an echocardiography or stress test may be done.

Pulmonary Function Tests

In patients with LTS, the flow volume loops may show a lot of anomalies including a delay in reaching peak expiratory flow, a truncation of peak expiratory and peak inspiratory flow, or a sudden drop of expiratory flow at the end of expiration. It may be noted that pulmonary function tests do not offer more specific information regarding the stenosis than what is gained from imaging. However, the flow-volume loops give information about the functional status of the patient and may be helpful in monitoring for restenosis after intervention. It is imperative to mention that pulmonary function test (PFT) lacks sensitivity, and proper inspiratory and expiratory loops can be appreciable only when the tracheal lumen is reduced to 6–8 mm.[11]

Imaging

A radiograph of the chest often provides valuable information regarding the tracheal air column. Anteroposterior and lateral plain neck radiography is required to assess the soft tissues and airway narrowing if present since it gives specific information about the glottic and subglottic air column. Fluoroscopy may be performed in children with symptoms of airway obstruction to diagnose lesions of the larynx and trachea. A barium-enhanced oesophagram may be required to rule out vascular malformations and gastroesophageal reflux disease (GERD). If a definitive intervention is planned to correct the stenosis, coronal and sagittal views of either computed tomography (CT) scan or MRI are useful to evaluate the stenotic lesion. A CT with thin cuts (1 mm) will evaluate the entire airway. Multiplanar reformations (MPR) along with virtual bronchoscopy helps in deciding the type of intervention required for correcting the stenosis. MRI is an alternative to CT and provide better soft tissue details and allows better visualization of the stenotic lesion by sagittal and coronal reconstructions.[12,13] However, most of the patients that require surgery have respiratory distress and excessive secretions and it is cumbersome for these patients to lie in the MRI gantry for prolonged time. Therefore, in most centers a CT with thin cuts is preferred over MRI for imaging. Preoperative imaging often underestimates the caliber and length of the stenosis in pediatric patients.[14]

Bronchoscopy and Direct Laryngoscopy

Direct laryngoscopy and bronchoscopy are the standard criterion for evaluation of the airway. Bronchoscopy remains the primary procedure in the diagnostic workup of tracheal stenosis as it helps in defining the characteristic features, extent, and location of the stenosis. Performing a fiberoptic bronchoscopy in an awake patient allows the physician to examine vocal cord function to determine if recurrent laryngeal nerve damage is present; it also allows for the evaluation of dynamic airway collapse with respiration. When used together, bronchoscopy and CT helps in extremely accurate preoperative planning and good prediction of postoperative outcome.[15] The findings of bronchoscopy in various conditions associated with LTS are enumerated in Table 2.

TREATMENT OPTIONS

There is no definitive medical therapy to treat the disease process found in LTS. Underlying infectious and inflammatory cause should be treated. Aggressive

Table 2: Bronchoscopy findings in conditions associated with laryngotracheal stenosis (LTS)	
Conditions causing LTS	Bronchoscopy findings
Post intubation Stenosis	Circumferential luminal narrowing Thin membrane that extends into the lumen Long segment of eccentric soft tissue thickening
Tuberculosis	Granulation tissue with friable and ulcerated mucosa Raised, cobblestoned appearance of the mucosa
Wegener granulomatosis	Inflammatory ulcers, plaques, or granulomatous tissues
Amyloidosis	Thickened tracheal segments corresponding to areas of amyloid deposits

treatment of gastroesophageal reflux disease is mandatory for ensuring good surgical results as well as to minimize the rate of restenosis that can occur following surgical repair. The only definitive therapy for LTS is surgical correction.

Surgical Management

Milder forms of LTS are managed by endoscopic procedures (dilatation and/or use of a carbon dioxide laser). Moderate to severe forms of LTS require surgical reconstruction. The main procedures for surgical reconstruction are the anterior cricoid split, single-stage or multistage laryngotracheal reconstruction, or cricotracheal resection; of these the most commonly performed are laryngotracheal reconstruction and cricotracheal resection. The goal and measure of success of surgical procedures is the decannulation rate. Laryngotracheal reconstruction (LTR) is chosen for grade 2 and less severe grade 3 stenosis, while cricotracheal resection is typically the preferred surgical option for patients with severe grade 3 or grade 4 stenosis. Laryngotracheal reconstruction has the advantage of being less invasive. The decannulation rates are similar in patients with severe forms of LTS (severe grade 3 and grade 4) with both the techniques. But even then, cricotracheal resection is preferred in these patients since comparatively more patients treated with LTR require a second surgery to achieve decannulation.

Use of Stents

Stents are used to maintain airway patency in patients prior to surgery or chemoradiation, and as palliation in patients who have failed endoscopic management and are medically unsuitable for open procedures or therapeutic endoscopies. They are also used in patients with benign lesions but extensive strictures. Stenosis that are more than 4 cm in length are commonly associated with postoperative anastomotic leaks and in patients with trachea destroyed by multiple reconstruction attempts.[16] Sometimes they are used as an adjunct to surgery to stabilize the newly anastomosed trachea. Stents commonly used are made up of either silicone or metal. Silicone stents are associated with the problem of stent migration and elimination of mucociliary clearance. The greatest disadvantage of metal stents is build-up of granulation tissue at the edge of these stents and the incidence reported is as high as 18%.[17] The average functional life of metal stents is around 12 months.[18]

Because of the formation of granulation tissue, metallic stents are ideally used in cases of malignant strictures, and silicone stents are reserved for use in the treatment of benign strictures. All stents can be inserted and removed endoscopically. This can be done by using topical anesthesia and sedation or under general anesthesia.

The various treatment options in patients with LTS are enumerated in Table 3. In general, the strictures that are less than 2–3 cm in length can be treated endoscopically, and strictures that are more than 2–3 cm are generally treated surgically.

The surgical approach and position of the patient during surgery depends on the site of stenosis as detailed in Table 4.

ANESTHETIC MANAGEMENT

We as anesthesiologists are called for our services during endoscopic procedures like stent placement, laser dilatation and for corrective reconstruction procedures. The choice of anesthesia will differ depending on the procedure and surgical technique. Endoscopic procedures (balloon dilatation, laser) and stenting are more commonly done as compared to major surgical reconstructions. The anesthetic management for surgical reconstruction is discussed separately.

Anesthesia for Dilatation, Laser Therapy and Stent Placement

Initial bronchoscopy can be possible with the use of local anesthetics. Sedation can be provided without airway compromise using dexmedetomidine and/or ketamine. Dilatation or laser therapy and stent placement needs to be done under general anesthesia.

Premedication

Sedative premedication should be avoided as far as possible and should be used only for very anxious patients because of the danger of hypoventilation and

Table 3: Treatment modalities in patients with laryngotracheal stenosis[19,20,21]	
Procedure	Patient criteria
Endoscopic treatment	<ul><li>No external compression, tracheomalacia or significant collapse</li><li>Grade I and II stenosis</li><li>Length of stenosis less than 2–3 cm</li><li>Identifiable airway lumen</li><li>If tracheostomy present, the entry should not be adjacent to the site of stenosis</li></ul>
Stenting	<ul><li>Failed endoscopic management</li><li>Medically unsuitable for open procedures</li><li>Have 5–8 mm length of "normal" airway below vocal folds</li></ul>
Surgical options	<ul><li>Grade III and IV stenosis</li><li>Failure of endoscopic and/or stent treatments</li><li>No identifiable lumen</li><li>Length greater than 3 cm</li><li>Tracheomalacia</li></ul>

Table 4: Surgical approach and position [22-24]

Location	Approach	Position
High and mid tracheal lesion	Collar incision with/without an upper sternotomy	Supine with arms by the side and neck in full extension
Low tracheal lesion	Right posterolateral thoracotomy	Supine with arms by the side and neck in full extension or Left lateral decubitus position with neck flexed
Carinal lesions	Right posterolateral thoracotomy or bilateral submammary trans-sternal thoracotomy for extensive carinal involvement	Left lateral decubitus position with neck flexed

further airway obstruction. An antisialagogue (glycopyrrolate) may be given to decrease excessive airway secretions.

Preoxygenation

A partially obstructing lesion can completely obstruct the airway under anesthesia or sometimes by a bronchoscope entering the stenotic area. Therefore, it is imperative to preoxygenate the patient before starting the procedure. Because of altered airflow, preoxygenation will take longer time than usual.

Induction and Intubation

Induction of anesthesia needs to be tailored to the patients' lesions and their medical history. Both intravenous and inhalational induction may be used, though most centers use intravenous drugs for induction and maintenance (TIVA). Propofol and fentanyl are commonly used though, if available, remifentanyl is the ideal opioid to be used. It is recommended to avoid neuromuscular blockade and maintain a patient ventilating spontaneously till the airway is secured. Once the airway is secured, then atracurium or vecuronium are used.

The location of stenosis and its extent are the most important determinant about the options of continuing with spontaneous or controlled ventilation and placing a laryngeal mask airways (LMA) or an endotracheal tube (ETT). Subglottic stenosis just below the vocal cords may cause difficulty in placement of the endotracheal tube. In these cases, awake sedated bronchoscopy leading to control of the airway is recommended.

In proximal lesions, LMAs can be placed to allow ventilation, oxygenation and access for fiberoptic bronchoscopy. In mid-tracheal lesions, it is possible to place the ETT slightly proximal to the stenosis. After placement of ETT, jet ventilation can then be performed from above the stenosis. It is imperative to mention here that jet ventilation across the stenosis can be associated with stacking of the gases. The gradual decrease in blood pressure after starting of the positive pressure ventilation, with the associated decrease in the saturation of the patient should raise the doubt of air stacking in addition to the differential diagnosis of tension pneumothorax or myocardial infarction intraoperatively as well as 6–8 hours postoperatively.

Maintenance of Anesthesia

Anesthesia for stent positioning can be maintained using inhalational agents like sevoflurane but is more commonly maintained using total intravenous anesthesia using short-acting agents like propofol and remifentanil or fentanyl. Intravenous agents can deepen the plane of anesthesia during the periods of suctioning, airway dilatation, and stenting when ventilation is interrupted. Patients may be ventilated with intermittent positive pressure ventilation, jet ventilation, or high-frequency ventilation.

It needs to be stressed that before any laser or cautery use in the airway, typical safety precautions need to occur. These include lowering the FiO_2 to below 30% and ensuring that the endotracheal tube (ETT) or other combustible materials are away from the laser and also wearing of laser protective glasses.

Extubation

Regardless of the type of anesthetic agent used during a case, the trachea must be extubated at the end of the procedure, once the patient is fully awake with intact airway reflexes.

Anesthesia for Tracheal Resection/Reconstruction

Like most airway surgeries, anesthesia for tracheal reconstruction surgery requires planning and collaboration between the surgeon and the anesthesiologist, since the airway is "shared". Appropriate equipment such as multiple sizes of endotracheal tubes (ETT) or emergency tracheotomy kits should be readily available, even if the initial airway examination was reassuring. The anesthetic intraoperative course for open surgical correction of this disease can be divided into five phases.[25]

1. Induction and intubation
2. Surgical dissection
3. Open airway
4. Surgical closure
5. Emergence and extubation.

The most challenging phases for the anesthesiologist are induction and intubation; open airway, and the emergence and extubation phases.

Premedication and Anxiolysis

The premedication should be approached in the same way as that for stent placements. Preoperative medications to limit or prevent gastroesophageal reflux may be given. However, the use of benzodiazepines or opiates is controversial, which are best avoided. In most cases, a calm and caring demeanour, together with a clear and confident anesthetic and surgical plan relayed to the patient, are usually sufficient to allay any anxiety.

IV Access and Monitoring

Two peripheral intravenous (IV) lines (one in each lower extremity, since both the upper extremities are tucked and inaccessible) are usually enough. Central venous access is not necessary in most cases. Monitoring includes standard ASA monitors (ECG, SpO_2, blood pressure, temperature and capnography). A left radial arterial line should be used to monitor blood pressure and for intraoperative blood gas analysis. In these patients the innominate artery may get compressed during surgery, thereby making pressure readings in the right arm inaccurate. Similarly, the pulse oximeter should be placed on the right hand to alert to the presence of innominate artery compression. A warming blanket, nasogastric tube and a urinary catheter are also used additionally.

Induction and Intubation

One of the main challenges during induction is establishing an airway in the presence of stenosis, with the possibility of a total airway occlusion. This may be further compounded by the inability to use the usual options like transtracheal ventilation, tracheostomy, or other surgical airways, which we use in a usual difficult airway scenario because of the pathology found in laryngotracheal stenosis. One must be cautious since these patients may be breathing comfortably when awake, and can have collapsed airway after induction. Therefore, an otolaryngologist should be present during induction along with his armamentarium, prepared to take a surgical airway if required.

Both inhalational and intravenous induction may be chosen. The advantages of an inhalational induction are preservation of spontaneous ventilation and maintaining a patent airway. Sevoflurane is ideal for inhalational induction. One must be prepared for longer onset because of prolonged passage due to airway stenosis. For airway manipulation a MAC of at least 1.1 to 1.3 may be desired and this may cause hypotension.

Intravenous induction with propofol is the more commonly used technique. Propofol provides ideal conditions for laryngoscopy and intubation but has the potential to abolish spontaneous ventilation, which may cause total airway obstruction. However, it has the advantage of rapid onset and ease of titration, so that it can be used along with a short acting opioid like remifentanyl to give total intravenous anesthesia (TIVA).

In most of the patients, laryngoscopy and intubation with a reinforced tube is possible. Depending upon the location of the lesion, an ETT can be placed above the lesion or through the lesion with a small ETT if a proximal lesion is present. Great care should be exercised during intubation as tissue dislodgement, bleeding, and edema can quickly occur. Awake intubation with regionally blocked airway can be one alternate technique in case of a difficult airway scenario and if the patient is cooperative.

In certain extreme cases where the lesion is mobile and airway can collapse at the time of induction, it is prudent to take up the patient for a tracheostomy prior to taking up for reconstructive surgery.[26,27] Irrespective of the choice of induction, it is always safe to secure the airway before giving a muscle relaxant. Once a secure airway is established, maintenance of anesthesia can be done with sevoflurane and an intermediate-acting muscle relaxant, or by TIVA. If available, then remifentanyl is the ideal opioid that should be used. Otherwise fentanyl can also be used.

Ventilating the Open Airway

Besides induction, the other challenge that the anesthesiology team encounters is ventilation through an open airway. It is important to discuss the plan with the surgeon before the induction of anesthesia. Gas exchange during this portion is challenging and can be performed in one of four ways discussed further.

a. **Jet ventilation:** The jet ventilation catheter is inserted through the ETT and passed into the distal trachea. The advantages of this technique are that it is a simple procedure providing a surgical field unobstructed by the ETT and adequate control of gas exchange. However, it has a potential to cause barotrauma and hypercarbia due to hypoventilation.
b. **Distal tracheal intubation and intermittent positive pressure ventilation (IPPV):** This technique is probably the most common method of ventilation during the open airway phase of the surgery. Here, the ETT is pulled back above the lesion (if not already in that location), and a new ETT is inserted into the distal trachea by the surgeon (Fig. 1). The tip of this tube lies in the trachea in high and mid-tracheal lesions. In low tracheal or carinal lesions the tip is placed in either main stem bronchus followed by single lung ventilation. The trachea is again intubated prior to anastomosis by the surgeon either by pulling the proximal ETT or by inserting new one into the trachea past the anastomotic site.
c. **Spontaneous ventilation:** There are few case reports where the patients are allowed to breathe spontaneously throughout the surgery, with oxygen flowing through the endotracheal tube or through a catheter passed through the stoma.[28]
d. **Cardiopulmonary bypass:** Cardiopulmonary bypass (CPB) and percutaneous extracorporeal membrane oxygenation (ECMO) has allowed for safe management of patients at risk of total airway obstruction while simultaneously permitting surgical repair of lesions previously considered unresectable. They allow gas exchange while completely bypassing the stenotic lesion.[29]

Extubation and Associated Issues

Prompt extubation at the conclusion of the procedure is the preferred goal since mechanical ventilation has the potential for disrupting the anastomosis. The process of extubation and emergence has to be very smooth. The neuromuscular blocking agent needs to be reversed and confirmed with a nerve stimulator.

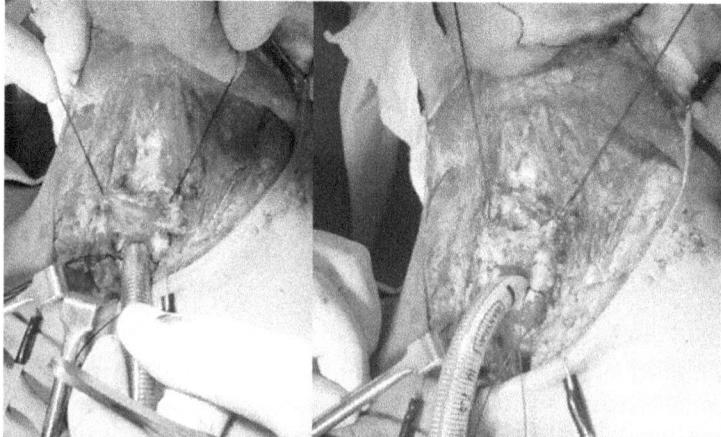

Fig. 1: Endotracheal tube placed in distal trachea by the surgeon.

If TIVA is used, it can be stopped a few minutes prior to emergence and be replaced with nitrous oxide to allow for a predictable, rapid, and controlled emergence at the appropriate time. Similarly, the volatile agent should be stopped. Nitrous oxide should be stopped only after confirming adequate reversal of the neuromuscular agent. Small doses of opioids may be given about 15 minutes before the end to optimize the analgesia and post operative pain, and antiemetics should be administered in the last 30 minutes to prevent postoperative nausea and vomiting.

Certain patients may require elective postoperative mechanical ventilation because of concerns of airway edema or the need for continued ventilator support. This can be achieved by using a small endotracheal tube, tracheostomy tube, or a T-tube. In most cases a tracheostomy tube is connected to a T-tube and humidified oxygen is provided. Even if we go for elective ventilation because of some reason, the plan should be early extubation. A chin stitch is taken to keep the neck in flexion during closure. It is important to maintain this position during emergence and it always helps if the patient has been educated about this preoperatively. One must test for the presence of an air leak to ascertain absence of significant airway edema, before extubating the trachea. Nebulization with racemic adrenaline may be done if airway edema is suspected.

Postoperative Management

The patient must be kept under strict supervision in the intensive care unit (ICU) or the high dependency unit (HDU) since the immediate postoperative period is such a perilous time in terms of airway compromise for these patients. The head end should be propped up at 30° and the neck flexion should be maintained (either with the help of the chin stitch or by using custom made orthopedic corsets). Regardless of the presentation to the ICU, all of these patients are administered humidified oxygen in an attempt to minimize the risk of anastomotic disruption. The pattern and effort of breathing should be constantly assessed to detect problems with the reconstructed airway. Clinical evaluation is supplemented with periodic arterial blood gases (ABGs). The patient may have frequent secretions that need to be addressed by aggressive pulmonary toilet. Adequate analgesia is imperative and to achieve this, a combination of intermittent intravenous paracetamol and fentanyl infusion at a rate of 0.5–1.0 µg/kg/h may be given.

REGIONAL ANESTHESIA FOR LARYNGOTRACHEAL STENOSIS SURGERY

Some centers advocate the use of regional anesthesia for surgery in patients with LTS. It is a combination of local/topical anesthesia along with cervical epidural catheter and sedation. The epidural in these patients allows the patient to breath spontaneously throughout the case, be awake and also provide analgesia after surgery. In a prospective feasibility study, 20 patients with subglottic or upper trachea stenosis were operated upon under a combined neuraxial and local anesthetic technique. All patients tolerated the procedure, with excellent or good functional outcome. In these patients, a cervical epidural catheter was placed at C7-T1 level and sedation was provided with propofol and remifentanil infusion.[30]

CONCLUSION

The perioperative management of patients with laryngotracheal stenosis requires close collaboration and communication between anesthesiologists, surgeons and the nursing staff. A well-structured, coordinated plan is the key to successful management of these patients. These patients are at particularly high-risk of catastrophic events during induction and prior to the establishment of a definitive airway. Advances in techniques, both surgical and anesthetic in recent years make this procedure relatively safe and worthwhile in carefully selected and appropriate patients. The main goals for the anesthesia provider during these cases should be having a variety of options for gaining and maintaining control of the airway, providing adequate anesthesia while maximizing surgical field exposure, and being able to extubate the patient at the end of the procedure.

REFERENCES

1. Miller R, Murugu S. Evaluation and classification of laryngotracheal stenosis. RAMR. 2014;4:344-7.
2. Hartley BEJ, Cotton RT. Pediatric airway stenosis: laryngotracheal reconstruction or cricotracheal resection? Clin Otolaryngol. 2000;25:342-9.
3. Grillo HC, Donahue DM. Postintubation tracheal stenosis. Semin Thorac Cardiovasc Surg. 1996;8:370-80.
4. CosanoPovedano A, Muñoz Cabrera L, CosanoPovedano FJ, et al. Endoscopic treatment of central airway stenosis: five years' experience. Arch Bronconeumol. 2005;41(6):322-7.
5. Freitag L, Ernst A, Unger M, et al. A proposed classification system of central airway stenosis. The European respiratory journal. 2007;30:7-12.
6. McCaffrey TV. Classification of laryngotracheal stenosis. The Laryngoscope. 1992;102:1335-40.
7. Grundfast KM, Morris MS, Bernsley C. Subglottic stenosis: retrospective analysis and proposal for standard reporting system. The Annals of otology, rhinology, and laryngology. 1987;96:101-5.
8. Lano C, Duncavage JA, Reinisch L, et al. Laryngotracheal reconstruction in the adult: a ten year experience. The Annals of otology, rhinology, and laryngology. 1998;107:92-7.
9. Nouraei S, Nouraei S, Upile T, et al. A proposed system for documenting the functional outcome of adult laryngotracheal stenosis. Clinical Otolaryngology. 2007;32:407-9.
10. Pinsonneault C, Fortier J, Donati F. Tracheal resection and reconstruction. Can J Anaesth. 1999;46:439-55.
11. Miller RD, Hyatt R. Evaluation of obstructing lesions of the trachea and larynx by flow-volume loops. The American review of respiratory disease. 1973;108:475-81.
12. Gomez-Caro A, Morcillo A, Wins R, et al. Surgical management of benign tracheal stenosis. Multimed Man Cardiothorac Surg. 2011;2011 (1111):mmcts.2010.004945.
13. Berry MF; Friedberg JS. Techniques of Tracheal Resection. In: Sugarbaker DJ (ed). Adult Chest Surgery Textbook (2nd ed). New York: McGraw Hill; 2014;57:460-8.
14. Chiu PPL, Kim PCW, Forte V, et al. The airway Reconstruction Team. Recent challenges in the management of congenital tracheal stenosis : an individualized approach. Journal of Pediatric Surgery. 2005;40:774-80.
15. Rangananath N, Arathi BHR, Ramamani PV, et al. Anaesthetic considerations for tracheal resection in oncological thyroid surgeries. Indian J Anaesth. 2015;59(3):188-90.

16. Wright CD, Grillo HC, Wain JC, et al. Anastomotic complications after tracheal resection: Prognostic factors and management. The Journal of thoracic and cardiovascular surgery. 2004;128:731-9.
17. Walser EM. Stent placement for tracheobronchial disease. Eur J Rad. 2005;55:321-30.
18. Eller RL, Livingston WJ, Morgan CE, et al. Expandable tracheal stenting for benign disease: worth the complications. Ann Otol Rhinol Laryngol. 2006;115(4):247-52.
19. Rosen CA. Glottic and Subglottic stenosis: Evaluation and surgical planning. In: Simpson B, Rosen CA (eds). Operative Techniques in Laryngology. Springer, Berlin, Heidelberg. 2008;(Chapter 6):37-42
20. McCaffrey TV. Management of subglottic stenosis in the adult. Ann Otol Rhinol Laryngol. 1991;100:90-4.
21. Gardner GM, Courey MS, Ossoff RH. Operative evaluation of airway obstruction. Otolaryngol Clin North Am 1995;28:737-50.
22. Ossoff RH, Courey MS, Netterville JL. Laryngotracheal reconstruction in the adult: a ten-year experience. Ann Otol Rhino laryngol. 1998;107:92-7.
23. Pinsonneault C, Fortier J, Donati F. Tracheal resection and reconstruction. Can J Anesth. 1999;46(5 Pt 1):439-55.
24. Marks R, Tanner L, Wenlender B. Management of a tumour in the distal trachea while maintaining spontaneous ventilation. J Anesth. 2010;24:932-4.
25. Sandberg W. Anesthesia and airway management for tracheal resection and reconstruction. Int Anesthesiol Clin. 2000;38(1):55-75.
26. Mentzelopoulos SD, Romana CN, Hatzimichalis AG, et al. Anaesthesia for tracheal resection: a new technique of airway management in a patient with severe stenosis of the mid-trachea. Anesth Analg. 1999;89(5):1156-60.
27. Sandberg W. Anaesthesia and airway management for tracheal resection and reconstruction. International Anesthesiology Clinics. 2000;38(1):55-75.
28. Eller RL, Livingston WJ 3rd, Morgan CE, et al. Expandable tracheal stenting for benign disease: worth the complications. Ann Otol Rhinol Laryngol. 2006;115(4):247-52.
29. Chiu CL, Teh BT, Wang CY. Temporary cardiopulmonary bypass and isolated lung ventilation for tracheal stenosis and reconstruction. Br J Anaesth. 2003;91(5):742.
30. Macchiarini P, Rovira I, Ferrarello S. Awake upper airway surgery. Ann Thorac Surg. 2010;89:387-91.

CHAPTER 18

Perioperative Fibrinogen Supplementation: Safety and Efficacy

Anju Grewal, Nidhi Bhatia

KEY POINTS

- Fibrinogen is one of the critical proteins required for clot formation, as it provides a lattice essential for increasing the strength of the clot.
- In cases of major blood loss, fibrinogen reaches a critical value much earlier as compared to other procoagulatory factors or platelets.
- Fibrinogen levels < 150–200 mg/dL are often associated with increased tendency of perioperative bleeding.
- For controlling bleeding in the perioperative and trauma settings, recent European trauma guidelines recommend administration of fibrinogen concentrates when significant bleeding is accompanied by a plasma fibrinogen level of < 1.5–2.0 g/L or when thromboelastic signs or functional fibrinogen deficiency is observed.
- The therapeutic options that are available for repleting the decreased plasma fibrinogen levels are fresh frozen plasma (FFP), cryoprecipitate and fibrinogen concentrate. The safety, efficacy and infusion speed of all of these options are significantly variable

INTRODUCTION

Fibrinogen, a coagulation factor present in blood in greatest amounts, plays a main role in hemostasis.[1] It is a plasma glycoprotein synthesized by the liver, and a substrate for thrombin, plasmin and factor XIIIa, with a half-life of 3 to 5 days. Fibrinogen is one of the critical proteins required for clot formation, as it provides a lattice essential for increasing the strength of the clot.[2] Following injury, clot is formed and stabilized by genesis of fibrin from fibrinogen; and this conversion is catalyzed by thrombin. Soluble fibrin monomers create a net which entraps red blood cells to form a clot. Further the clot strength is improved by cross-linking fibrin polymers with factor XIIIa. In addition to this fibrinogen also binds to the platelet fibrinogen receptor, glycoprotein GPIIb/IIIa, which results in activation of platelets and its aggregation. Thus, fibrinogen is a critical component and substrate for clot formation, amplification and strength.[2-4]

Fibrinogen is important for the entire process of coagulation, and is being considered to be one of the main targets to achieve hemostasis during excessive perioperative bleeding.[5] Failure to control blood loss initiates a vicious cycle, with subsequent development of coagulopathy.[6] In order to limit excessive perioperative blood loss, it is important to maintain plasma fibrinogen concentration within normal limits.[7]

CRITICAL THRESHOLD VALUE OF FIBRINOGEN

In cases of major blood loss, fibrinogen reaches a critical value much earlier as compared to other procoagulatory factors or platelets. But the critical threshold value for fibrinogen, known to have a protective effect on the amount of blood loss, is still debatable. Though a threshold of 100 mg/dL is often recommended, fibrinogen levels < 150-200 mg/dL are often associated with increased tendency of perioperative bleeding.[8] Hypofibrinogenemia is defined as decrease in fibrinogen levels, with levels being between 0.5 g/L and 1.5 g/L (plasma fibrinogen levels of 1.5-4.5 g/L are considered normal).

WHEN DO WE NEED FIBRINOGEN REPLACEMENT THERAPY?

Current recommendations for fibrinogen supplementation include administering fibrinogen as a prophylactic measure as well as for treatment of hemorrhage in cases of acquired and congenital fibrinogen deficiency. Several studies observed higher pre- and postoperative fibrinogen concentrations to be associated with lower bleeding volumes.[2,4,5] Acquired fibrinogen deficiency is associated with massive blood loss, disseminated intravascular coagulation (DIC) and liver failure. Following massive blood loss, hypofibrinogenemia can occur due to hemodilution from volume replacement and due to DIC. Infusion of fibrinogen concentrate has a propensity to decrease postoperative bleeding volumes and transfusion requirements.[2,4,5,9,10]

DIAGNOSING FIBRINOGEN DEFICIENCY

Plasma fibrinogen concentrations can be measured using functional assays that determine clot formation using either spectroscopic or viscoelastic clot detection.[2] Thromboelastography (TEG) and thromboelastometry (ROTEM) are the viscoelastic point-of-care tests that can be used in the perioperative settings to determine functional fibrinogen levels.[2,11,12] In clinical practice, these tests simplify and improve coagulation point of care monitoring and management.

TARGET FIBRINOGEN LEVELS FOR REPLETION

In cases of congenital fibrinogen deficiencies, plasma fibrinogen levels of approximately 0.5-1.0 g/L are critical, as below this level patients are prone to develop profuse bleeding. However, this level is too low in perioperative settings. For controlling bleeding in the perioperative and trauma settings, recent European trauma guidelines recommended to administer fibrinogen concentrates when significant bleeding is accompanied by a plasma fibrinogen level of < 1.5-2.0 g/L or when thromboelastic signs or functional fibrinogen deficiency is observed.[2,10] In case of bleeding significant enough to require transfusion, fibrinogen concentrate (or cryoprecipitate) should be administered when the FIBTEM analysis (ROTEM device), detects the maximum clot firmness (MCF) below 10-12 mm or less than 7 mm at 10 minutes or both. In cases of non-availability of ROTEM monitoring, it is important to maintain plasma fibrinogen levels at 1.5-2.0 g/L.[8] It also needs to be emphasized that during severe bleeding, acquired hypofibrinogenemia may be associated with low plasma concentrations of all coagulation factors (not only fibrinogen) and inhibitors and so treatment with blood products containing coagulation factors should be considered (with or without administration of fibrinogen concentrate), with careful monitoring of the coagulation system.[10] In settings such as pregnancy, we may need to consider different therapeutic thresholds. In peripartum patients, fibrinogen levels increase to 5-6 g/L, and levels <2.0 g/L are considered to be greatly indicative of the risk of postpartum hemorrhage.[13,14]

FIBRINOGEN DOSING

Fibrinogen can be dosed based on bleeding levels and plasma fibrinogen concentration.[2] Fibrinogen therapy can also be guided by maximum clot firmness (MCF) values. Normal MCF values of 9-25 mm correlate with normal fibrinogen levels. Fibrinogen concentrates in a dose of 25-50 mg/kg or cryoprecipitate 8-10 units should be administered if MCF values are <6-8 mm at 10 minutes. The dose of fibrinogen concentrate to be administered can be calculated using the following formula:

Fibrinogen concentrates (g) = [Target MCF (mm) − Actual MCF (mm)] × [Body weight (kg)/70] × 0.5 g/mm.[2]

PRODUCTS USED TO REPLETE FIBRINOGEN LEVELS

In present times, the therapeutic options that are available for repleting the decreased plasma fibrinogen levels are fresh frozen plasma (FFP), cryoprecipitate and fibrinogen concentrate.[2,7,15] The safety, efficacy and infusion speed of all of these options are significantly variable.[15]

Fresh Frozen Plasma

Fresh frozen plasma (FFP), an allogenic blood product, is a fibrinogen source most widely available. It contains all the clotting factors as well as many other proteins, including all the constituents of human plasma.[2] Prior to its administration, FFP needs to undergo both AB compatibility testing and also needs to be thawed, as it is stored at −20°C. Different plasma preparations are available, including single donor FFP, plasma that is frozen within 24 hours of collection, and thawed plasma (to be used within 5 days of initial thaw).[2,7] These products are however not ideal sources of fibrinogen, as their fibrinogen concentrations vary from 1 to 3 g/L. The average fibrinogen concentration in FFP is approximately 2.5 g/L, which is marginally above the likely target concentration of 2 g/L. 12.2 mL/kg of FFP is known to increase plasma fibrinogen levels by only 0.4 g/L, whereas 33.5 mL/kg increases levels by 1.0 g/L. As fibrinogen concentration in FFP is low, large volumes are required for effective supplementation. Hence, infusion volumes required to achieve target fibrinogen levels are high, with the transfusion being slow. This results in extending the time required for infusion, with increased risk of volume overload. Further, as the concentration of coagulation factors in single-donor FFP is highly variable, its precise dosing is difficult. As FFP is also not virally inactivated, its use maybe associated with increased possibility of viral transmission. Other potential complications associated with its administration include immunological and allergic reactions and the risk of transfusion related acute lung injury (TRALI). Overall, the risk of circulatory overload and inability to optimally replete fibrinogen levels precludes FFP as an effective therapy for fibrinogen supplementation.[2,7,15]

Cryoprecipitate

Cryoprecipitate contains fibrinogen, factors VIII, XIII and Von Willebrand factor. Just like FFP, cryoprecipitate is also an allogenic product that needs to be cross-matched and thawed prior to its administration. It is obtained by thawing FFP at 1°C to 6°C centrifugation, and resuspending the precipitated proteins in a small volume of plasma (10–20 mL) and refreezing at –20°C.[2,4,7] As compared to FFP, the concentration of fibrinogen is higher in cryoprecipitate, typically around 15 g/L. However, similar to FFP, administration of cryoprecipitate is also associated with some disadvantages, including increased risk of viral transmission, variable fibrinogen concentration, time needed for thawing and requirement for blood group matching. Usually 4 to 6 units of cryoprecipitate needs to be administered. Approximately 29 units (140 mg/unit) are required (375 mL volume) to provide 4 g of fibrinogen. Although this decreases the fibrinogen concentration variability, but it also raises safety concerns due to exposure to 4 to 6 donors per transfusion. Further, though cryoprecipitate is widely used, evidence for its use is limited. Guidelines suggest that in cases of bleeding associated with low fibrinogen levels, use of cryoprecipitate should be avoided if specific factor concentrates are available.[2,4,7,15,16]

Fibrinogen Concentrates

Fibrinogen concentrate is a human-derived product, produced from pooled human plasma and does not contain relevant levels of other coagulation factors.[2,4] It is available as pasteurized, lyophilized product from pooled donors that undergo purification, viral inactivation, and do not require cross-matching. Fibrinogen concentrate is being increasingly used for treatment of both congenital and acquired fibrinogen deficiency. It is standardized and stored as lyophilized powder at room temperature. As it can be reconstituted in small volumes using sterile water, fibrinogen concentrates can be given rapidly without having to wait for thawing.[2,4,7,15] As compared to FFP or cryoprecipitate, the concentration of fibrinogen in fibrinogen concentrate (1 g/50 mL) is more consistent and it is known to increase plasma fibrinogen concentration in a dose-dependent manner. Approximately 4 units of fibrinogen concentrate (200 mL volume) are required to provide 4 g of fibrinogen. In addition to having a great deal of accuracy and consistency with regards to the doses that need to be given, as well as low infusion volumes needed, fibrinogen concentrate administration is associated with a very low-risk of viral transmission and no significant increase in thrombotic events. Further, antigens and antibodies are removed by additional purification, thus significantly decreasing the risk of allergic and immunological reactions.[2,4,7,15,17-19]

Efficacy of Fibrinogen Concentrates

Its administration is known to improve clot quality and attenuate bleeding. Numerous studies have shown that fibrinogen concentrates significantly improve coagulation in patients with acquired hypofibrinogenemia, such as in cases of traumatic bleeding, obstetric hemorrhage and cardiothoracic surgery. Fibrinogen concentrate can also be administered in patients with known thrombocytopenia; as it increases both the fibrinogen mediated platelet aggregation and the density of fibrin network.[6,10] The optimal level of plasma fibrinogen at which fibrinogen concentrate should be given is currently debatable. The 2015 American practice guidelines for perioperative blood management considered fibrinogen concentrate to be among other pharmacologic treatments used for excessive bleeding in the case of hypofibrinogenemia. But these guidelines failed to specify the plasma fibrinogen concentration that defines hypofibrinogenemia. The European Society of Anesthesiology guidelines for the management of severe perioperative bleeding recommend fibrinogen concentrate substitution if significant bleeding is associated with a suspected low fibrinogen concentration or function. It defines plasma fibrinogen concentration of <1.5–2.0 g/L as a trigger for fibrinogen substitution. However, it is important to keep in mind the fact that during perioperative bleeding the coagulation alterations are complex and multifactorial, and fibrinogen concentrates may not be efficacious in every case. Hence, its use must always be guided by point of care investigations.[6,10,15]

Safety of Fibrinogen Concentrates

Recent reports in literature have shown that administration of fibrinogen concentrate (median dose of 2 g), aiming at plasma fibrinogen levels of 2 g/L, is not associated with an increase in thromboembolic and cardiac events, while at the same time reducing mortality. The reasons for lack of increased thromboembolic risks following fibrinogen administration could be multifactorial:[5,6]

- The risk of giving an overdose of fibrinogen maybe counteracted by increased fibrinogen consumption during hemorrhage as well as by hemodilution.
- In hemodilution, fibrin clot structure is loose, less firm and more prone to undergo fibrinolysis.
- Fibrinogen assists in anticoagulant by binding thrombin and inhibiting thrombin-mediated factor V activation.

Thus, as compared to FFP and cryoprecipitate, fibrinogen concentrate is associated with numerous advantages for fibrinogen replacement therapy, i.e. consistent and accurate dosing, better safety profile and rapidity of administration. Though cryoprecipitate is cheaper than fibrinogen concentrate, the overall cost-effectiveness of both, including compatibility testing, thawing and administration, is similar.[4]

CONCLUSION

To conclude, in the perioperative period, massively bleeding patients have a high risk of developing low fibrinogen levels and abnormal fibrinogen polymerization, thus requiring fibrinogen supplementation. High circulating fibrinogen is known to exert a protective effect with regards to limiting blood loss. Current evidence suggests that in cases of massive perioperative bleeding, effective fibrinogen supplementation can significantly help in decreasing blood loss, reducing the need for transfusion of other blood components, thus restoring the normal coagulation status and reducing mortality. Of the available sources of fibrinogen (FFP, cryoprecipitate, fibrinogen concentrate), replacement with fibrinogen concentrate is highly safe and efficacious. Further, perioperative bleeding can be better managed by clarifying the fibrinogen levels at which therapy should be initiated and by using reliable tests for monitoring fibrinogen levels.

REFERENCES

1. Levy JH, Szlam F, Tanaka KA, et al. Fibrinogen and hemostasis: a primary hemostatic target for the management of acquired bleeding. Anesth Analg. 2012;114:261-74.
2. Levy JH, Goodnough LT. How I use fibrinogen replacement therapy in acquired bleeding? Blood. 2015;125:1387-93.
3. Weisel JW. Fibrinogen and fibrin. Adv Protein Chem. 2005;70:247-99.
4. Franchini M, Lippi G. Fibrinogen replacement therapy: A critical review of the literature. Blood Transfus. 2012;10:23-7.
5. Fassl J, Buse GL, Filipovic M, et al. Perioperative administration of fibrinogen does not increase adverse cardiac and thromboembolic events after cardiac surgery. Br J Anaesth. 2015;114:225-34.
6. Fominskiy E, Nepomniashchikh VA, Lomivorotov VV, et al. Efficacy and safety of fibrinogen concentrate in surgical patients: A meta-analysis of randomized controlled trials. J Cardiothorac Vasc Anesth. 2016;30:1196-204.
7. Sorensen B, Bevan D. A critical evaluation of cryoprecipitate for replacement of fibrinogen. Br J Haemat. 2010;149:834-43.
8. Fries D, Martini WZ. Role of fibrinogen in trauma-induced coagulopathy. Br J Anaesth. 2010;105:116-21.
9. Acharya SS, Dimichele DM. Rare inherited disorders of fibrinogen. Haemophilia. 2008; 14:1151-8.
10. Kozek-Langenecker SA, Afshari A, Albaladejo P, et al. Management of severe perioperative bleeding: Guidelines from the European Society of Anaesthesiology. Eur J Anaesthesiol. 2013;30:270-382.
11. Solomon C, Baryshnikova E, Tripodi A, et al. Fibrinogen measurement in cardiac surgery with cardiopulmonary bypass: analysis of repeatability and agreement of Clauss method within and between six different laboratories. Thromb Haemost. 2014; 112:109-17.
12. Ranucci M, Solomon C. Supplementation of fibrinogen in acquired bleeding disorders: experience, evidence, guidelines, and licences. Br J Anaesth. 2012;109:135-7.
13. Hansen AT, Andreasen BH, Salvig JD, et al. Changes in fibrin D-dimer, fibrinogen, and protein S during pregnancy. Scand J Clin Lab Invest. 2011;71:173-6.
14. Charbit B, Mandelbrot L, Samain E, et al. PPH Study Group. The decrease of fibrinogen is an early predictor of the severity of postpartum hemorrhage. J Thromb Haemost. 2007;5:266-73.
15. Rahe-Meyer N, Sorensen B. Fibrinogen concentrate for management of bleeding. J Thromb Haemost. 2011;9:1-5.
16. Nascimento B, Goodnough LT, Levy JH. Cryoprecipitate therapy. Br J Anaesth. 2014; 113:922-34.
17. Meyer NR, Solomon C, Hanke A, et al. Effects of fibrinogen concentrate as first-line therapy during major aortic replacement surgery: A randomized, placebo-controlled trial. Anesthesiology. 2013;118:40-50.
18. Solomon C, Pichlmaier U, Schoechl H, et al. Recovery of fibrinogen after administration of fibrinogen concentrate to patients with severe bleeding after cardiopulmonary bypass surgery. Br J Anaesth 2010;104:555-62.
19. Nascimento B, Callum J, Tien H, et al. Fibrinogen in the initial resuscitation of severe trauma (FiiRST): A randomized feasibility trial. Br J Anaesth. 2016;117:775-82.

CHAPTER 19

Pain, Agitation and Delirium in Adult Intensive Care Unit

SP Ambesh

KEY POINTS

- Pain, agitation and delirium (PAD) are the most common problems encountered in adult critically ill and mechanically ventilated patients in an Intensive care unit (ICU).
- Prolonged delirium, a manifestation of brain dysfunction, is one of the strongest independent predictors (risk factors) of mortality, morbidity, increased length of stay and cost of care in ICU. Prevention of delirium may improve the outcome.
- Pain evokes a stress response. Adequate analgesia (with opioid and adjuvants) and sedation is helpful in prevention of agitation and stress induced reactions.
- Administration of sedatives (benzodiazepines, propofol or $α_2$-adrenoceptor agonists) in ICU patients is universal in practice. However, poor safety record of sedatives and late realization of their adverse effects is a major concern.
- In order to obtain positives from the sedatives it is prudent to practice evidence and protocol-based approach in ICU. The article focuses on identification of problems of pain, agitation, sedation, and delirium through various scoring systems and their management through evidence-based clinical practice guidelines.

INTRODUCTION

Most critically ill patients in intensive care units (ICUs) are on invasive mechanical ventilation along with various intravascular monitoring lines and urinary catheter. These patients are likely to experience pain, anxiety, sleep deprivation and delirium. Many a times, ICU patients become very much agitated and risk to pull out endotracheal tube (ETT), urinary catheter or intravascular lines used for monitoring and administration of life-sustaining medications. Since long, the concept of the "ICU triad" of pain, agitation and delirium (PAD) has been recognized. However, despite appreciation of the concept of "ICU triad" and having strong epidemiologic body of knowledge about the use of certain drugs to guide the therapy, noticeable evolution still remains warranted. There may be a number of reasons for it: Firstly, most ICU patients' clinical condition remains dynamic and fluctuates rapidly that mandates frequent change in drug selection and dose adjustment according to changed clinical situations. Secondly, most ICUs use multidrug regimen (narcotics, benzodiazepines, propofol, $α_2$ adrenoreceptor agonists and antipsychotics) in an effort to provide pain relief and sedation, and each drug is administered dynamically in response to perceived target analgesia and sedation. Thirdly, there is significant variability in the quality of nursing care, medical care, and physiotherapy of a ICU patient and subsequently in analgesia and sedation practice worldwide. Finally, there is uncertainty in how best to diagnose an individual patient perceiving pain or suffering with delirium. It is now well-recognized that PAD if remain undetected and untreated for a prolonged time, is quite distressing to patients and is associated with increased length of hospital stay, morbidity and mortality.

PAIN IN ADULT ICU PATIENTS

Majority of ICU patients have pain and identify it as a great source of stress which has negative physiological as well as psychological consequences.[1] Pain is the long lasting unpleasant experience and is a leading cause of insufficient sleep in many patients. Critically ill patients may experience pain not only at rest but also related to surgical intervention, trauma, burns or cancer. Procedural pain is ubiquitous; and inadequate treatment remains a significant problem for many ICU patients. Unrelieved pain is the constant reminder of the disease and death that can preclude patients from participating in their ICU care (e.g. early mobilization and weaning from mechanical ventilation). Therefore, assessment of pain and provision of administration of analgesics is an essential component of ICU care. However, the assessment of pain in many critically ill patients is difficult as the patients may not be sufficiently interactive to give valid responses or may not be able to self-report their pain because of altered level of consciousness.

The International Association for the Study of Pain (IASP) states "the inability to communicate verbally does not negate the possibility that an individual is experiencing pain and is in need of appropriate pain-relieving treatment".[2] In such patients, the clinician must assess the pain by observing behavioral reactions of patient as surrogate measures of pain as long as their motor functions are intect.[3] A recently published study has shown that 82% (n = 75) of ICU discharged but still hospitalized patients remembered pain and discomfort due to endotracheal tube and 77% (n = 93) remembered experiencing moderate to severe pain during their stay in ICU.[4] In another study, 82% (n = 120) of cardiac surgery patients, one week after discharge from the ICU, reported pain as the most traumatic experience of their ICU stay; 38% patients, even after six months of discharge, recalled pain as the most distressing memory.[5]

Pain evokes a stress response that may have deleterious consequences for ICU patients. Due to increased level of circulating catecholamines, arterial vasoconstriction occurs which impairs tissue perfusion and tissue oxygen partial pressure.[6] Unrelieved pain also triggers catabolic hypermetabolism that may lead to hyperglycemia, lipolysis, and breakdown of muscle mass. Hypercatabolic state and hypoxemia also impair wound healing and increases the risk of wound infection. Pain also causes immunosuppression and decreases the number of cytotoxic T cells and neutrophil phagocytic activity.[7]

Assessment and Treatment of Pain in ICU Patients

Routine pain assessment and reassessment is essential for appropriate treatment. To effectively treat pain the clinician must have the ability to perform reproducible assessment of pain and must monitor patients over time to determine the adequacy of pain relief interventions. Pain being very subjective, self-report from the patient is most reliable and considered as "gold standard".

No objective pain monitor exists. A 0–10 numeric rating scale is most valid and feasible. When critically ill patient is unable to self-report his pain, the clinician must use structured, valid, reliable, and feasible tools that concentrate primarily on patient's behavior as indicator of pain.[8] Various studies have shown that implementation of behavioral pain scales improves both ICU pain management, clinical outcomes and helps in optimizing the use of analgesics and sedatives with shortened ICU stay.[9,10]

Intravenous opioids (fentanyl, morphine, remifentanil and methadone) are the primary analgesics in the management of pain in ICU patients. Nonsteroidal analgesics (Ketorolac, diclofenac, ibuprofen), local and regional anesthetics (e.g. bupivacaine, lignocaine), acetaminophen, and anticonvulsants can be used as adjunctive to reduce opioid requirements and their adverse effects. Intravenous acetaminophen in conjunction with opioids has been shown to be safe and effective. Regional or neuraxial blocks are the excellent modalities of pain relief in postsurgical patients.[11,12] Neuropathic pain is quite refractory and opioids alone are not effective in the treatment; however, it can be effectively treated with enterally administered gabapentin and carbamazepine in patients who have satisfactory gastrointestinal motility and absorption.[13,14] While selecting the opioids and other analgesics, the drug's pharmacokinetic, pharmacodynamic properties and safety profile must be considered in relation to an individual patient.

Several, complimentary and nonpharmacological methods for pain management (e.g. music therapy, massage therapy, relaxation techniques, etc.) are also quite popular as these are low cost, easy to provide, safe, opioid sparing and analgesia-enhancing. These interventions can be concomitantly used.

Statements and Clinical Practice Guidelines for Analgesia in Adult ICU[15]

Clinical practice guidelines that have been reviewed and endorsed by the American College of Chest Physicians and the American Association for Respiratory Care for treatment of pain in ICU patients are as under:[15]‡
1. Adult medical, surgical and trauma ICU patients experience pain both at rest and routine ICU care (B).
2. Women and cardiac surgery patients experience more pain (B). Procedural pain is also common in adult ICU patients (B). Therefore, it is recommended to routinely monitor pain in all adult ICU patients (+1B).
3. The behavioral pain scale (BPS) and the critical pain observation tool (CPOT) are the most valid and reliable pain scales for monitoring pain in medical, surgical or trauma (non-brain injury) patients in ICU who are not able to self-report, and in whom motor function is intact and behavior is observable (B).

(‡The quality of evidence for each statement and recommendation are ranked as high (A), moderate (B), or low/very low (C). The strength of recommendations are ranked as strong (1) or weak (2), and either in favor of (+) or against (−) an intervention. For all strong recommendations, the phrase "recommend ..." is used throughout. For all weak recommendations, the phrase "suggest ..." is used throughout. In the absence of sufficient evidence, or lack of group consensus, no recommendation (0) are made.)[15]

4. Vital signs monitoring alone for assessment of pain is not suggested (–2C). However, vital signs may be used as a cue to begin further assessment of pain in such patients (+2C).
5. Use of preemptive analgesia and/or nonpharmacological interventions (e.g. relaxation) is recommended to alleviate pain in adult ICU patients prior to chest tube removal (+1C). Administration of same therapy is also suggested for other types of invasive and potentially painful procedures (+2C).
6. Intravenous opioids are recommended as first line drug class of choice to treat non-neuropathic pain in critically ill patients (+1C).
7. The use of enteral gabapentin or carbamazepine, in addition to intravenous opioids, is recommended for the treatment of neuropathic pain (+1A).
8. Addition of non-opioid analgesics (acetaminophen, ketamine, cyclo-oxygenase inhibitors, etc.) are suggested to decrease the dose of opioids administered and their related adverse effects (+2C).
9. It is recommended to consider use of thoracic epidural anesthesia/analgesia for postoperative pain relief in patients undergoing abdominal aortic surgery (+1B). The guidelines provide no recommendation for using a lumbar epidural over parenteral opioids for postoperative analgesia for patients undergoing abdominal aortic aneurysm surgery (0, A). Thoracic epidural analgesia is suggested for patients with traumatic rib fractures (+2B).

AGITATION IN ADULT ICU PATIENTS

Most ICU patients suffer with agitation and anxiety which can adversely affect the clinical outcomes.[16,17] To counteract the agitation, sedation is commonly used. It is prudent to promptly diagnose and treat possible underlying cause of agitation (e.g. pain, delirium, hypoxemia, hypoglycemia, dehydration, hypotension, drug withdrawal, fever, etc.). Frequent reorientation, and optimization of environment must be done to maintain normal sleep. Continuous deep sedation is advocated for reasons such as the treatment of severe respiratory failure, refractory status epilepticus, intracranial hypertension, and prevention of awareness in patients treated with neuromuscular blocking agents.[18] However, sedatives should only be administered after putting the efforts to reduce anxiety, agitation and provision of adequate analgesia and optimization of the environment to maintain normal sleep pattern.

It is well-recognized now that maintaining deep sedation for a prolonged period has negative consequences while light sedation levels in ICU patients have been proven beneficial.[19,20,21] Studies have demonstrated that patients whose routine daily sedation was interrupted, received less sedatives overall and spent fewer days on mechanical ventilation and in ICU with significantly increased rate of survival.[22,23] Further, a prospective, multicenter, longitudinal cohort study has shown that the depth of sedation is independently associated with the duration of mechanical ventilation, in-hospital mortality, and rates of death within 180 days.[24] The use of lighter sedation resulted in more ventilation-free and ICU-free days[25] and did not increase the rate of short-term adverse events and long-term psychiatric outcome.[26,27,15] To guide and minimize the sedatives use various sedation scales are designed.

Sedation Scales

A number of subjective sedation scales are available to monitor depth of sedation and agitation in adult ICU patients receiving mechanical ventilation.[15]
1. Observer's Assessment of Alertness/Sedation Scale (OAA/S)
2. Ramsay Sedation Scale (Ramsay)
3. New Sheffield Sedation Scale (Scheffield)
4. Sedation Intensive Care Score (SEDIC)
5. Motor Activity Assessment Scale (MAAS)
6. Adaptation to the Intensive Care Environment (ATICE)
7. Minnesota Sedation Assessment Tool (MSAT)
8. Vancouver Interaction and Calmness Scale (VICS)
9. The Riker Sedation-Agitation Scale (SAS)[28] (Table 1)
10. The Richmond Agitation-Sedation Scale (RASS)[29] (Table 2).

Based on analysis of various properties (cumulative psychometric properties and quality of evidence inter-rater reliability, convergent or discriminant validation, providing consensus target on goal directed delivery of sedative agents, limitations of use and demonstration of feasibility of its use) SAS and RASS yielded highest psychometric scores, inter-rater reliability, and ability to discriminate different sedation levels in various clinical situations.[15] Therefore, SAS and RASS are most valid and reliable, and are presented below.

In SAS, the appropriate target of sedation score is 3 to 4 on a scale from 1 to 7. Score 4 denotes a calm, easily rousable patient who responds to commands. Below 4, lesser the score deeper the sedation; and above 4, higher the score greater the agitation.

The RASS has 10 points, ranging from −5 to +4. At a score of 0 to −2, the patient is calm and cooperative. As the score decreases towards negative the level of

Table 1: Riker sedation–agitation scale (SAS)[28]

Score	Term	Description
(Score 7)	Dangerous agitation	Trying to pull out endotracheal tube, urinary catheters, climbing over bed rail, thrashing from side to side or striking at staff
(Score 6)	Very agitated	Requiring restraint and frequent verbal reminding of limits, biting endotracheal tube
(Score 5)	Agitated	Anxious or physically agitated, calming at verbal instruction Calm, easily rousable, but follows commands
(Score 4)	Calm and cooperative	Calm, easily rousable, follows commands
(Score 3)	Sedated	Difficult to arouse but awakens to verbal stimuli or gentle shaking; follows simple commands but drifts off again
(Score 2)	Very sedated	Rouses to physical stimuli but does not communicate or follow commands, may move spontaneously
(Score 1)	Cannot be aroused	Minimal or no response to noxious stimuli, does not communicate or follow commands

Table 2: Richmond agitation-sedation scale (RASS)[29]

Score	Term	Description
+4	Combative	Overtly combative, violent, immediate danger to staff
+3	Very agitated	Pulls or removes tubes or catheters; aggressive
+2	Agitated	Frequent non-purposeful movement, fights ventilator
+1	Restless	Anxious but movements not aggressive or vigorous
0	Alert and calm	Alert and calm
−1	Drowsy	Not fully alert but has sustained awakening (eye opening or eye contact) to voice (≥10 sec)
−2	Light sedation	Briefly awakens with eye contact to voice (<10 sec)
−3	Moderate sedation	Movement or eye opening to voice but no eye contact
−4	Deep sedation	No response to voice but movement or eye opening to physical stimulation
−5	Unarousable	No response to voice or physical stimulation

sedation deepens and if the score increases towards positive, the level of agitation increases.

Guidelines for SAS Assessment

- Agitated patients are scored by their most severe degree of agitation as described.
- If patient is awake or awakens easily to voice, assign SAS of 4 (calm and appropriate, might even be napping).
- If more stimuli (e.g. shaking) is required to awaken, assign SAS of 3.
- If patient arouses to stronger physical or noxious stimuli but never awakens to the point of responding or following commands, assign SAS of 2.
- Little or no response to noxious physical stimuli represents SAS of 1.

Characteristics of SAS

- Increased differentiation for agitation and sedation compared to RASS
- Symmetric range of levels for agitation and sedation.

Guidelines for RASS Assessment

- Observe the patient
  - Patient is alert, restless, or agitated **(score 0 to +4)**
- If not alert: state patient's name and say to open eyes and look at speaker.
  - Patient awakens with sustained eye opening and eye contact **(score −1)**
  - Patient awakens with eye opening and eye contact, but not sustained **(score −2)**
  - Patient has any movement in response to voice but no eye contact **(score −3)**
- When no response to verbal stimulation or physical stimulation of patient by shaking shoulder and/or rubbing sternum
  - Patient has any movement to physical stimulation **(score −4)**
  - Patient has no response to any stimulation **(score −5)**
- If RASS is −4 or −5, then stop and reassess patient at later time.

Characteristics Common to SAS and RASS

Both SAS and RAS are useful as a screening instrument to determine eligibility for delirium assessment. They are considered the most valid and reliable sedation scales. However, using these scales it is difficult to categorize patients who are sedated but are aroused in an agitated state when stimulated (recommend scoring based on behavior when aroused). They are not suitable for patients who have significant auditory or visual impairments. Also, patients administered neuromuscular blockers are not assessable using these scales.

Statements and Clinical Practice Guidelines for ICU Sedation[15]

1. Maintaining light levels of sedation in adult ICU patients is associated with improved clinical outcomes (e.g. shorter duration of mechanical ventilation, and shorter ICU stay) (B).
2. Maintaining light levels of sedation increases the physiologic stress response, but is not associated with an increased incidence of myocardial ischemia (B).
3. Sedatives should be titrated to maintain a light rather than a deep level of sedation, unless clinically contraindicated (+1B).
4. The RASS and SAS scales, both are the most valid and reliable sedation assessment tools for measuring quality and depth of sedation in adult ICU patients (B).
5. No recommendation for the use of objective measures of brain function [e.g. auditory evoked potentials (AEPs), bispectral index (BIS), narcotrend index (NI), patient state index (PSI), or state entropy (SE)] are made as the primary method to assess depth of sedation in noncomatose nonparalyzed adult ICU patients. These monitors are inadequate substitutes for subjective sedation scoring system (−1B).
6. It is suggested that ICU patients who are ventilated and are receiving neuromuscular blocking agents, objective measures to assess brain function (e.g. AEPs, BIS, NI, PSI, or SE) be used as an adjunct to subjective sedation assessments (+2B).
7. EEG monitoring is recommended to monitor nonconvulsive seizure activity in adult ICU patients with either known or suspected seizures or to titrate electrosuppressive medication to achieve burst suppression in adult ICU patients with elevated intracranial pressure (+1A).
8. Practice analgesiafirst sedation for intubated and mechanically ventilated ICU patients (2B).
9. Sedation strategies using nonbenzodiazepines (propofol or dexmedetomidine) be preferred over benzodiazepines (midazolam or lorazepam) to improve clinical outcomes in mechanically ventilated adult ICU patients (+2B).

DELIRIUM IN ICU PATIENTS

Delirium is a major health problem in critically ill and mechanically ventilated ICU patients with an incidence varying from 16%[30] to 89%.[31] Despite a high prevalence, delirium is commonly overlooked. It is a syndrome characterized by the acute onset of cerebral dysfunction with a change or fluctuation in baseline mental status, inattention, and either disorganized thinking or an altered level of consciousness.[15] National Institute of Health (NIH) has defined delirium as "sudden severe confusion and rapid changes in brain function that occur with physical or mental illness". Four domains of delirium have been described[32]: (i) disturbance of consciousness, (ii) change in cognition, (iii) development over a short period and (iv) fluctuation. During the delirium, patients are often inattentive. However, the delirium is generally reversible that appears while recovering from a sedated or over-sedated state. Delirium, as a manifestation of acute brain dysfunction, is an important independent predictor of negative clinical outcomes in ICU patients. Magnetic resonance imaging studies of ICU patients have shown that longer the duration of delirium higher the risks of developing cerebral atrophy as well as cerebral white matter disruption.[33,34] Prolonged delirium is associated with increased mortality, length of stay in ICU, cost of care and long-term cognitive dysfunction consistent with a dementia-like state.

Two distinctive forms of delirium have been identified: the hypoactive and the hyperactive (or agitated). During hypoactive delirium the patients are inattentive, have disordered thinking and a decreased level of consciousness. There is no agitation. Pure hyperactive delirium, though rare (<2%),[35] has agitation and at times associated with violent movements of limbs. Individual patient may suffer with both the forms of delirium, intermittently. The mortality is high in patients who suffer with hypoactive delirium; however, those who survive have better functional status than hyperactive or mixed delirium.[36] Though there are no evidence that specific treatment may improve the outcome; European ICU surveys have shown that the depth of sedation frequently goes unmonitored.[37] Evidence suggests that maintaining light depth of sedation and prevention of over-sedation with its routine monitoring may have improved patients' outcomes.[38]

Identification of Delirium in Adult ICU Patients

One of the main problems in accurately addressing the delirium has been its under-recognition. Delirium may be a disease induced syndrome as a consequence of organ dysfunction in severe sepsis. Early identification of iatrogenic causes (e.g. excessive sedatives and opioids medication, prolonged immobilization, lack of natural lights, etc.) of delirium in ICU patients is very important. This will help in timely management of the pathological or iatrogenic cause and reduction in the incidence, severity, and duration of delirium. It is important to realize that a critically ill ICU patient may develop delirium due to withdrawal of various drugs/alcohol which he has been taking chronically. Abrupt discontinuation of sedatives/opiates/dexmedetomidine in ICU patient have been associated with drug withdrawal symptoms manifesting as anxiety, agitation, tremors, headaches, sweating, insomnia, hyperactive delirium, muscle cramps, myoclonus, nausea, vomiting and at times seizures.[39,40]

In routine ICU practice, diagnosis of delirium is not that easy. It requires active screening and continuous monitoring of the patient by the attending ICU nurses and the clinicians as the severity of illness can rapidly fluctuate in patients who receive multiple analgesics and sedatives. Currently, there are two most commonly used methods for identifying the delirium that otherwise frequently goes undiagnosed.[41]

Flowchart 1: Confusion assessment method for the CAM-ICU.

1. Acute change or fluctuating course of mental status:
- Is there an acute change from mental status baseline? or
- Has the patient's mental status fluctuated during the past 24 hours?

—No→ CAM-ICU negative no delirium

↓ Yes

2. Inattention:
- "Squeeze my hand when I say the letter 'A'"
Read the following sequence of letters:
S A V E A H A A R T or C A S A
B L A N C A or A B A D B A D A A Y
Errors: No squeeze with 'A' and squeeze on letter other than 'A'
- If unable to complete letters→ pictures

—0–2 errors→ CAM-ICU negative no delirium

↓ >2 errors

3. Altered level of consciousness
Current RASS level

—RASS other than zero→ CAM-ICU positive delirium present

↓ RASS = zero

4. Disorganized thinking:
1. Will a stone float on water?
2. Are there fish in the sea?
3. Does one pound weigh more than two?
4. Can you use a hammer to pound a nail?
Command: "Hold up this many finger" (Hold up 2 fingers)
"Now do the same thing with the other hand"
(Do not demonstrate)
or "Add one more finger" (If patient unable to move both arms)

—> 1 error→ (CAM-ICU positive delirium present)
—0–1 error→ CAM-ICU negative no delirium

Source: Reproduced from the chapter Sedation, Analgesia Delirium in ECMO patient; "Extracorporeal Membrane Oxygenation-Advances in Therapy; Edited by Michael S, published by INTECH (2016) under Creative Commons for free distribution and use of content.[43]

1. The confusion assessment method of the ICU (CAM-ICU)[42]
2. Intensive care delirium screening checklist (ICDSC)[30]

Both the methods require assessment of sedation scale in order to distinguish hyperactive from hypoactive delirium. The CAM-ICU (Flowchart 1) is a dichotomous assessment at a single time point. It is an excellent diagnostic tool in critically ill ICU patients as it is easy, rapid to administer and can be performed with minimal training (Table 3). Since delirium is characterized by a fluctuating course, the 'spot' nature of the CAM-ICU may miss an episode of delirium. Therefore, assessment frequency of every 4–12 hours gives better idea of patient's mental status. It can be used in patients with hearing and visual disturbances and is easily reproducible.

The ICDSC requires longer assessment period and therefore may lead to increased false positive screens for delirium. The ICDSC relies on clinical

Table 3: The confusion assessment method for ICU patients (CAM-ICU)[42]

Features and descriptions	Absent	Present
I. Acute onset or fluctuating course*		
A. Is there evidence of an acute change in mental status from the baseline?		
B. Or, did the (abnormal) behavior fluctuate during the past 24 hours, that is, tend to come and go or increase and decrease in severity as evidenced by fluctuation on RASS or the Glasgow Coma Scale		
II. Inattention†		
Did the patient have difficulty focusing attention as evidenced by a score of less than 8 correct answers on either the visual or auditory components of the attention screening examination (ASE)		
III. Disorganized thinking		
Is there evidence of disorganized or incoherent thinking as evidenced by incorrect answers to 3 or more of the 4 questions and inability to follow the commands? Questions: 1. Will a stone float on water? 2. Are there fish in the sea? 3. Does 1 pound weigh more than 2 pounds? 4. Can you use hammer to pound a nail? Commands: 1. Are you having unclear thinking? 2. Hold up this many fingers (Examiner holds 2 fingers in front of the patient) 3. Now do the same thing with other hand (without holding 2 fingers in front of the patient)		
IV. Altered level of consciousness		
Is the patient's level of consciousness anything other than alert, such as being vigilant or lethargic or in a stupor or coma? **Alert:** Spontaneously fully aware of environment and interact appropriately **Vigilant:** Hyper-alert **Lethargic:** Drowsy but easily aroused, unaware of some elements in the environment or not spontaneously interacting with the interviewer, becomes fully aware and appropriately interactive when prodded minimally **Stupor:** Difficult to arouse, unaware of some or all elements in the environment or not spontaneously interacting with the interviewer, becomes incompletely aware when prodded strongly; can be aroused only by vigorous and repeated stimuli and as soon as the stimulus ceases, stuporous subject lapses back into unresponsive state		

Contd...

Contd...

Features and descriptions

	Absent	Present
Coma: Unarousable, unaware of all the elements of environment with no spontaneous interaction or awareness of the interviewer so that the interview is impossible even with maximum prodding		
Overall CAM-ICU assessment (Features 1 and 2 and either features 3 or 4):	Yes ...	No ...

*RASS consists of 10-point score that ranges from a high of 4 (combative) to a low of –5 (deeply comatose and unresponsive). Patients who are spontaneously alert, calm, and not agitated are scored at 0 (neutral zone). Anxious or agitated patients receive a range of scores depending on their level of anxiety: 1 for anxious, 2 for agitated (fighting ventilator), 3 for very agitated (pulling on or removing catheters), or 4 for combative (violent and a danger to staff). The scores –1 to –5 are assigned for patients with varying degrees of sedation based on their ability to maintain eye contact: 1. for more than 10 seconds, 2. for less than 10 seconds, and –3 for eye opening but no eye contact. If physical stimulation is required, then the patient is scored as either –4 for eye opening or movement with physical or painful stimulation or –5 for no response to physical or painful stimulation (Flowchart 1).

†In completing the visual ASE, the patient is shown 5 simple pictures at 3-second intervals and is asked to remember them. Immediately the patient is shown 10 subsequent pictures and asked to nod "yes" or "no" to indicate whether he had or had not just seen each of the pictures. Since 5 pictures had been shown to him already, for which the correct response was to nod "yes," and 5 others were new, for which the correct response was to nod "no,". The patient scores perfectly if he achieves 10 correct responses. Scoring accounted for either errors of omission (indicating "no" for a previously shown picture) or for errors of commission (indicating "yes" for a picture not previously shown). In completing the auditory ASE, patient is asked to squeeze the rater's hand or lift his hand/finger whenever he hears the letter "A" during the recitation of a series of 10 letters. The rater then reads 10 letters (S, A, H, E, V, A, A, R, A, T) in a normal tone at a rate of 1 letter per second;. A scoring method similar to that of the visual ASE is used for the auditory ASE testing.

experience and observational methods to detect inattention, disorientation, hallucinations, presence of sleep, and inappropriate speech or mood (Table 4). It may be difficult to detect these symptoms particularly in nonverbal mechanically ventilated patients.

Prevention and Treatment of Delirium

Delirium prevention strategies can be divided into: Nonpharmacological, pharmacological and combined pharmacologic/nonpharmacologic approaches. Various nonpharmacological interventions (e.g. outside the ICU, repeated reorientation, reduction in noise, cognitive stimulation, use of vision and hearing aids, adequate hydration and early mobilization) have shown the reduction in the incidence of delirium in hospitalized patients.[45] During the period of sedation-interruption, early mobilization has shown the reduction in delirium to almost half.[46] Dexmedetomidine as well as benzodiazepines have shown the reduction in incidence of delirium in ICU patients. In a multicenter, prospective trial, dexmedetomidine or midazolam was used to keep the sedation target in the range of -2 to +1 on the RASS; those patients who received dexmedetomidine had lower risk of delirium and spent less days on mechanical ventilation.[47] A multicenter European trial has shown superiority of dexmedetomidine over propofol or midazolam in the rates of composite end point of agitation, anxiety and delirium.[48] However, there is little evidence to treat established delirium.

Statements and Clinical Practice Guidelines for Delirium in ICU[15]

1. Routine monitoring of delirium should be performed in all ICU patients (+1B).
2. CAM-ICU and ICDSC both are recommended as the most valid and reliable delirium monitoring tools in adult ICU patients (A).
3. Pre-existing dementia, history of baseline hypertension and/or alcoholism and the high severity of illness at the time of admission have been identified as risk factors for development of delirium in ICU patients (B). Further, coma is an independent risk factor for delirium (B).
4. Early mobilization of ICU patient, whenever feasible, is suggested in order to reduce incidence and duration of delirium (+1B).
5. Promote sleep in ICU patients by controlling light and noise and minimizing the stimuli to the patient in night (1C).
6. In the absence of compelling evidences, there is no suggestion or recommendation for the use of pharmacological drugs (haloperidol or other antipsychotics) to prevent, delirium (0, C).
7. Use of combined nonpharmacological and pharmacological delirium prevention protocol has no evidence in reducing incidence of delirium in adult ICU patients (0, C).
8. In the absence of evidence, prophylactic use of haloperidol or atypical antipsychotics to prevent delirium in adult ICU patients is not suggested (–2C).
9. Continuous IV infusions of dexmedetomidine rather than benzodiazepines is suggested for sedation (if required) in patients with delirium unrelated to alcohol or benzodiazepine withdrawal) (+2B).

Table 4: Intensive care delirium screening checklist (ICDSC)[30]

- Scoring of patient is done over the entire shift.
- A focused bedside patient assessment is required for components #1 through #4. This cannot be completed if the patient is deeply sedated or comatose (i.e., SAS = 1 or 2; RASS = –4 or –5).
- Components #5 through #8 are based on observations throughout the entire shift. Information from the prior 24 hours (i.e., from prior 1–2 nursing shifts) should be obtained for components #7 and #8.

1. **Altered level of consciousness** — No 0   1 Yes
   Deep sedation/coma over entire shift (SAS = 1, 2; RASS = –4,–5)
   = Not assessable
   Agitation (SAS = 5, 6, or 7; RASS = 1–4) at any point
   = 1 point
   Normal wakefulness (SAS = 4; RASS = 0) over the entire shift
   = 0 points
   Light sedation (SAS = 3; RASS= –1, –2, –3):
   = 1 point (if no recent sedatives)
   = 0 points (if recent sedatives)

2. **Inattention** — No 0   1 Yes
   Difficulty following instructions or conversation, patient easily distracted by external stimuli.
   Will not reliably squeeze hands to spoken letter A: S A V E A H A A R T

3. **Disorientation** — No 0   1 Yes
   In addition to name, place, and date, does the patient recognize ICU caregivers? Does patient know what kind of place they are in? (list examples: dentist's office, home, work, hospital)

4. **Hallucination, delusion, or psychosis** — No 0   1 Yes
   Ask the patient if they are having hallucinations or delusions. (e.g. trying to catch an object that is not there). Are they afraid of the people or things around them?

5. **Psychomotor agitation or retardation** — No 0   1 Yes
   Either:
   a. Hyperactivity requiring the use of sedative drugs or restraints in order to control potentially dangerous behavior (e.g. pulling IV lines out or hitting staff)
   OR
   b. Hypoactive or clinically noticeable psychomotor slowing or retardation

6. **Inappropriate speech or mood** — No 0   1 Yes
   Patient displays: inappropriate emotion; disorganized or incoherent speech; sexual or inappropriate interactions; is either apathetic or overly demanding

7. **Sleep-wake cycle disturbance** — No 0   1 Yes
   Either: Frequent awakening/< 4 hours sleep at night OR sleeping during much of the day

8. **Symptom fluctuation** — No 0   1 Yes
   Fluctuation of any of the above symptoms over 24 hours period

Total Shift Score: 0........8

Score 0: Normal   **1–3:** Subsyndromal delirium   **4–8:** Delirium

The ICDSC was designed in 2001 as a quick-to-administer instrument to screen patients for delirium even when communication is compromised. The ICDSC has 8 items that are based on Diagnostic and Statistical Manual (DSM)-IV criteria. Rating the items is based on observations of the patient over an 8-hour shift or a 24-hour period. Administration of the ICDSC takes less than 5 minutes and has moderate sensitivity with good specificity.

*Adapted and modified from : Bergeron et al. Intensive Care Med. 2001;27:859-64.[30]
: Quimet et al. Intensive Care Med. 2007;33:1007-13.[44]

CONCLUSION

The ICU patients with various invasive monitoring suffer pain, agitation, sleep deprivation and delirium. Significant advances have been made in our understanding of ICU sedation, pain and delirium as well as in methods to provide physical and psychological comforts. There is no dearth of publications showing consistent use of methods (use of sedatives, sedation score, sedation interruption, adequate analgesia with fentanyl/sufentanil, delirium score monitoring and prevention of delirium) that can lead to decrease in days on mechanical ventilation and length of ICU stay. However, only a small proportion of ICUs have established and written protocol for sedation and analgesia or a scoring system for the monitoring of analgesia, sedation and delirium. A successful strategy is to implement an evidence-based, institutionally specific, integrated pain, agitation and delirium protocol to assess, treat and prevent PAD, using an interdisciplinary team approach. A protocolized approach can significantly improve patient outcomes and serve as a guide for quality assurance efforts.

REFERENCES

1. Stein-Parbury J, McKinley S. Patients' experiences of being in an intensive care unit: a select literature review. Am J Crit Care. 2000;9:20-7.
2. International association for the study of pain | IASP taxonomy. Available at: http://www.iasp.pain.org/AM/Template.cfm?Section=Pain_Defi...isplay.cfm&ContentID=1728#Pain.
3. Anand KJ, Craig KD. New perspectives on the definition of pain. Pain. 1996;67:3-6; discussion 209.
4. Gélinas C. Management of pain in cardiac surgery ICU patients: Have we improved over time? Intensive Crit Care Nurs. 2007;23:298-303.
5. Schelling G, Richter M, Roozendaal B, et al. Exposure to high stress in the intensive care unit may have negative effects on health-related quality-of-life outcomes after cardiac surgery. Crit Care Med. 2003;31:1971-80.
6. Akça O, Melischek M, Scheck T, et al. Postoperative pain and subcutaneous oxygen tension. Lancet. 1999;354:41-2.
7. Peterson PK, Chao CC, Molitor T, et al. Stress and pathogenesis of infectious disease. Rev Infect Dis. 1991;13:710-20.
8. Puntillo K, Pasero C, Li D, et al. Evaluation of pain in ICU patients. Chest. 2009; 135:1069-74.
9. Chanques G, Jaber S, Barbotte E, et al. Impact of systematic evaluation of pain and agitation in an intensive care unit. Crit Care Med. 2006;34:1691-9.
10. Payen JF, Bosson JL, Chanques G, et al. DOLOREA Investigators: Pain assessment is associated with decreased duration of mechanical ventilation in the intensive care unit: A post Hoc analysis of the DOLOREA study. Anesthesiology. 2009;111:1308-16.
11. Bernards CM, Shen DD, Sterling ES, et al. Epidural, cerebrospinal fluid, and plasma pharmacokinetics of epidural opioids (part 2): Effect of epinephrine. Anesthesiology. 2003;99:466-75.
12. Richman JM, Liu SS, Courpas G, et al. Does continuous peripheral nerve block provide superior pain control to opioids? A meta-analysis. Anesth Analg. 2006;102:248-57.
13. Pandey CK, Bose N, Garg G, et al. Gabapentin for the treatment of pain in Guillain-Barré syndrome: A double-blinded, placebo-controlled, crossover study. Anesth Analg. 2002;95:1719-23.

14. Pandey CK, Raza M, Tripathi M, et al. The comparative evaluation of gabapentin and carbamazepine for pain management in Guillain-Barré syndrome patients in the intensive care unit. Anesth Analg. 2005;101:220-25.
15. Barr J, Fraser GL, Puntillo K, et al. Clinical practice guidelines for the management of pain, agitation, and delirium in adult patients in the intensive care unit. Crit Care Med. 2013;41:263-306.
16. Fraser GL, Prato BS, Riker RR, et al. Frequency, severity, and treatment of agitation in young versus elderly patients in the ICU. Pharmacotherapy. 2000;20:75-82.
17. Atkins PM, Mion LC, Mendelson W, et al. Characteristics and outcomes of patients who self-extubate from ventilatory support: A case-control study. Chest. 1997;112:1317-23.
18. Reade MC, Finfer S. Sedation and delirium in the intensive care unit. N Engl J Med. 2014;370:444-54.
19. Kress JP, Pohlman AS, O'Connor MF, et al. Daily interruption of sedative infusions in critically ill patients undergoing mechanical ventilation. N Engl J Med. 2000;342:1471-77.
20. Kollef MH, Levy NT, Ahrens TS, et al. The use of continuous IV sedation is associated with prolongation of mechanical ventilation. Chest. 1998;114:541-8.
21. Treggiari MM, Romand JA, Yanez ND, et al. Randomized trial of light versus deep sedation on mental health after critical illness. Crit Care Med. 2009;37:2527-34.
22. Kress JP, Pohlman AS, O'Connor MF, et al. Daily interruption of sedative infusions in critically ill patients undergoing mechanical ventilation. N Engl J Med. 2000;342:1471-7.
23. Girard TD, Kress JP, Fuchs BD, et al. Efficacy and safety of a paired sedation and ventilator weaning protocol for mechanically ventilated patients in intensive care (Awakening and Breathing Controlled trial): a randomised controlled trial. Lancet 2008;371:126-34.
24. Shehabi Y, Bellomo R, Reade MC, et al. Early intensive care sedation predicts long-term mortality in ventilated critically ill patients. Am J Respir Crit Care Med. 2012;186:724-31.
25. Treggiari MM, Romand JA, Yanez ND, et al. Randomized trial of light versus deep sedation on mental health after critical illness. Crit Care Med. 2009;37:2527-34.
26. Kress JP, Gehlbach B, Lacy M, et al. The long-term psychological effects of daily sedative interruption on critically ill patients. Am J Respir Crit Care Med. 2003;168:1457-61.
27. Strøm T, Stylsvig M, Toft P. Long-term psychological effects of a no-sedation protocol in critically ill patients. Crit Care. 2011;15:R293.
28. Riker RR, Picard JT, Fraser GL. Prospective evaluation of the Sedation-Agitation Scale for adult critically ill patients. Crit Care Med. 1999;27:1325-9.
29. Sessler CN, Gosnell MS, Grap MJ, et al. The Richmond Agitation-Sedation Scale: validity and reliability in adult intensive care unit patients. Am J Respir Crit Care Med. 2002;166:1338-44.
30. Bergeron N, Dubois MJ, Dumont M, et al. Intensive care delirium screening checklist: Evaluation of a new screening tool. Intens Care Med. 2001;27:859-64.
31. Ely EW, Girard TD, Shintani AK, et al. Apolipoprotein E4 polymorphism as a genetic predisposition to delirium in critically ill patients. Crit Care Med. 2007;35:112-7.
32. Diagnostic and statistical manual of mental disorders, 4th ed. text rev.: DSM- IV-TR. Arlington, VA: American Psychiatric Association, 2011.
33. Gunther ML, Morandi A, Krauskopf E, et al. The association between brain volumes, delirium duration, and cognitive outcomes in intensive care unit survivors: the VISIONS cohort magnetic resonance imaging study. Crit Care Med. 2012;40:2022-32.
34. Morandi A, Rogers BP, Gunther ML, et al. The relationship between delirium duration, white matter integrity, and cognitive impairment in intensive care unit survivors as

determined by diffusion tensor imaging: the VISIONS prospective cohort magnetic resonance imaging study. Crit Care Med. 2012;40:2182-9.
35. Peterson JF, Pun BT, Dittus RS, et al. Delirium and its motoric subtypes: a study of 614 critically ill patients. J Am Geriatr Soc. 2006;54:479-84.
36. Van den Boogaard M, Schoonhoven L, Evers AW, et al. Delirium in critically ill patients: impact on long-term health-related quality of life and cognitive functioning. Crit Care Med. 2012;40:112-8.
37. Soliman HM, Melot C, Vincent JL. Sedative and analgesic practice in the intensive care unit: the results of a European survey. Br J Anaesth. 2001;87:186-92.
38. De Jonghe B, Bastuji-Garin S, Fangio P, et al. Sedation algorithm in critically ill patients without acute brain injury. Crit Care Med. 2005;33:120-7.
39. Cammarano WB, Pittet JF, Weitz S, et al. Acute withdrawal syndrome related to the administration of analgesic and sedative medications in adult intensive care unit patients. Crit Care Med. 1998;26:676-84.
40. Hospira Inc: FDA package insert for dexmedetomidine. Available at: http://www.precedex.com/wp-content/uploads/2010/11/Prece-dex_PI.pdf.
41. Jackson DL, Proudfoot CW, Cann KF, et al. The incidence of sub-optimal sedation in the ICU: a systematic review. Crit Care. 2009;13:R204.
42. Ely EW, Inouye SK, Bernard GR, et al. Delirium in mechanically ventilated patients: validity and reliability of the Confusion assessment method for the intensive care unit (CAM-ICU). JAMA. 2001;286:2703-10.
43. Satyapriya SV, Lyaker ML, Rozycki AJ, Papadimos. Sedation, analgesia delirium in the ECMO patient. In: Firstenberg MS (Ed). Extracorporeal Membrane Oxygenation- Advances in Therapy. Croatia: InTech. 2016.
44. Ouimet S, Riker R, Bergeron N, et al. Subsyndromal delirium in the ICU: evidence for a disease spectrum. Intensive Care Med. 2007;33(6):1007-13.
45. Vidán MT, Sanchez E, Alonso M, et al. An intervention integrated into daily clinical practice reduces the incidence of delirium during hospitalization in elderly patients. J Am Geriatr Soc. 2009;57:2029-36.
46. Schweickert WD, Pohlman MC, Pohlman AS, et al. Early physical and occupational therapy in mechanically ventilated, critically ill patients: a randomised controlled trial. Lancet 2009;373:1874-82.
47. Riker RR, Shehabi Y, Bokesch PM, et al. Dexmedetomidine VS midazolam for sedation of critically ill patients: a randomized trial. JAMA. 2009;301:489-99.
48. Jakob SM, Ruokonen E, Grounds RM, et al. Dexmedetomidine vs midazolam or propofol for sedation during prolonged mechanical ventilation: two randomized controlled trials. JAMA. 2012;307:1151-60.

CHAPTER 20

Perioperative Atrial Fibrillation: A Perioperative Physician's Outlook

Priya R Menon, Akshaya Rai

KEY POINTS

- Atrial fibrillation (AF) is the commonest rhythm abnormality seen in the perioperative period.
- AF is self-limiting in 98% of patients with no major consequence. In 2% patients AF may persist postoperatively (POAF) and has high morbidity especially in form of stroke and higher long-term mortality.
- Prevention strategies are important and perioperative monitoring is a must.
- More careful attention and planning is required for patients who are >65 years, undergoing cardiac, thoracic and abdominal surgeries.
- The underlying pathology should be corrected before attempting to cardiovert an asymptomatic or minimally symptomatic patient.
- Statins, ACEI and ARB and rate control drugs should be continued till day of surgery to suppress arrhythmia after noncardiac surgery.
- Ventricular rate should be controlled with pharmacological or electric cardioversion preoperatively in patients with chronic AF.
- When perioperative AF (POAF) occurs, cardioversion is preferred in unstable patients and amiodarone is the most commonly used medication.
- As the new onset PAOF is transient, anticoagulation should be avoided due to risk of postoperative hemorrhage.
- For patients on chronic anticoagulation, its continuation should be based on risk of bleeding outweighing the risk of thromboembolism.

INTRODUCTION

With the increase in life expectancy of the general population over time due to improving medical facilities, our confrontation with patients in geriatric age group has increased considerably. Thus, due to the increasing number of surgeries being performed in the elderly, the incidence of new onset perioperative atrial fibrillation (POAF) is also showing a rising trend. POAF is seen more in cardiac surgeries with the incidence being as high as 60% in combined coronary artery bypass graft (CABG) and valve surgery. In noncardiac surgeries, the incidence depends on the age of the patient, comorbidities and also on the type of surgery. Thoracic surgeries have an incidence of around 30%, while colorectal surgery have around 13% and ophthalmic surgery around 0.37%.[1] This means that the anesthesiologist must be able to identify and deal with this arrhythmia, which can be a major reason for hemodynamic instability in the operation room (OR) and in the postoperative period. A rapid ventricular rate does not allow adequate diastolic filling time and the coronary flow is unable to meet the high myocardial oxygen demand. Thus, the patient is at risk of developing myocardial ischemia. The presence of AF increases the risk of stroke, thromboembolic episodes and heart failure, leading to higher health expenses but a poor quality of life. The aim of this chapter is to briefly throw light on the pathophysiology, treatment and prevention of POAF.

DEFINITION, DIAGNOSIS AND CLASSIFICATION

The American Heart Association (AHA) defines atrial fibrillation (AF) as rapid oscillation and/or fibrillation of the atria due to irregular electrical activity which varies in amplitude, shape and timing, whereas the atrioventricular conduction remains intact.[2]

Diagnosis of AF is based on ECG which shows irregular R-R interval, no distinct P wave and short atrial cycle (interval between 2 atrial activation) of 200 ms or less (>300 Beats/min).

New onset AF means development of an irregularly irregular heart beat which needs either a pharmacological or electrical cardioversion. Very rarely AF may present as bradyarrhythmia which can be dangerous in patient with fixed cardiac output. Classification of AF is listed in Table 1.

RISK FACTORS

The risk factors for AF can be classified as:
- Patient related factors
- Surgery related factors
- Reversible factors

Patient related risk factors are listed in Table 2. Black race is associated with a lower risk.[4]

But the most consistent factor is old age.[5]

Incidence of AF is higher (up to 60%) in cardiac surgeries especially combined CABG and valvular surgeries, while less among off pump CABG and transcatheter procedures. In noncardiac surgeries the incidence is less than 1% in minor surgeries but may go up to 30% in colorectal surgeries.[6] In thoracic surgeries incidence is less in minimally invasive but higher in major lung and esophageal surgeries.[6]

Lone AF patients are under 60 years of age with no structural heart problems but have AF due to genetic mutation. This shows that genetics also plays an important role in the development of this arrhythmia.[7]

Table 1: Classification of atrial fibrillation[3]	
Classification	Presented pattern of first detected episode
Paroxysmal	Lasting for ≤ 48 hours, usually terminating spontaneously
Persistent	Lasting for >7 days, cardioversion may be needed Long standing persistent: lasting for >1 year, cardioversion failed or not attempted
Permanent	Long-term atrial fibrillation, no pursuit of rhythm control

Table 2: Risk factors for atrial fibrillation

Patient factors	Reversible factors
- Male - Old age - Smoker - ASA class III or IV - Hypertension - Ischemic heart disease - Valvular heart disease - Diabetes mellitus - COPD - OSAS - LVH - C_2H_5OH abuse - Genetics	- K^+ imbalance due to large fluid shifts causes changes in resting membrane potential, excitability - Hypomagnesemia - Hypocalcemia - Metabolic acidosis - Hypovolemia - Hypoxia - Preoperative and postoperative intake of beta blocker and ACEI is shown to decrease POAF

(ASA: American Society of Anesthesiologists; COPD: Chronic obstructive pulmonary disease; OSAS: Obstructive sleep apnea syndrome; LVH: Left ventricular hypertrophy; ACEI: Angiotensin-converting enzyme inhibitor).

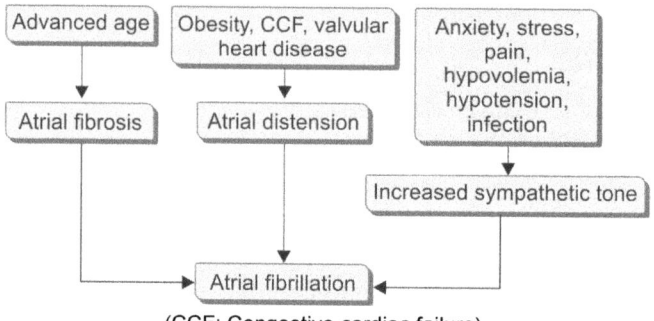

Flowchart 1: Pathophysiology of atrial fibrillation.[8]

(CCF: Congestive cardiac failure).

PATHOPHYSIOLOGY

The pathophysiology of AF is incompletely understood. The atrial remodeling due to the advancing age leading to fibrotic atria, is thought to make the atria vulnerable to POAF. Other comorbidities like hypertension, chronic obstructive pulmonary disease and ischemic heart disease make the patient vulnerable to POAF[9] and then the perioperative factors further add to these risk factors (Flowchart 1).

Does this mean that one does not see AF in young patients? Data remains unclear, but in a study done on asymptomatic, young noncardiac surgery patients, an AF requiring medication was seen in 2% patients before and 6% patients after surgery[10] due to anxiety, stress, pain, all which lead to sympathetic stimulation.

Obesity causes diastolic dysfunction and increase in left atrium (LA) size, a predisposition to POAF. Patients with congestive cardiac failure or valvular disorders also have chronically enlarged atria which is also a substrate for arrhythmia.[11] Thus, left sided diastolic dysfunction should alert the anesthesio-logist about the heightened risk of AF perioperatively. Prolonged PR interval is implicated in POAF after coronary artery bypass grafting. Equally implicated in the development of POAF are various factors in form of pain, hypovolemia, hypoxia and infection which cause sympathetic stimulation which in turn leads to arrhythmia.[12]

Few studies have tried to link POAF to loss of parasympathetic stimulation on atrium and not the increasing sympathetic tone. These studies have concluded that epidural infusion of opioids is better than local anesthetic infusions in reducing POAF.[13]

In patients undergoing cardiac surgery there may be an added role of surgery itself while other factors may be as follows:
- Handling of the heart during surgery
- Direct injury to the atria by cannulation causing stimulation of inflammatory process
- Ventricular stunning leading to rise in LA pressure
- Improper cooling of the heart
- Activation of inflammatory cascade due to cardiopulmonary bypass leading to POAF
- Acute stretching of the atria due to fluid overloading done to maintain hemodynamics after the cross clamp is off
- Sympathomimetics administered while coming off cardiopulmonary bypass (CPB).

From these one can conclude that the patients who tend to have AF peri and postoperatively have the substrate for it due to alteration of the atrial architecture either due to cardiac disease itself or due to the various comorbidities making the atria more prone to POAF. Such patients should have a good monitoring to handle the problem before it becomes hemodynamically relevant.

PREDICTORS OF POAF AFTER SURGERY

The factors which can predict the onset of POAF are:
- A raised preoperative brain natriuretic peptide (BNP) value.
- A less negative P-wave in aVR and a more positive or more negative P-wave in V1 are predictive features on ECG.
- LV diastolic dysfunction on echocardiogram or angiographic evidence of RCA stenosis.
- Electrolyte imbalance with postoperative raised WBC.

Predictors postcardiac surgery are:
- Age more than 65 years
- LA size >41 mm
- Mitral valve disease
- Chronic renal insufficiency.

PREVENTION

New onset POAF is seen normally between 2nd and 4th postoperative day. As shown in the etiology and pathophysiology, various causes are preventable. Those such as reversible factors are also the surgical factors.

Nonpharmacological Methods

Adequate analgesia will reduce the incidence of AF. Pain causes stimulation of sympathetic outflow and triggers POAF. Good analgesia in form of epidural opioids, regional anesthesia has shown to reduce incidence of POAF. The sympathetic blockade caused reduces the release of catecholamines and its negative chronotropic effect and also decreases sensitivity of the myocardium to the released catecholamines. General anesthesia combined with regional anesthesia has shown to decrease the incidence of POAF as compared to patients who were administered general anesthesia alone.[14]

Anti-inflammatory measures to reduce systemic inflammatory response syndrome (SIRS) which has been proven to play a major role in POAF. Various markers of inflammation like IL-6, CRP, WBC and TNF-alpha are raised and they reflect the degree of surgical stress which in turn increases local and systemic inflammation and plays a pivotal role in precipitating AF. Antioxidant administration in the perioperative period can help reduce the incidence of POAF as they decrease the level of these oxidative free radicals. Statins and N-acetylcysteine have been shown to decrease the vulnerability of the heart to the free radicals and thus diminishing the incidence of POAF. Some studies on cardiac surgical patients have reported decreased incidence of POAF in patients treated with vitamin C in the perioperative period.[15]

Polyunsaturated fatty acids (PUFAs) have shown to significantly reduce both atrial and ventricular rhythm abnormalities in patients with ischemic heart disease (IHD) and implanted defibrillators.[16] Administration of PUFAs in CABG patients was shown to reduce POAF significantly.

Perioperative continuous venovenous hemofiltration (CVVH) has been thought to reduce the inflammatory markers and thus maybe beneficial in reducing the incidence of POAF in cardiac surgical patients but the timing of when to start the patient on CVVH is unclear and some recent studies have refuted the claim.[17] Its use in noncardiac surgical patients is debatable and needs further research.

Euvolemia in perioperative period diminishes the risk of POAF. Anesthetic agents along with hypovolemia and blood loss decrease the cardiac output due to decrease in venous return which in turn cause tissue hypoxia. Tissue hypoxia stimulates the sympathetic system to maintain tissue perfusion. This adrenergic stimulation causes increased chronotropic activity, ultimately causing rhythm disturbance. In postsurgical patients, a new onset AF is a sign of hypovolemia which may be due to a masked bleeding. Not only the tissue hypoperfusion but also the ischemia of cardiac cells leads to conduction abnormalities which can be seen as POAF. Large volume overloading and huge fluid shifts also trigger POAF by reducing the compliance of the overtly dilated atria. This is seen especially in 48 hours postcardiac surgery where the patients with positive net fluid balance show higher incidence of POAF.[18]

Optimal oxygenation in subjects who suffer from chronic respiratory failure will prevent PAOF. Chronic hypoxia seen in obese patients or ones suffering from chronic obstructive pulmonary disease (COPD) are at heightened risk of POAF. Due to chronic hypoxia, there is change in the pulmonary vascular resistance which leads to increase in RV afterload. This leads to RV and RA dilatation, so the stretch on atrial cells predisposes to POAF. Patients with obstructive sleep apnea not using nocturnal CPAP are predisposed to POAF due to this chronic hypoxia.[19]

Acute hypoxia peri and postoperatively leads to increase in adrenergic activity as there is tissue hypoxia. Sympathetic stimulation leads to increase in heart rate and supraventricular tachyarrhythmias (SVT). Hypoxia also leads to change in the electric properties of the conducting cells triggering SVT. Thus, optimization of tissue oxygenation both in patients with acute and chronic respiratory failure is mandatory to prevent POAF. The possible maneuvers in chronic respiratory failure are noninvasive ventilation (NIV), spirometry and vigorous chest physiotherapy.

Hemoglobin optimization is important as perioperative anemia triggers POAF by stimulating sympathetic system and the conducting tissue ischemia leads to arrhythmia but there is no defined level of hemoglobin which can prevent POAF. In fact various studies in postcardiac surgery patients have shown that patients received for transfusion are prone to higher incidence of POAF.[20] So the transfusion trigger for each patient should be individualized depending on the type of surgery, the clinical status so that tissue oxygen delivery does not suffer.

Metabolic status during the perioperative period can be the trigger for POAF. Metabolic acidosis due to whatever reason leads to surge in intrinsic catecholamine synthesis predisposing the myocardium to arrhythmia. Hypoglycemia is a strong stimulus for adrenergic activity leading to arrhythmia. In a diabetic patient with a new onset AF postoperatively, hypoglycemia should be ruled out.[21] Hyperglycemia is equally detrimental as high blood glucose levels lead to cell membrane damage and so the electrophysiological properties are also altered causing POAF. High blood sugars also cause inflammatory reaction leading to release of inflammatory mediators and oxidative species.

Thyroid status should be evaluated for patients who are planned for surgery especially cardiac surgery as low levels of T3 is associated with altered ion transport, specially calcium, in myocardial cells making the heart prone to rhythm abnormalities.

Electrolyte balance should be maintained within normal levels to prevent POAF. Both K^+ and Mg^{++} deficiency can trigger POAF.[22] Mg^{++} should be given as infusion as an antiarrhythmic in postcardiac patients provided the patient has low Mg^{++} as it would not be effective if patient is normomagnesemia.

Temperature management is crucial in prevention of POAF. Hypothermia leads to increased adrenergic activity especially in noncardiac surgery. In cardiac surgery POAF is seen when patients are cooled actively to 28°C. Mild hypothermia (33°C) is advocated in cardiac surgery patients to prevent POAF but in noncardiac surgery normothermia should be employed.[23]

Pharmacological Prevention

Preoperative

The subset of patients who have risk factors which can trigger POAF, should such susceptible patients be the ones in whom the pharmacological prevention should started, is a big dilemma. It is difficult to recommend if prophylactic administration of rate regulating drugs will improve clinical outcomes. Before contemplating the rate control drugs for AF, one should look at the correctable factors like electrolyte imbalance, hypoxia or hyperglycemia to name a few. Medications like beta blockers, amiodarone, calcium channel blockers, sotalol and digoxin have been studied and used as preventive measures for POAF.

Beta blockers: From large studies and meta analyses, it was deciphered that use of beta blockers perioperatively in cardiac surgical patients does decrease the incidence of AF and also decreases mortality. So, it should be used as prophylaxis unless contraindicated.[24,25]

The preoperative beta blocker use has been put forward as a Class I recommendation (ACC/AHA/ESC) for the prevention of POAF after cardiac surgery.[3]

Perioperative ischemic evaluation (POISE) trial enrolled over 8000 patients who underwent major noncardiac surgery. Patients were randomized to metoprolol succinate or placebo. The primary end point was a composite outcome of nonfatal cardiac arrest, cardiovascular death and nonfatal MI at 30 days after surgery. Clinically significant new POAF was recorded in 2.2% of patients in the metoprolol group versus 2.9% in the placebo group. This infers that preoperative metoprolol administration may prevent new onset POAF, but this intervention also heightened the risk of mortality and stroke.[26]

After this trial, there was a change in the guidelines in perioperative care of patients posted for noncardiac surgery. Now it is recommended that the patients should continue beta blockers till the day of surgery (Class I indication ACC AHA ESC) and it should be restarted early postoperatively to decrease the incidence and complications of AF.

Nondihydropyridine calcium channel blockers: These are used if beta blockers are contraindicated. Its use as prophylaxis in preoperative period is associated with reduced incidence of POAF after cardiac surgery.[27]

Preoperative use of calcium channel blockers have been put forward as a Class I recommendation for the prevention of POAF after cardiac surgery.[28] Though effective, these have their own share of complications in form of heart block and heart failure and should be used only if beta blockers cannot be administered.

Amiodarone: This is a Class III antiarrhythmic agent as per the Williams-Vaughan classification. Preoperative amiodarone is a Class IIa recommendation (ACC/AHA/ESC) for the prevention of POAF after cardiac surgery.[29] It should be used in patients in whom beta blockers cannot be used.

Amiodarone is recommended for prevention of AF in high-risk patients and also in acute postoperative period (LOE A, Class IIa) but it can cause life-threatening bradycardia and hypotension, especially if given more than a gram per day and as a parenteral medication.[30]

Sotalol: It is an anti-arrhythmic which has been compared with beta blockers in many large meta-analysis and has been shown to be more effective than beta blockers in preventing POAF.[31] Its safety profile is questionable due to prolongation of QT interval and the threat of Torsade des pointes. Due to these reasons, it can be given under vigilant monitoring and is a Class IIb recommendation (ACC/AHA/ESC).[3]

Statins: These have anti-inflammatory and pleiotropic effects and thus help in reducing POAF without much drug related side effects. Numerous large controlled trials have shown that patients who were given preoperative prophylaxis of statins showed lesser incidence of POAF and also postoperative MI.[32]

Magnesium: Administration of magnesium in the perioperative period can reduce the incidence of POAF just as the other rhythm controlling drugs. Few meta-analysis have shown that patients who were administered magnesium showed lesser incidence of POAF especially in cardiac surgery.[33]

Corticosteroids: Steroids have been shown to reduce incidence of POAF but the danger of superadded infections is a deterrent. Recent studies have shown that low dose of steroids help in decreasing the incidence of POAF without adding the risk of infection.[34]

Various theories which attribute this property of steroids to its anti-inflammatory function and also that they help absorption of other rate limiting drugs like beta blocker. Patients who develop POAF show higher levels of CRP and WBC as compared to those who do not. Administering steroids reduces the levels of these inflammatory mediators and may thus reduce POAF.

Nonsteroidal anti-inflammatory drugs: Ibuprofen and ketotifen have been shown to reduce POAF incidence as compared to placebo but are best avoided due to side effects in form of nephrotoxicity in the perioperative period especially in the higher age group patients.[35]

Colchicine: This is an anti-inflammatory drug, is being evaluated in preventing POAF in cardiac surgery.[36] Digitalis is not effective as a preventive tool in PAOF as it decreases the ventricular rate as it acts on the vagal tone.[37]

MANAGEMENT OF ATRIAL FIBRILLATION

The goal is to restore sinus rhythm and maintain stable hemodynamics. As AF is mostly transient, it may not require any intervention. Therapy is indicated if the patient is hemodynamically unstable and has symptoms of cardiac failure, AF duration is >48 hours or the patient is at risk of thromboembolism.

The basic step in managing POAF is to determine the cause. In majority of cases once the cause is identified like electrolyte imbalance, hypoxia, etc. and managed the arrhythmia settles. The AF can be persistent, paroxysmal or permanent and on the type of AF would depend if one needs to manage it in the operation room (OR) conservatively or not.

The next step is to determine if the AF is hemodynamically significant or not. If it is hemodynamically significant then should one control the rate or the rhythm? AFFIRM trial was one of the trials which compared rate or rhythm control in nonsurgical patients and it was seen that patients in whom rhythm control was the goal, they had higher incidence of complication like Torsades de pointes, bradycardia, gastric complications.[38]

In whom to control the rhythm? The rhythm should be controlled in patients:
- ❑ Who remain symptomatic in spite of rate control
- ❑ Who cannot tolerate the medications, and
- ❑ In whom the rate remains uncontrolled despite maximum doses.

Should it be treated with drugs or electrical cardioversion?
- If patient is symptomatic, e.g. has spells of unconsciousness, chest pain or is hemodynamically unstable, then direct current cardioversion should be performed immediately.[39]
- If patients are young, having AF for the first time, there is no structural cardiac problems and there is no atrial enlargement, then electric or pharmacological cardioversion should be done.

If the AF is present for >48 hours or the duration is unknown, then the focus should be on controlling the rate. A heart rate of around 90-115 bpm should be aimed at if the patient is hemodynamically stable. Then, one should control the ventricular rate using rate control drugs. If the patient was previously on a beta blocker or a CCB, it should be restarted. If already restarted, then the dose or the frequency should be increased. Whether to administer rate control drug orally or intravenously depends on if the patient is symptomatic or not (Table 3).

The algorithm depicting the management of AF and decision-making regarding the choice of drug is shown in Flowchart 2. Beta blockers, CCB, amiodarone and digoxin are the drugs which are used to control heart rate. A beta blocker is the first choice provided the systolic function is normal. Metoprolol and esmolol are the best drugs to use in the perioperative period as they can be given intravenously. Also, esmolol has a short half-life of 9 minutes so its action can be titrated. It is always better to start the same beta blocker which the patient was taking in the preoperative period and change its dose or frequency as required.

Table 3: Medication regime for rate control drugs[40]		
Drug	Intravenous	Oral
Metoprolol	5 mg every 5 mins up to 3 doses. If response is inadequate another 5 mg IV every 5 mins could be administered maximum 3 doses	12.5–25 mg/ 6 hourly. Titrated dose.
Esmolol	500 mcg/kg loading dose over 1 minute followed by maintenance of 25–300 µg/kg/min IV (titrate by 50 µg/kg/min)	
Atenolol	2.5 mg over 5 mins, repeated every 10 min up to a maximum dose of 10 mg	
Diltiazem	2 doses of 0.15 mg/kg each can be given 15 mins apart followed by maintenance infusion. If response is inadequate increase the rate	30 mg every 6th hourly to a maximum dose of 360 mg
Digoxin	Loading dose 10–15 µg/kg followed by maintenance dose 62.5 – 250 µg. Serum levels should be <2 ng/mL and, 1 ng/mL in chronic cardiac failure patients	Same dose as IV
Amiodarone	150 mg slow IV over 10 mins followed by 1 mg/kg dose over 6 hours followed by 0.5 mg/kg doses in the next 18 hours	If stable with 0.5 mg/kg dose then convert to oral dose. 400 mg/TDS for 4 days then convert to 200 mg OD

Flowchart 2: Practical management of postoperative atrial fibrillation after noncardiac surgery.[40]

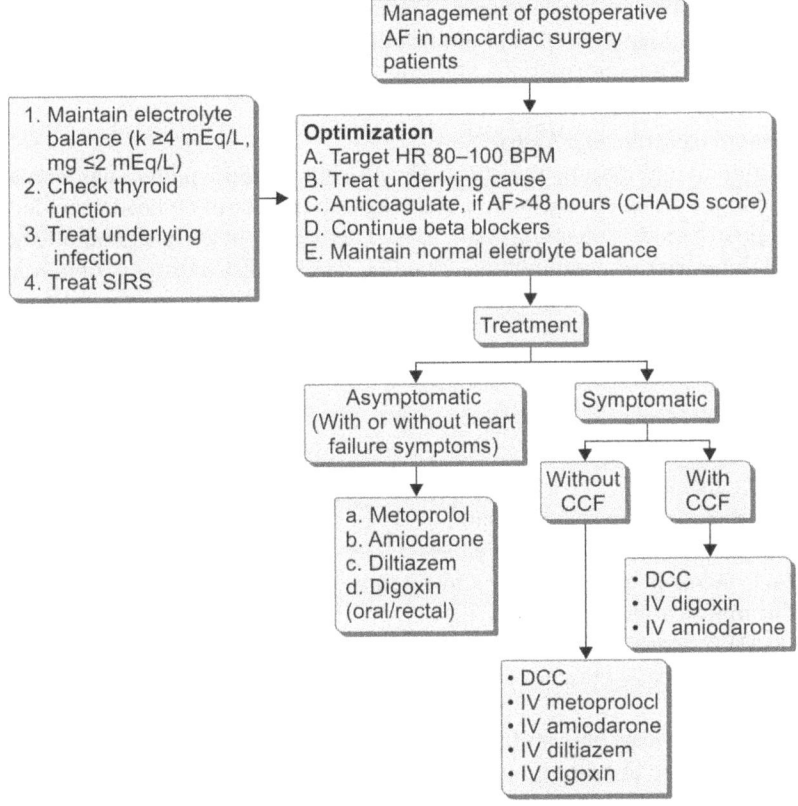

(IV: Intravenous; CCF: Congestive cardiac failure; DCC: Direct current cardioversion; AF: Atrial fibrillation; SIRS: Systemic inflammatory response syndrome).

Nondihydropyridine CCB verapamil and diltiazem are used for rate control but they have a higher incidence of hypotension and negative inotropicity. It should be used with caution, especially if patient is having WPW syndrome as it will decrease the ventricular rate. Due to this reason it is used only when the beta blockers or amiodarone cannot be use as the conversion of supraventricular tachycardia (SVT) to sinus rhythm is higher with beta blockers than with CCB.

Amiodarone has CCB action, beta blocking action as well as it is an antiarrhythmic. However, it has a long half-life of 4–80 hours after a single dose and has a very erratic oral bioavailability. Therefore, it should be given intravenously as the loading dose, the effect of which can be seen in 1–30 min and action may last up to 60–180 min. It can be used in low ejection fraction patients but due to it pulmonary and thyroid toxicity it should not be use in young patients who may need a long-term therapy.

Digoxin has no role in POAF as it is a state of high sympathetic drive, but if the patient is in CCF then digoxin can be employed to manage SVT. It can be safely administered to patients with systolic heart failure because of its positive inotropic properties.

Ibutilide is a class III antiarrhythmic agent of William-Vaughan classification and has been used for management of acute AF after cardiac surgery. The results have been promising but few patients had VT, which may be due to electrolyte abnormality. Thus normal K^+ and Mg^{++} levels should be maintained and defibrillator should be kept ready.

In whom to use anticoagulants?
In addition to maintaining the rate, if AF >48 hours or if the patient has an history of thromboembolic episodes then anticoagulation should be used provided the risk of postoperative bleeding is not high. The benefit of anticoagulation should outweigh the risk of postoperative bleeding. HAS-BLED scoring system may be used to determine the bleeding risk. It consists of 7 factors:
- Hypertension
- Abnormal renal/liver function
- Stroke
- Bleeding history
- Predisposition
- Labile INR
- Elderly (age older than 65 years)
- Drugs/alcohol concomitantly.

Each factor is given 1 point and a score of ≥3 should be a closely guarded antithrombotic therapy.[41]

CHADS2 scoring system is used to calculate the risk of thromboembolism. Higher score means greater risk of thromboembolism for the patient. It consists of 5 factors:
- Congestive heart failure (1 point)
- Hypertension (1 point)
- Age older than 75 years (1 point)
- Diabetes mellitus (1 point)
- Stroke (2 points).

The maximum score is 6

Score 0   No risk

Score 1   Intermediate risk. Can be anticoagulated with aspirin or oral anticoagulation

Score ≥ 2   High risk. Needs oral anticoagulation

CHA2DS2-VASc scoring system has two more variables added to these five, i.e. sex and vascular disease, and thus has improved predictive ability. In addition, age between 65 to 74 years has been added and given 1 point, whereas age 75 years or older is given 2 points.[42]

European guidelines recommend CHA2DS2-VASc scoring system while American chest physician recommend CHA2DS2.

Oral anticoagulation treatment is efficacious in stroke prevention.[43]

Proposed algorithm for the management of patients with recent onset AF with emphasis on preventing thromboembolic events is depicted in Flowchart 3.

Medications Used for Anticoagulation

Vitamin K antagonists: Warfarin is the commonest drug from this group. Stroke prevention due to AF needs PT-INR in the range of 2.0–3.0.

Flowchart 3: Proposed algorithm for the management of patients with recent onset AF with emphasis on preventing thromboembolic events.

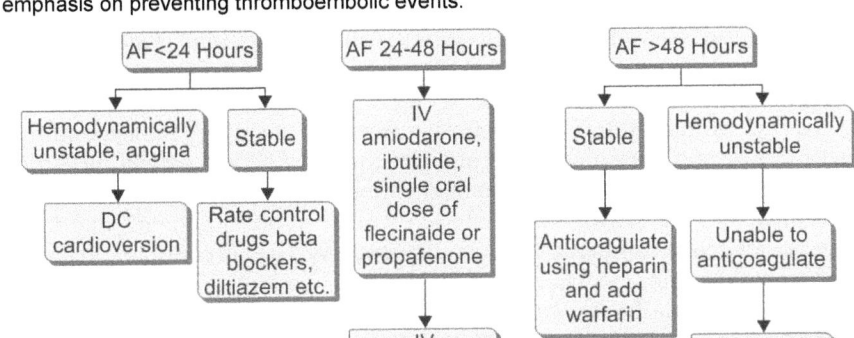

(ECHO: Echocardiogram; IV: Intravenous; DC: Direct current).

New direct oral anticoagulants: Examples—dabigatran, rivaroxaban, apixaban, edoxaban. They have a short half-life therefore limited monitoring is needed. They have a highly predictable pharmacokinetic profile.

As the risk of postoperative bleeding is high, the pros and cons of each drug should be kept in mind before initiation of the therapy.

Patients who need electrical cardioversion with AF > 48 hour duration need to be anticoagulated irrespective of scores as the risk of stroke is high.

Cardiology consultation should be sought if:
- AF with rapid ventricular response and difficult-to-control heart rate
- Hemodynamically unstable patient
- Persistent POAF of > 24 hours or recurrent episodes
- Patients with WPW syndrome and if electric cardioversion or antiarrhythmic drugs are being considered
- Complications of AF as a thromboembolic episode, cardiac ischemia, acute cardiac failure.[8]

CONCLUSION

Atrial fibrillation is the most common postoperative rhythm disorder observed between preoperative period to postoperative day 4, the pathophysiology of which is incompletely understood. It is associated with a high postoperative morbidity, leading to increase length of hospital stay and higher expenditure. AF in the long-term can lead to complications such as stroke, thromboembolism, renal insufficiency, heart failure. In cardiac surgery, AF may need intra-aortic balloon pump (IABP) implantation and other complications like deep sternal wound infections are also seen. So, the aim should be to identify the high-risk patients in the preoperative visits and use prophylaxis measures to prevent it.

In the prevention of POAF, beta blockers and amiodarone are effective and have been recommended. Almost 50% of POAF will subside after 24 hours and so a rate control measure during this period will suffice. Amiodarone, ibutilide, flecainide, propafenone, dofetilide are recommended for pharmacologic cardioversion. Direct-current cardioversion is employed if drug therapy fails. Beyond this if POAF continues or if AF develops after weeks of surgery the patient may need more strong measures like prolonged monitoring, antiarrhythmic drugs and anticoagulation to prevent the complications.

AF has been extensively researched in cardiac surgical patient's due to its higher incidence as compared to noncardiac surgery. Lack of continuous cardiac monitoring after noncardiac surgeries once the patient is shifted from the recovery unit maybe the reason that postoperative AF may remain undetected in noncardiac surgeries thus showing lower incidence.

REFERENCES

1. Bhave PD, Goldman LE, Vittinghoff E, et al. Incidence, predictors, and outcomes associated with postoperative atrial fibrillation after major noncardiac surgery. Am Heart J. 2012;164:918-24.
2. AFFIRM Investigators. Atrial Fibrillation Follow-up Investigation of Rhythm Management. Baseline characteristics of patients with atrial fibrillation: the AFFIRM Study. Am Heart J. 2002;143(6):991-1001.
3. Fuster V, Ryden LE, Cannom DS, et al. ACCF/AHA/HRS focused updates incorporated into the ACC/AHA/ESC 2006 guidelines for the management of patients with atrial fibrillation: a report of the American College of Cardiology Foundation/American Heart Association Task Force on practice guidelines. Circulation. 2011;123:e269-3677.
4. Sun X, Hill PC, Robert L, et al. Comparison of frequency of atrial fibrillation after coronary artery bypass grafting in African Americans versus European Americans. Am J Cardiol. 2011;108(5):669-72.
5. Amar D, Zhang H, Leung DHY, et al. Older age is the strongest predictor of postoperative atrial fibrillation. Anesthesiology. 2002;96:352-56.
6. Maesen B, Nijs J, Maesen J, et al. Postoperative atrial fibrillation: a maze of mechanisms Europace. 2012;14(2):159-74.
7. Philip I, Berroeta C, Leblanc I. Perioperative challenges of atrial fibrillation. Current opinion in Anesthesiolgy. 2014;27:344-52.
8. Amar D. Perioperative atrial tachyarrhythmias. Anesthesiolgy. 2002.97;1618-23.
9. Murphy GJ, Ascione, Caputo M, et al. Operative factors that contribute to postoperative atrial fibrillation: Insights from a prospective randomized trial. Card Electrophysiol Rev. 2003(2):136-9.
10. Polanczyk CA, Goldmann, Edward R, et al. Supraventricular arrhythmia in patients having noncardiac surgery. Clinical correlates and effect on length of stay. Ann Intern Med. 1998;129:279-85.
11. Melduni RM, Suri RM, Seward JB, et al. Diastolic dysfunction in patients undergoing cardiac surgery: A pathophysiological mechanism underlying the initiation of new onset postoperative atrial fibrillation. J Am Coll Cardiol. 2011;58(9):953-61.
12. Chelazzi C, Villa G, De Gaudio AR. International Scholarly Research network, ISRN Cardiology Vol 2011, Article ID. 203179,1-10.
13. Jiang Z, Dai JQ, Shi C, et al. Influence of patient controlled IV analgesia with opioids on supraventricular arrhythmias after pulmonary resection. Br J Anaesth. 2009;103(3):364-68.
14. Creswell LL, Alexander JC, Lisbon A, et al. Intraoperative interventions: American College of Chest Physicians for the prevention and management of postoperative atrial fibrillation after cardiac surgery. Chest. 2005;128,(2 Suppl):24S-27S.

15. Baker WL, White CM. Postcardiothoracic surgery atrial fibrillation: a review of preventive strategies. Ann Pharmacother. 2007;41(4):587-98.
16. Leaf A, Albert CM, Josephson M, et al. Fatty Acid Antiarrhythmia Trial Investigators. Prevention of fatal arrhythmias in high risk subjects by fish oil n-3 fatty acid intake. Circulation. 2005;112(18):2762-68.
17. Mauermann WJ, Nuttall GA, David DJ, et al. Hemofiltration during cardiopulmonary bypass does not decrease the incidence of atrial fibrillation after cardiac surgery. Anesth Analg. 2010;110(2):329-34.
18. Kalus JS, Caron MF, White CM, et al. Impact of fluid balance on incidence of atrial fibrillation after cardiothoracic surgery. Am J Cardiol. 2004;94(11):1423-5.
19. Patel D, Mohanty P, Biase LD, et al. Safety and efficacy of pulmonary vein antral isolation in patients with obstructive sleep apnea syndrome: Impact of continuous positive airway pressure. Circ Arrhythm Electrophysiol. 2010;3(5):445-51.
20. Sood N, Colemann CI, Kluger J, et al. The association among blood transfusions, white blood cell count and the frequency of postcardiothoracic surgery atrial fibrillation: A nested cohort study from atrial fibrillation suppression trials I, II and III. J Cardiothorac Vasc Anesth. 2009;23(1):22-7.
21. Celebi S, Celebi OO, Aydogdu S, et al. A peculiar medical cardioversion of atrial fibrillation with glucose infusion—a rare cause of atrial fibrillation: hypoglycemia. Am J Emerg Med. 2011;29(1):134.e1-3.
22. Walsh SR, Tang T, Wijewardena C, et al. Postoperative arrhythmias in general surgical patients. Ann R Coll Surg Engl. 2007;89(2):91-5.
23. Kurz A. Thermal care in the perioperative period. Best Pract Res Clin Anaesthesiol. 2008;22(1):39-62.
24. Omorphos S, Hanif M, Dunningl J. Are prophylactic beta blockers of benefit in reducing the incidence of AF following coronary artery bypass grafting? Interactive Cardiovascular and Thoracic Surgery. 2004;3(4):641-6.
25. Arsenault KA, Yusuf AM, Crystal E, et al. Interventions for preventing postoperative atrial fibrillation in patients undergoing heart surgery. Cochrane Database Syst Rev. 2013;1:CD003611.
26. Devereaux PJ, Yang H, Yusuf S, et al. Effects of extended-release metoprolol succinate in patients undergoing noncardiac surgery (POISE trial): a randomised controlled trial. Lancet. 2008;371:1839-47.
27. Wijeysundera DN, Beattie WS, Rao V, et al. Calcium antagonists reduce cardiovascular complications after cardiac surgery: a meta-analysis. J Am Coll Cardiol. 2003;41:1496-505.
28. Mitchell LB. CCS Atrial Fibrillation Guidelines Committee. Canadian Cardiovascular Society atrial fibrillation guidelines. Prevention and treatment of atrial fibrillation following cardiac surgery. Can J Cardiol. 2010;2011(27):91-7.
29. Fuster V, Ryden LE, Cannom DS, et al. 2011 ACCF/AHA/HRS focused updates incorporated into the ACC/AHA/ESC 2006 guidelines for the management of patients with atrial fibrillation: a report of the American College of Cardiology Foundation/American Heart Association Task Force on practice guidelines. Circulation. 2011;123:e269-367.
30. Patel AA, White CM, Gillespie EL, et al. Safety of amiodarone in the prevention of postoperative atrial fibrillation: a meta-analysis. Am J Health Syst Pharm. 2006;63:829-37.
31. Burgess DC, Kilborn MJ, Keech AC. Interventions for prevention of postoperative atrial fibrillation and its complications after cardiac surgery: a meta-analysis. Eur Heart J. 2006;27:2846-57.
32. Bhave PD, Goldman LE, Vittinghoff E, et al. Statin use and postoperative atrial fibrillation after major noncardiac surgery. Heart Rhythm. 2012;9(2):163-9.
33. Miller S, Crystal E, Garfinkle M, et al. Effects of magnesium on atrial fibrillation after cardiac surgery: a meta-analysis. Heart. 2005;91:618-23.

34. Ho KM, Tan JA. Benefits and risks of corticosteroid prophylaxis in adult cardiac surgery: a dose–response meta-analysis. Circulation. 2009;119(14):1853-66.
35. Cheruku KK, Ghani A, Ahmad F, et al. Efficacy of nonsteroidal anti-inflammatory medications for prevention of atrial fibrillation following coronary artery bypass graft surgery. Prev Cardiol. 2004;7:13.
36. Imazio M, Brucato A, ferrazzi P, et al. Colchicine reduces postoperative atrial fibrillation: results of the colchicine for the prevention of the postpericardiotomy syndrome (COPPS) atrial fibrillation sub study. Circulation. 2011;124: 2290-5.
37. Podrid PJ. Prevention of postoperative atrial fibrillation: what is the best approach? J Am Coll Cardiol. 1999;34:340-2.
38. Wyse DG, Waldo AL, Di Marco JP, et al. A comparison of rate control and rhythm control in patients with atrial fibrillation. Engl J Med. 2002;347:1825-33.
39. European Heart Rhythm Association, European Association for Cardio-Thoracic Surgery, Camm AJ, Kirchhof P, Lip GY, et al. ESC Committee for Practice Guidelines. Guidelines for the management of atrial fibrillation: The Task Force for the Management of Atrial Fibrillation of the European Society of Cardiology (ESC). Europace 2010;12:1360-420.
40. Danelich IM, Lose JM, Wright SS, et al. Practical Management of Postoperative Atrial Fibrillation after Noncardiac Surgery. J Am Coll Surg. 2014;219(4):831-41.
41. Pisters R, Lane DA, Nieuwlaat R, et al. A novel user-friendly score (HAS-BLED) to assess 1-year risk of major bleeding in patients with atrial fibrillation: the Euro Heart Survey. Chest. 2010;138:1093-1100.
42. Odum LE, Cochran KA, Aistrophe Ds, et al. The CHADS2 versus the new CHA2DS2-VASc scoring systems for guiding antithrombotic treatment of patients with atrial fibrillation: review of the literature and recommendations for use. Pharmacotherapy. 2012;32:285-96.
43. Hylek EM, Go AS, Chang Y, et al. Effect of intensity of oral anticoagulation on stroke severity and mortality in atrial fibrillation. N Engl J Med. 2003;349:1019-26.

CHAPTER 21

Perioperative Medication Errors

Lakshmi Kumar, Keerthi Nandakumar

KEY POINTS

- Perioperative drug errors are poorly reported in our country but they can be a tool for assessment of quality of care to patients undergoing surgery.
- Drug errors result from system errors like poor labeling and identification, sound alike and look alike medications, wrong doses and omission to administer a drug.
- Introduction of advanced drug delivery systems although safe, need supervision as wrong programming or incorrect use could result in wrong doses being administered.
- Physician supervised drug orders, nurse's education, color coding and organized drug locations and second checks of drugs could potentially minimize errors.
- Drug errors could result in no impact on patient to major disability and even death.
- Receptive and blame free approach to error reporting and sharing information with a view to create awareness and improve vigilance could contribute in improvements.
- A nationwide database of incidents in the future may improve our knowledge and protocols in minimizing such errors.

INTRODUCTION

Quality in healthcare delivery encompasses safety, efficiency, outcome and satisfaction of patient and relatives. Ensuring quality in the perioperative setting is complex as it involves multidisciplinary involvement, need for prompt interventions, high-intensity environment and significant work force turnover. Ensuring safety in drug administration is one of the indices of quality in health care.

Perioperative medication errors are preventable complications that if allowed to occur can result in undesirable and even catastrophic outcomes for the patient. In the United States of America this has been reported as a third most common killer after heart diseases and cancer, claiming around 400,000 lives per year.[1] Although literature on drug errors is available from other countries,[2-5] it is largely underreported in our country.

RESPONSIBILITY TO THE PATIENT

A medication error is defined as an error in drug administration irrespective of the presence or absence of adverse consequences.[6] Every patient is entitled to the 5 rights of medication, *the right patient, the right drug, the right dose, the right time and the right route.* An adverse drug event (ADE) differs from drug error as not all medication errors result in ADE. A medication error can be either due to omission or due to an act of commission.[7] A recent study evaluating perioperative medication errors reported as much as 193 events in 277 operations of which 79.3% were medication errors and 47.2% adverse drug events.[8] Among specialties, anesthesia involves prescription, labeling of medications and administration at short time notice. These processes are often conducted without the supervision of a second person and create a potential environment for errors.

BACKGROUND FOR THE OCCURRENCE OF DRUG ERRORS

In a perioperative setting, the time from dispensing to administration of a medicine cannot be more than a few seconds or sometimes a few minutes. The anesthetist often has to multitask by monitoring the patient, documenting, keeping an eye on the surgical proceedings and recognizing the need to administer multiple medications often simultaneously. The process of mixing and administering medications while continuing care in stressful situations creates numerous opportunities for reducing attentiveness to drugs being drawn. This places operating theaters at a high-risk for adverse events (47.7–50.3%).[9]

Highly stressful situations, handling of multiple issues, fatigue and inexperience contribute to the risk. The use of infusion pumps of similar sounding drugs, target controlled infusion pumps also have contributed to many errors from miscalculations, malfunction or simply operator inefficiency.

INCIDENCE AND CLASSIFICATION OF DRUG ERRORS

Webster has classified drug errors as:
- Omission to administer a drug
- Substitution of one drug for another
- Incorrect dose and mode of administration
- Insertion and repetition.

The estimated incidence of medication error in anesthetic practice ranges from 0.33% to 0.73%.[3,10] The incidence of drug errors is estimated to be between 1 in 203 anesthetics[10] in a study by Cooper and similar incidences have been reported by Llewellyn[11] and Khan et al.[12]

Majority of drug errors were noted at induction, maintenance and a very small number was reported at recovery. The chance of an error in an ASA physical status III patient was higher than in ASA grades I and II (0.81% vs. 0.28% reporting incidence). More than two thirds of drug errors (61.5%) were due to substitution and incorrect dosages accounting for two of the largest categories.

PATTERN OF MEDICATION ERRORS

Erdmann et al.[13] studied the consequences and prevalence of medication errors through a questionnaire. Nearly 91.8% respondents acknowledged to medication errors amounting to a mean rate of 4.7% per person. Most of these drug errors occurred due to replacement of the drug for another (68%) followed by dosing errors (49.1%) and omission (35%).

Neuraxial drug errors were reported in only 7% of responses. Most of the errors (47.8%) occurred without any harm to the patient, while 1.75% resulted in severe harm or morbidity. The commonest causes were distraction and fatigue (64.9%) and misreading of syringes, ampoules and labels (54.4%).

In an analysis in Japan over 400,000 anesthetics were analyzed over a 4 year period.[14] They reported an incidence of 18.27 errors per 100,000 anesthetics. Drug errors led to cardiac arrest in 2.21 per 100,000 anesthetics. Their analysis showed that maximum errors happened due to overdose or error in selection of non-anesthetic drugs (42.1%). Other causes included overdose of anesthetics (28.7%), high spinal that was inadvertent (17.9%), toxicity of local anesthetics (6.4%) ampoule or syringe swap (4.3%), and blood mismatch (0.6%). Mortality following these incidents was 0.44/100,000. Highest incidence of such events (88%) were in ASA I and II patients undergoing straight forward surgical procedures and resulted from an overdose or a wrong selection of a nonanesthetic drug.[14] Drugs commonly involved were vasoactive drugs, opioids, muscle relaxants, sedatives and local anesthetics. In a similar analysis, Yamamoto et al.[5] in an 8 year period follow-up of such events investigated drug errors that accounted for 26.2% of the total critical incidents reported. Medication overdosage (25%), substitution (23%) and omission (21%) were the most frequently recorded errors and involved antibiotics and muscle relaxants. A questionnaire directed at practitioners revealed that 85% had experienced a drug error or at least a near miss. Majority of such errors (n = 1038,98%) were of minor consequence but four deaths were also reported. Commonest errors reported were a swap of relaxants instead of reversal agents. Choosing a wrong syringe or 'swapping' (70.4%) and misreading labels (46.8%) were most commonly involved. Majority of anesthesiologists (97.6%) reported 'reading' the label most of the time although they felt that the color of the label was also an indicator. More than 50% of them felt they would report the error, if a reporting program existed and most agreed that there should be better standards for drug labels.[15]

Sakaguchi et al.[4] in the same year published his study of 64,285 cases where wrong medication was the most common type of drug error (48%). Administering an overdose (38%), underdosing (4%), omission (2%), and incorrect administration route (8%) were the common reported errors. Drugs most frequently implicated were opioids, cardiac stimulants, and vasopressors. Syringe swap occurred in 42%, drug ampoule swap occurred in 33%, and the wrong choice of drug was made in 17% amongst reported drug errors. Overdose resulted from misunderstanding the dose (53%), incorrect pump use (21%) and dilution error (5%). The most common error reported by Zhang et al.[3] was however, omission and it is possible that an omission is less likely to be admitted as an error by the anesthesiologist.

In a study evaluating the ability of anesthesiologists to correctly calculate the infusion dose for children, only 15% could provide correct calculations. The extent of drug errors varied from drug concentrations 50 times too low up to 56 times too high.[16] Errors arising out of wrong dose preparations were found to deviate significantly from the desired concentration.[17]

LOOK-ALIKE, SOUND-ALIKE (LASA) AND SIMILAR PACKAGING

Accidental injection of potassium chloride instead of sodium bicarbonate is reported in a patient undergoing coronary artery bypass graft (CABG) resulting in hyperkalemic arrest due to similar looking ampoules of drugs.[18] At our institution, the accidental use of succinylcholine instead of midazolam at the time of sedation due to similar vials has occurred. Another situation involving look alike drugs occurred when mannitol bottle was mistaken for normal saline during caudal injection. Administration of wrong drugs in intrathecal and epidural spaces can result in grave consequences. Accidental intrathecal injection of potassium chloride mistaken for bupivacaine had presented with seizures and myoclonus although this patient was treated with lavage and had a complete recovery.[19] Tranexamic acid has been administered accidentally intrathecally instead of bupivacaine due to similar looking vials of the drugs with no lasting effects.[20,21] The accidental infusion of paracetamol into the epidural space in a 45-year-old woman has also been reported.[22]

ERROR PREVENTION IN THEATER SETTING

The traditional methods of drug administration in anesthesia are highly prone to error given the human factors involved. The need for new systems and technology to assist and organize anesthetic drug delivery has been recognized. Jensen et al.[23] in 2004 had suggested measures based upon one general and five evidence-based strategies to reduce the incidence of drug errors in anesthetic practice. Countermeasures mandate that the label on any drug or ampoule must be carefully read before a drug is drawn up or injected.

Optimization of the legibility and label content should be in accordance to agreed standards, syringes should always be labeled, formal organization of drug drawers and workspaces that allow prepositioned site for drugs should be practiced. Recommendations are for drug labels to be checked by a second person or with device before a drug is drawn up or administered.

Khan SA[24] used a prototype device that resulted in safe drug administration behavior amongst experienced anesthetists. This required the user to scan the drug to generate a label for the syringe and secondly scan the labeled syringe with a bar code scanner. The name of drug intended was checked twice before use thereby eliminating opportunities for error arising from similar looking syringes or ampoules.

The anesthesia patient safety foundation (APSF)[25] brought forth recommendations to include safety that include the use customized drug trays, standard dilutions of high alert drugs, use of barcode medication administrations (BCMA), use of prefilled syringes and premixed preparations of medicines, and electronic documentation methods for anesthesia record. They found that when users complied with the system's principles, the incidence drug errors reduced by 21%. The foundation also speaks for the establishment of a receptive environment for reporting errors (including near misses) and discussion of lessons learned. The foundation has also recommended to develop a culture of education, understanding, and accountability via curriculum-based medical education activity and to establish a culture of cooperation and recognition between institutions, professional organizations and accreditation agencies.

The American Society of Anesthesiologists (ASA) and International Standards Organisation (ISO) supports the labeling of drugs, meeting specific standards with reference to the color coding, font, label content of vials and ampoules. ASA also introduced bar codes and tall man letters (recommendation to reduce errors between look alike and sound alike medications).

Merry AF[26] recommends using ampoules and vials having preprinted flag labels for syringes, provided the drug dose accuracy has been checked, double checking of drug names on drawing drugs into these syringes, labeling of all lines and catheters and avoiding use of unlabeled syringes and fluid.

Most participants in a study believed that a computerized system to calculate infusion rates, especially in pediatric population was necessary to avoid errors in drug dosing.[16] Newer intravenous fluid delivery systems include the VEINROM[27] (Vasopressors, Emergency drugs, Induction agents, Reversal agents, Opioids and Miscellaneous drugs). In addition to barcoding, color and texture coding and specific labeling, this also has a unique lock and key mechanism, a separate syringe port for each of the separate drug syringes, thus eliminating errors arising out of wrong drugs in infusions.

The European Board of Anaesthesiology[28] recommends that labels never be put on to empty syringes and that syringes should be labeled immediately after the drug has been drawn into them and before they leave the operator's hand. An analysis of use of atropine prefilled syringes (PFS) compared to conventionally filled syringes revealed that even though the former was more costly, the regular use of PFS resulted in a major cost savings by decreasing the medication errors and the related expenses and by preventing the wastage resulting from regularly preparing the drug for all cases.[29] Since the need for new anesthetic drug administration systems were realized, many new systems have been developed.

Webster et al.[30] desiged a method of anesthesia administration with color coding, and labeling of syringes that could reduce medical error. This reduced drug errors in comparison with conventional methods with a relative risk reduction of 35%. Fewer parenteral drug errors occurred with the new system than with conventional methods, a relative reduction of 35%. No major adverse outcomes from these errors were reported with the new system.

A patented multimodal system (SAFER Sleep) was designed to reduce errors in the recording and administration of drugs in anesthesia. This system utilized customized drug trays and purpose designed drug trolley drawers and pre-filled syringes for commonly used anesthetic drugs. This system also incorporated large legible color coded drug labels, a computer that read all barcodes, and a computer touch screen that allowed, automatic auditory and visual verification of selected drugs, computerized anesthetic record, antibiotic administration warning and scanning drug labels. It was compared with the conventional practice in drug administration with a manually compiled anesthetic record. The overall mean rate of drug errors per 100 administrations was 9.1 with the new system (one in 11 administrations) versus 11.69 with conventional methods (one in nine administrations). The reduction in drug errors were however not significant. Drug error rates were lower when both checks incorporated in the new machine were applied, namely scanning bar code. The anesthesia records were also more legible and preferred by the anesthesiologists. Targeted simple, blame free system wide interventions at the proximal level to reduce targeted drug errors have also been found to be effective.

White et al.[31] in order to decrease elevated serum potassium levels post potassium chloride administration devised drug request forms designed to reduce any errors in the drug administration. The introduction of the drug request forms reduced errors of postinfusion elevation of potassium decreased to 0 from 7.7%.

Complex steps involving the programming and setting up of PCA infusions can result in errors in administration of intravenous or epidural infusions.

They are mainly operator-related or machine malfunctioning-related. Data from the US FDA's manufacturer and user facility device experience (MAUDE) database indicate that operator error was the cause in 6.5% of these PCA related events. It appeared that pump misprogramming resulted in 81% errors and 50% patient morbidity. Device malfunction accounted for 76.4% of adverse events.[32-34] Introduction of improved PCA pump designs-based on ergonomic and cognitive engineering principles, the use of barcode technology with safety features incorporated in the pump as well as multimodal postoperative pain management may help in reducing the future incidence and severity of PCA medication error.[34]

An analysis was conducted to systemically evaluate each medication handling process step and score possible failure modes to quantify areas of risk. A set of five targeted counter measures were identified and implemented over 12 months. These included improvements in syringe labeling, standardization of medication organization in the anesthesia workspace and two-provider infusion checks. Reporting improved during the project and continued to remain so. Median medication error rate decreased from 1.56 to 0.95 per 1000 anesthetics delivered.[35]

The University of Washington created the anesthesia medication template (AMT). This was to assess the ability to reduce perioperative medication errors by anesthesia providers. Following its implementation, the mean monthly error rate fell from 1.24 to 0.654 per 1000 reported anesthetic deliveries. The mean monthly error rate of reported swap, preparation, miscalculation, and timing errors also decreased from 0.97 to 0.35 errors per 1000 anesthetics. However, medication errors that resulted in patient harm did not change even after implementation of the AMT.[36]

MEDICATION ERRORS IN THE ICU

Perioperative errors extend to ICU care of patients also. Execution of 80–200 steps are involved in the process of administering one critically ill-patient with a single dose of medication.[37,38] In an ICU environment, this complex process is executed many times over every single day on sick patients who need urgent attention from multidisciplinary professionals. The use of high-risk substances and varied routes of administration is also more prevalent and these events occur in the setting of busy and high-pressure environment. Administration of the drug is fraught with the possibility of drug errors although errors can occur at any point in the process of management. The administration phase is the most critical and can involve timing, omission, incorrect method, route or dose.[39,40] O'Shea claimed that nurses are solely responsible for drug administration, while Armitage and Knapman suggested this task accounts for 40% of nurses' clinical care.[41,42] Incidence of medication errors is most commonly reported in the ICU as errors per 1000 patient days.[43]

Rothschild found that drug therapy errors accounted for 78% of all medical errors in US ICUs, and that patients experienced an average of 1.75 errors a day during their ICU stay. Around 20% of these errors risked patients' lives, while 40% required treatment.[44] Using the method of direct observation for detection, an average of one medical error was documented for every five doses of medication administered, and among medical errors 23% were errors by omission.[45]

The critical care safety study reported an overall rate of 80.5 medication errors associated with harm/1,000 patient-days in medical and coronary-care patients.[44] In the recent worldwide sentinel event evaluation (SEE) study, the rate of parenteral medication errors was 745/1,000 patient-days.[46] With medications given by continuous infusion, the rate was 105/1,000 patient-days.[47]

In an ICU setting, the most frequently reported errors were erroneous infusion rate (40.1%), omission of the drug (14.4%), improper dosing (11.7%) and incorrect timing (13.9%).[48] Intravenous route carries the highest risk of severe adverse effects that are difficult to reverse, while the cardiovascular and gastrointestinal drugs are the most common culprits.[49,50]

LOOPHOLES IN REPORTING OF ERRORS AND HOW TO INCREASE THE REPORTING?

The use of forms to encourage reporting of drug errors may not be always a foolproof option, if we do not have the means to record all the anesthetics delivered. In a system like ours, which is still lacking in automated systems that can process and automatically capture information, it may not be possible to really document all anesthetics delivered, which is needed to assess actual error rates per anesthetic delivered. So until bar coded machines, prefilled syringes and automated solutions are not made available, we can only see the tip of the iceberg. Developing a blame free, noncritical and encouraging environment is also necessary to improve the reporting of such medication errors, if we have to improve.

SYSTEMS IMPROVEMENT IN ICU

Emphasis should be given instead to improve the system factors wherein the work conditions are designed to reduce the risk of errors and also develop a safety culture. The UK Health and Safety Commission defines safety culture as 'the product of individual and group values, attitudes, perceptions, competencies and patterns of behavior that determine the commitment to, and the style and proficiency of, an organization's health and safety management'.[51]

Multiple system-based interventions like computerized physician order entry, changes in work schedules, intravenous systems, staff education, medication reconciliation, pharmacist involvement, protocols and guidelines and support systems for clinical decision-making, have been introduced over the years to prevent medication errors.

However, when these systems were reviewed only computerized physician order entry, staff education, medication reconciliation, and protocols and guidelines (PG) demonstrated any effect in reducing medication errors.[52] Another method to improve the robustness of the system is continuous auditing and evaluation of the quality-of-care against predetermined benchmark indicators that reflect structures, processes, or outcomes. The national or hospital body could ensure surveillance of these indicators. The WHO, European and American and UK position papers and reporting systems are examples of the reporting systems and infrastructure at international and national levels. At a hospital level, medical review boards, voluntary or mandatory reporting systems and auditing serve this purpose. Such processes require the development of a transparent work culture where errors are reported without fear of blame or punitive repercussions and where identification of errors are seen as an opportunity to learn and improve.

MANAGEMENT OF ERRORS IN OPERATION THEATER AND ICU

The two main approaches to managing adverse events are addressing the human and system factors. Human factors involve identifying negligence or incompetence of the operator. If this is present rectifying measures should be instituted and involves focus on improving knowledge and individual training.

System factors focuses on the conditions in which errors occur, and is regarded as a systems failure, or a result of the interaction between human elements, technology and social skills. In this case, prevention considers process restructuring and identification of problems 'hidden' in the system.[53]

The need to make a truthful disclosure of the error to the patient's family remains an ethical imperative. However, surveys conducted show that only 17–30% of physicians inform their patients a medical error has occurred.[54-56] An appropriate time to communicate with the patient's family is when the patients safety and care has been ensured and as soon as possible after the insult. This should be done in a room that allows privacy and a quiet atmosphere for communications. One needs to use simple unambiguous words understood by the lay person. It is important to extend a feeling of sympathy to the patient. The physician should allow sufficient time for questions from the family and record these details in the medical records.

Major adverse outcomes vary from morbidity in the form of disability, increased hospitalization costs to mortality. The impact of major disability and death can be devastating to families and may also erode public confidence in health care services.

CONCLUSION

Anesthesia specialty is vulnerable for perioperative medication errors. Awareness of situations that it could occur and established protocols for drug loading, cross checks and administration could minimize errors. More sophisticated drug administration systems and directed training programs could contribute to reduction in these critical incidents for the future.

ACKNOWLEDGMENT

The authors wish to acknowledge the contributions from Dr Zubair Umer Mohamed, Consultant Intensive Care, towards his contributions on the section on medication errors in the ICU.

REFERENCES

1. James JT. A new, evidence-based estimate of patient harms associated with hospital care. J Patient Saf. 2013;9(3):122-8.
2. Webster CS, Merry AF, Larsson L, et al. The frequency and nature of drug administration error during anaesthesia. Anaesth Intensive Care. 2001;29(5): 494-500.
3. Zhang Y, Dong YJ, Webster CS, et al. The frequency and nature of drug administration error during anaesthesia in a Chinese hospital. Acta Anaesthesiol Scand. 2013;57(2): 158-64.
4. Sakaguchi Y, Tokuda K, Yamaguchi K, et al. Incidence of anesthesia-related medication errors over a 15-year period in a university hospital. Fukuoka Igaku Zasshi. 2008;99(3):58-66.

5. Yamamoto M, Ishikawa S, Makita K. Medication errors in anesthesia: an 8-year retrospective analysis at an urban university hospital. J Anesth. 2008;22(3):248-52.
6. Kothari D, Gupta S, Sharma C, et al. Medication error in anaesthesia and critical care: A cause for concern. Indian J Anaesth. 2010;54(3):187-92.
7. Pronovost PJ, Thompson DA, Holzmueller CG, et al. Defining and measuring patient safety. Crit Care Clin. 2005;21(1):1-19.
8. Nanji KC, Patel A, Shaikh S, et al. Evaluation of perioperative medication errors and adverse drug events. Anesthesiology. 2016;124(1):25-34.
9. Brennan TA, Leape LL, Laird NM, et al. Incidence of adverse events and negligence in hospitalized patients: results of the Harvard medical practice study I. 1991. Qual Saf Health Care. 2004;13(2):145-51; discussion 151-2.
10. Cooper L, Digiovanni N, Schultz L, et al. Influences observed on incidence and reporting of medication errors in anesthesia. Can J Anaesth 2012;59(6):562-70.
11. Llewellyn RL, Gordon PC, Wheatcroft D, et al. Drug administration errors: a prospective survey from three South African teaching hospitals. Anaesth Intensive Care. 2009;37(1):93-8.
12. Khan FA, Hoda MQ. Drug related critical incidents. Anaesthesia. 2005;60(1):48-52.
13. Erdmann TR, Hamilton J, Garcia S, et al. Profile of drug administration errors in anesthesia among anesthesiologists from Santa Catarina. Rev Bras Anestesiol. 2016;66(1):105-10.
14. Irita K, Tsuzaki K, Sawa T, et al. Subcommittee on surveillance of anesthesia-related critical incidents. Critical incidents due to drug administration error in the operating room: an analysis of 4,291,925 anesthetics over a 4 year period. Masui. 2004;53(5): 577-84.
15. Orser BA, Chen RJB, Yee DA. Medication errors in anesthetic practice: a survey of 687 practitioners. Can J Anesth 2001;48(2):139-46.
16. Avidan A, Levin PD, Weissman C, et al. Anesthesiologists' ability in calculating weight-based concentrations for pediatric drug infusions: an observational study. J Clin Anesth. 2014;26(4):276-80.
17. Stucki C, Sautter A-M, Wolff A, et al. Accuracy of preparation of IV medication syringes for anesthesiology. Am J Heal Pharm. 2013;70(2):137-42.
18. Kumar A, Gupta K, Gupta M, et al. Fatal drug errors in anaesthesia: can we override? Indian J Anaesth. 2014;58(6):785-6.
19. Dias J, Lages N, Marinho A, et al. Accidental spinal potassium chloride injection successfully treated with spinal lavage. Anaesthesia. 2014;69(1):72-6.
20. Butala B, Bhosale G, Shah V, et al. Medication error: subarachnoid injection of tranexamic acid. Indian J Anaesth. 2012;56(2):168.
21. Mohseni K, Jafari A, Nobahar MR, et al. Polymyoclonus seizure resulting from accidental injection of tranexamic acid in spinal anesthesia. Anesth Analg. 2009;108(6):1984-6.
22. Charco Roca LM, Ortiz Sánchez VE, del Pino Moreno AL. Inadvertent epidural infusion of paracetamol. Rev Esp Anestesiol Reanim. 2014;61(8):457-9.
23. Jensen LS, Merry AF, Webster CS, et al. Evidence-based strategies for preventing drug administration errors during anaesthesia. Anaesthesia. 2004;59(5):493-504.
24. Khan SA, Khan S, Kothandan H. Simulator evaluation of a prototype device to reduce medication errors in anaesthesia. Anaesthsia. 2016;71(10):1186-90.
25. APSF Hosts Medication Safety Conference Consensus Group Defines Challenges and Opportunities for Improved Practice. http://www.apsf.org/newsletters/html/2010/spring/01_conference.htm. Accessed June 16, 2017.
26. Merry AF, Shipp DH, Lowinger JS. The contribution of labeling to safe medication administration in anesthetic practice. Best Pract Res Clin Anaesthesiol. 2011;25(2): 145-59.
27. Tewari A, Palm B, Hines T, et al. VEINROM: A possible solution for erroneous intravenous drug administration. J Anaesthesiol Clin Pharmacol. 2014;30:263-6.

28. Whitaker D, Brattebo G, Trenkler S, et al. European Section and Board of Anaesthesiology of the UEMS. The European Board of Anaesthesiology recommendations for safe medication practice. Eur J Anaesthesiol. 2017;34(1):4-7.
29. Benhamou D, Piriou V, De Vaumas C, et al. Ready-to-use pre-filled syringes of atropine for anaesthesia care in French hospitals — a budget impact analysis. Anaesth Crit Care Pain Med. 2017;36(2):115-21.
30. Webster CS, Larsson L, Frampton CM, et al. Clinical assessment of a new anesthetic drug administration system: a prospective, controlled, longitudinal incident monitoring study. Anaesthesia. 2010;65(5):490-9.
31. White JRM, Veltri MA, Fackler JC. Preventing adverse events in the pediatric intensive care unit: prospectively targeting factors that lead to intravenous potassium chloride order errors. Pediatr Crit Care Med. 2005;6(1):25-31.
32. Hicks RW, Sikirica V, Nelson W, et al. Medication errors involving patient-controlled analgesia. Am J Heal Pharm. 2008;65(5):429-40.
33. Hankin CS, Schein J, Clark JA, et al. Adverse events involving intravenous patient-controlled analgesia. Am J Heal Pharm. 2007;64(14):1492-9.
34. Schein JR, Hicks RW, Nelson WW, et al. Patient-controlled analgesia-related medication errors in the postoperative period: causes and prevention. Drug Saf. 2009;32(7):549-59.
35. Martin LD, Grigg EB, Verma S, et al. Outcomes of a failure mode and effects analysis for medication errors in pediatric anesthesia. Cravero J, ed. Pediatr Anesth. 2017;27(6):571-80.
36. Grigg EB, Martin LD, Ross FJ, et al. Assessing the impact of the anesthesia medication template on medication errors during anesthesia. Anesth Analg. 2017;124(5):1617-25.
37. Pharmacy-nursing shared vision for safe medication use in hospitals: executive summary session. Am J Health Syst Pharm. 2003;60:1046-52.
38. Bates DW, Cullen DJ, Laird N, et al. The ADE prevention study group. Systems analysis of adverse drug events. JAMA. 1995;274:35-43.
39. Krahenbuhl-Melcher A, Schilienger R, Lampert M, et al. Drug-related problems in hospital: a review of the recent literature. Drug Safety. 2007;30(5):379-407.
40. Bowdle T. Drug administration errors from the ASA closed claims project. ASA Newsletter. 2004;67(6):11-3.
41. O'Shea E. Factors contributing to medication errors: a literature review. J Clin Nur. 1999;8:496-504.
42. Armitage G, Knapman H. Adverse events in drug administration: a literature review. J Nur Manag. 2003;11(2):130-40.
43. Garrouste-Orgeas M, Timsit JF, Vesin A, et al. OUTCOMEREA Study Group. Selected medical errors in the intensive care unit: results of the IATROREF study: parts I and II on behalf of the Outcomerea study group. Am J Respir Crit Care Med. 2010;181:134-42.
44. Rothschild JM, Landrigan CP, Cronin JW, et al. The critical care safety study: The incidence and nature of adverse events and serious medical errors in intensive care. Crit Care Med. 2005;33:1694-700.
45. Kopp BJ, Erstad BL, Allen ME, et al. Medication errors and adverse drug events in an intensive care unit: direct observation approach for detection. Crit Care Med. 2006; 34:415-25.
46. Valentin A, Capuzzo M, Guidet B, et al. Research group on quality improvement of European Society of Intensive Care Medicine; Sentinel events evaluation study investigators. Patient safety in intensive care: results from the multinational Sentinel events evaluation (SEE) study. Inten Care Med. 2006;32:1591-98.
47. Herout PM, Erstad BL. Medication errors involving continuously infused medications in a surgical intensive care unit. Crit Care Med. 2004;32:428-32.
48. Calabrese AD, Erstad BL, Brandl K, et al. Medication administration errors in adult patients in the ICU. Intensive Care Med. 2001;27:1592-8.

49. Di Simone E, Tartaglini D, Fiorini S, et al. Medication errors in intensive care units: nurses' training needs. Emergency Nurse. 2016;24(4):24-9. Available from https://doi.org/10.7748/en.2016.11577 (Accessed 20 June 2017).
50. MacFie CC, Baudouin SV, Messer PB. An integrative review of drug errors in critical care. J Inten Care Soc. 2016;17(1):63-72.
51. Gadd S, Collins A. Safety culture: a review of the literature. 2002. Available from http://www.hse.gov.uk/research/hsl_pdf/2002/hsl02-25.pdf (Accessed 20 June 2017).
52. Manias E, Williams A, Liew D. Interventions to reduce medication errors in adult intensive care: a systematic review. Br J Clin Pharmacol. 2012;74(3):411-23.
53. Ministry of Health (2004). Risk Management in Health. The Problem of Errors. www.salute.gov.it/imgs/c_17_pubblicazioni_583_allegato.pdf (Last accessed: 16 June 2016.)
54. Gallagher TH, Waterman AD, Ebers AG, et al. Patients' and physicians' attitudes regarding the disclosure of medical errors. JAMA. 2003;289:1001-7.
55. Blendon RJ, DesRoches CM, Brodie M, et al. Views of practicing physicians and the public on medical errors. N Engl J Med. 2002;347:1933-40.
56. Lehmann LS, Puopolo AL, Shaykevich S, et al. Iatrogenic events resulting in intensive care admission: frequency, cause, and disclosure to patients and institutions. Am J Med. 2005;118:409-13.

CHAPTER 22

Prognostication after Cardiac Arrest

Suman D Chaudhry, Murali Pandurangan

KEY POINTS

- High-quality cardiopulmonary resuscitation (CPR), early defibrillation, targeted temperature management (TTM) and early coronary revascularization have been in prominence of attention from the perspective of cerebral vulnerability ensuing cardiac arrest.
- Despite best convention and adherence to latest guidelines, many patients submit to hypoxic-ischemic brain injury (HIBI) and post cardiac arrest syndrome as primary reasons for mortality and poor long-term prognosis.
- Regional heterogeneity produces different brain injury phenotypes and secondary injuries described as "Two Hit" model consequent to return of spontaneous circulation (ROSC).
- Prohibition of secondary injury remains the most crucial determinant of ultimate outcome nevertheless it is superimposed on different patient characteristics and prevailing individual comorbidities.
- In depth understanding of pathophysiology of CA along with serum biomarker assays in last 2 years is a new paradigm in prognostication. This is adopted for stratification and targeted therapies for patients with HIBI.
- Delayed multimodal neurologic prognostication and post acute care are evidence-based interventions pivotal to affirmative and acclamatory neurologic outcomes; early neurologic prognostication can substantially contribute to avoidable mortality and premature withdrawal of life supporting treatment.
- Various new scoring systems applicable from immediate post ROSC phase up until rehabilitation help stratify patients for management strategy and prognosis.

INTRODUCTION

New clinical evidences and the use of better technology in the practice of resuscitation and post resuscitation care have played an important role in the overall outcome of patient suffering cardiac arrest. The awareness of resuscitation amongst the public, use of automated defibrillators and enrolling wider members of the hospital on resuscitation courses have augmented the efforts to improve outcome. Better understanding the pathophysiology of phase following return of spontaneous circulation (ROSC) has enabled clinicians in prognosticating the patients. Multimodal approach combining clinical examination with other diagnostic methods, consisting of electrophysiology, blood biomarkers and brain imaging improves the accuracy. Proper multimodal assessment of coma is critical to avoid premature withdrawal of life support resulting in death.

The pattern of brain injury that remains after intensive care varies from mild to severe, with some brain regions being particularly susceptible despite the best possible management.

Cardiac arrest, a disastrous event, is associated with mortality rates more than 90%.[1] Out of the 28,000 cases of out of hospital cardiac arrest resuscitated by the Emergency Medical Services in England only 20% patients were in a shockable rhythm at the time of arrival of the EMS.[2] Shockable rhythm was found to have a better outcome. The 2017 census in United States (2017) revealed that out-of-hospital cardiac arrest constitutes 80 patients per 100,000 persons every year. The advances in resuscitation techniques have not improved the outcome in a big way. Only 10% of patients survive until hospital discharge while only 5% experience full neurologic recovery.[3]

Certain interventions improve survival rates from out of hospital cardiac arrest, the main being bystander cardiopulmonary resuscitation (CPR). CPR restores circulation to vital organs and increases the chances of the heart to remain in a shockable rhythm rather than deteriorating to a non-shockable rhythm. This increases the probability of patients being defibrillated soon after. Thus, delivering effective CPR promptly is crucial both until defibrillator arrives and subsequent to successful defibrillation. The principle assigns to both in-hospital and OHCA.

The Department of Health in the cardiovascular disease outcomes strategy (2013) identified that the Resuscitation Council (UK), the British Heart Foundation and NHS England have made improving survival rates from out of hospital cardiac arrest as their prority.[2] After achieving return of spontaneous circulation following successful resuscitation after CA, the crucial factor that determines the prognosis is the severity of post-cardiac arrest syndrome and hypoxic ischemic brain injury (HIBI).[3] These are pathophysiological changes characterized by myocardial dysfunction, systemic ischemia/reperfusion response and brain injury.[4,5] The cause of CA, the duration of the CA and the extent of the ischemic injury determine the severity of the disorders. Bearing this causative factor, the concept of cardiocerebral resuscitation (CCR) was introduced in 2009.[6,7]

Cardiocerebral resuscitation consists of three components. First one is the continuous or uninterrupted chest compressions or CPR from bystanders. The second is a different and more effective Advanced Cardiac Life Support (ACLS) algorithm for Emergency Medical System. The third is the post-resuscitation care. Resuscitation Guidelines UK and ACLS (Advanced Cardiac Life support) guidelines 2015 stress on these three components. The post ROSC care affirms therapeutic hypothermia or targeted temperature management (TTM) and early cardiac catheterization/intervention. Patients are deeply sedated, paralyzed and cooled and prognostication done at varied intervals subsequently.

PATHOPHYSIOLOGY OF CARDIAC ARREST

Hypoxic ischemic brain injury after cardiac arrest leads to pathophysiological changes which have been described as 'two-hit model'. The 'two-hit model consists of a primary and secondary injury (Fig. 1).[3] Similar to the head injury management protocol the primary injury is nonreversible while the secondary injury which results from cerebral reperfusion is potentially reversible. The brain is extremely sensitive to hypoxia and the cessation of cerebral oxygen delivery encroaches on neuronal oxygen reserves within 20 seconds of circulatory arrest,

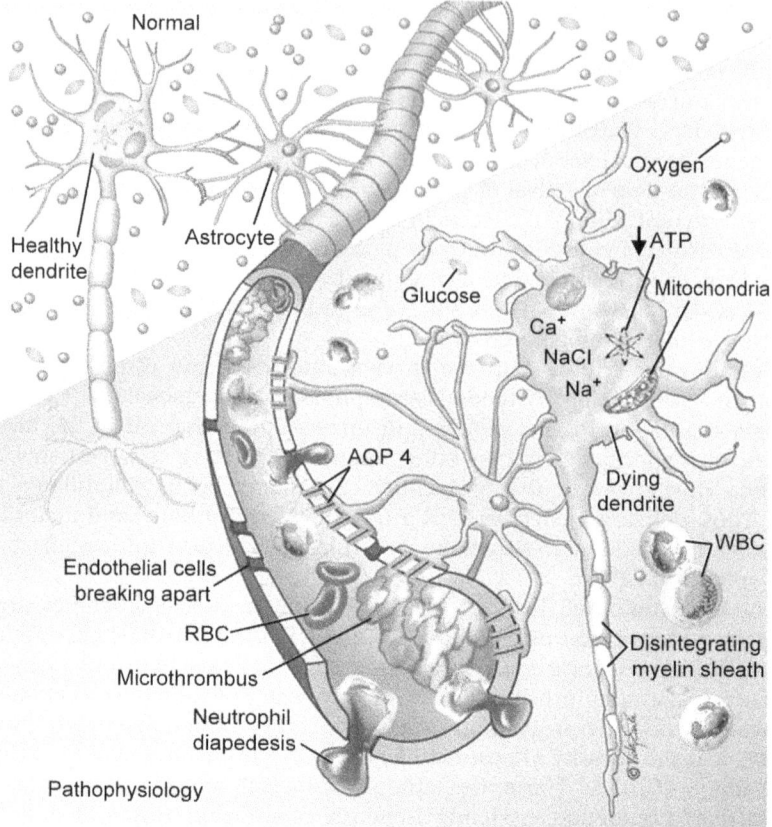

Fig. 1: Microvascular and cellular pathophysiological changes seen during the primary and secondary injury in hypoxic ischemic brain injury (HIBI).
(AQP 4: Aquaporin-4; RBC: Red blood cells; WBC: White blood cells).

with resultant neuron ischemia and cell death. This culminates in altered sensorium or unconsciousness.[8] The cerebrum is dependent on the cardiac output for supply of nutrients. Nearly 20 to 25% of cardiac output is required to maintain normal function of brain.[3] Activation of harmful protease cascades, calcium homeostasis disturbance, free radical formation, and cell death signaling mechanisms are due to depletion of ATP stores. Early resuscitation along with use of automatic defibrillators and insertion of implantable cardioverter defibrillators have helped in limiting primary injury. Ironically restoration of cerebral blood flow via successful resuscitation causes ATP regeneration with devastating further free radical formation and the secondary cerebral injury.[8]

Secondary injury of HIBI could take place within hours of resuscitation and days following the initial cardiac arrest and reperfusion. Cell death continues to happen due to apoptosis and necrosis. Cerebral autoregulation is impaired and cerebral edema develops with continuing inflammatory processes leading to further neuronal dysfunction.[9] The cerebrovascular endothelium function is now disrupted, and biomarkers of cerebrovascular endothelial injury are released into circulation.[10] Incidentally this ischemia/reperfusion response is just not confined to brain but extends throughout the body like systemic inflammatory response syndrome (SIRS). Biomarkers from the pathophysiological reactions can be detected after cardiac arrest and are associated with adverse outcomes in HIBI. These are also indicators of the severity of injury and predictors of long-term outcomes.[11] They add to the list of most recent prognostic indicators and is dealt with later in this chapter.

Systematic approach of prognosticating patients comprises of evaluating at scene of cardiac arrest; after ROSC; periodically after admission to the critical care and during long-term rehabilitation. What is often obliterated by the critical care and treating physicians is the founded fact that the ongoing pathophysiological mechanisms of HIBI[12] are overcast on the background of patient's usual health, concomitant physiology, comorbidities and bodily functional reserve.

Every single patient who suffers cardiac arrest would score differently when all above stated factors are considered. This score would determine the extent and quality of post-resuscitation care and prognostication. Based on this ideology several scoring systems have evolved over years. Only the recent ones are discussed in this chapter and they reinforce the multimodal paradigm of prognostication of cardiac arrest survivors.

NEUROLOGICAL OUTCOME AFTER CARDIAC ARREST

In prognostication studies, investigators usually dichotomize neurological outcome as good or poor. The cerebral performance categories (CPC) 4 or 5 corresponds to vegetative state or death respectively, and represent a poor outcome.[13] Most trials to date have relied on gross measures of functional or neurologic impairment such as modified Rankin Scale Score (mRS) or cerebral performance category (CPC) as a primary outcome.[14] In awake patients, CPC and mRS represent different aspects of functional recovery across levels, and are influenced not only by the severity of illness, but also by environmental and personal factors that modify the interplay between neurologic disability (e.g. arm paresis), ability to carry out activities of daily living, and ability to return to work. Most of the studies conducted after 2005 include CPC 3 among poor outcomes and dichotomize CPC as 1–2 vs. 3–5.[15, 16]

A CPC = 5 does not necessarily coincides with a poor neurological outcome at the time of death when no distinction is made between death due to neurological causes, as brain death, and death due other causes such as cardiac arrhythmias or multiorgan failure. To avoid this dilemma, when reporting neurological outcome, the best CPC achieved during the patient's hospital stay should be reported.[15] It is important to recognize that most of the deaths due to severe brain injury occur indirectly, i.e. because of withdrawal of life sustaining treatment (WLST). The exact cause of death, as neurological, cardiac. renal, sepsis, MODS or other should be reported clearly for medicolegal reasons.[15] Prognostication in patients treated with controlled temperature may result in action of sedative agents and muscle relaxants to be prolonged, hence residual effects must be excluded.[17]

MULTIMODAL PARADIGM OF PROGNOSTICATION

Under the multimodal paradigm, clinical examination is combined with other investigations for accuracy of prognostication. Clinical examination reveals vital and immediate information on the prognosis of patients following cardiac arrest. It should involve assessment of Glasgow Coma Score, pupillary response to light, corneal reflex, and presence of seizures. Biochemical markers have gained importance recently. Neuron Specific Serum Enolase (NSE) and other biomarkers are used to help to assess outcome in cardiac arrest patients with hypoxic ischemic brain injury and SIRS. Advanced bedside neurophysiological studies such as somatosensory evoked potentials (SSEPs) and electroencephalography (EEG) can give valuable information within short time. These predictors have the highest specificity and less than 5% false positive results with 95% confidences interval of less than 5% in patients treated with controlled temperature and have been documented in more than 5 studies from at least three different groups of investigators.

Clinical Examination

Clinical examination during the initial 72 hours may reveal findings which may be secondary to recovery from the cardiac arrest, prolonged actions of the resuscitation drugs and due to hypothermia. Absence of bilateral pupillary light reflex at 72 hours following ROSC predicts poor outcome. To avoid interobserver variation pupillary size should be measured quantitatively with the help of pupilometer.[18] Pupillary reaction is a very specific sign with a false positive result of 0% and the sensitivity is about 19% in predicting bad outcome. Only 20% of patients will have fixed dilated pupils by 72 hours.[19] Absence of corneal reflex also follows similar pattern of presentation as the pupillary reaction.[20]

Absence of motor response or an extensor motor response to pain following ROSC is very sensitive in predicting the poor outcome. This high sensitivity makes it a valuable clinical assessment to predict the neurological status and help triage patients. A 75% sensitivity makes it a good tool for screening but the false positive rate of 27% makes it less reliable. It can be used in conjunction with other clinical findings in improving the prognostication of the patient's outcome.

Neuromuscular blocking drugs suppress the motor response to the reflexes. It is mandatory to rule out effects of neuromuscular drugs before eliciting the corneal and motor responses.[21] Prolonging observation of these clinical signs beyond 72 h from ROSC should be standardized to minimize the risk of obtaining false positive results.

Myoclonus[22] is described as sudden, brief, involuntary jerks caused by muscular contractions or inhibitions. Status myoclonus is a prolonged duration of continuous and generalized myoclonic jerks. The presence of myoclonic jerks after ROSC is not always associated with poor outcome (FPR 9%). Onset of status myoclonus starting within 48 hours after resuscitation is closely associated with a poor prognosis (FPR 0% [95% confidence interval (CI) 0–5%]; sensitivity 8–16%). It is important to assess patients after the influence of the sedative medicines are ruled out. EEG recording can be useful to identify signs of awareness, reactivity and diagnose coexistent epileptiform activity.

Thus, predictors of poor outcome based on clinical examination are inexpensive, easy to use but potentially subject to interobserver bias. They are often unreliable in the first 2–3 days after resuscitation. In therapeutic hypothermia (TH)-treated patients' examination is usually postponed until rewarming and cessation of sedation 72 hours after ROSC. In both therapeutic hypothermia treated and non-therapeutic hypothermia treated patients the most accurate clinical-based predictor at ≥72 hours from ROSC is the absence of pupillary reflex to light with false positive result of 0%. Absence of pupillary reflex with false positive result up to 5% is more specific than absence of corneal reflex.

Electroencephalography

Changes in EEG could be mere absence of EEG reactivity. The absence of background reactivity to a loud noise or a painful stimulus such as tracheal suction suggests a dismal outcome. Absence of EEG background reactivity is a highly specific in predicting poor outcome with a FPR of 0–2% (upper 95% CI of about 7%).[23] Standardization of stimulus and reduction in inter-observer variability will overcome the limitation of EEG reactivity.

Status Epilepticus

When patients develop status epilepticus in therapeutic temperature management (TTM) treated patients it is almost invariably followed by poor outcome (FPR 0–6%). This is further reinforced by presence of an unreactive or discontinuous EEG background.

Burst-Suppression

Burst suppression can be loosely described as an isoelectric line with well separated burst of electrical activity. It is defined as more than 50% of the EEG record consisting of periods of EEG voltage <10 µV, with alternating bursts. It is a transient finding in comatose survivors of cardiac arrest. Burst-suppression may be compatible with neurological recovery. It is important to assess burst suppression 72 hours after the return of spontaneous circulation. When it is present it is consistently associated with poor outcome. EEG is helpful in comatose survivors of cardiac arrest during therapeutic hypothermia and after rewarming to help assess the level of consciousness, help to detect and treat non-convulsive seizures, which occur in 1 out of 4 comatose survivors of cardiac arrest.

Electrophysiology

Somatosensory evoked potentials (SSEPs) are among the most prevalent and robust predictors in post hypoxic coma. Bilateral absence of the N20 SSEP wave predicts death or vegetative state in post arrest comatose patients with cerebral performance score of 4–5. It invariably predicts poor outcome as early as 24 hours from ROSC in non-TH-treated patients.[4] Bilateral absence of N20 SSEP has been used as a criterion for deciding on withdrawal of life-sustaining treatment (WLST). It has high reliability with false positive ratio 0–2% and upper 95% CI of about 4%. In TH-treated patients SSEP also perform well when recorded after rewarming. The sensitivity of SSEPs is around 50% when recorded after rewarming and only 25% during therapeutic hypothermia (TH). N20 wave may be present during TH and subsequently disappear after rewarming partly in some patients with poor outcome.[4] It is important to maximize signal/noise ratio when recording SSEPs in these patients as the SSEPs are prone to interference coming from muscle contractions and electrical equipment connected to the patient.

Imaging

Imaging studies are not affected by sedation and paralysis and provide a topographic description of hypoxic brain injury. On the downside, their interpretation is more complex, less standardized and subject to interobserver variability. Execution of a MRI is cumbersome in unstable patients. Considering the limited availability of quality literature, caution must be exercised in use of imaging studies for prognostication after cardiac arrest.[24] Currently they are recommended only in centers with that specific experience.

Computer Tomography (CT) of Brain

To exclude further causes of coma brain CT is often performed in resuscitated comatose patients. The CT finding of global anoxic-ischemic cerebral insult following cardiac arrest is cerebral edema and an attenuation of the gray matter/white matter (GM/WM) interface. Cerebral edema appears as a reduction in the depth of cerebral sulci (sulcal effacement). Decreased density of the GM is quantitatively measured as the ratio (GWR) between the GM and the WM densities.[25] The GWR threshold for prediction of poor outcome with 0% FPR in prognostication studies ranged between 1.10 and 1.22.

Magnetic Resonance Imaging (MRI)

In contrast to brain CT, MRI provides a better spatial definition and a high sensitivity for identifying ischemic brain injury (Fig. 2).[26] However, it can be problematic in clinically unstable patients. MRI can reveal extensive changes when SSEPs are normal. All studies on prognostication after cardiac arrest using imaging have a low precision, and a very low quality of evidence.

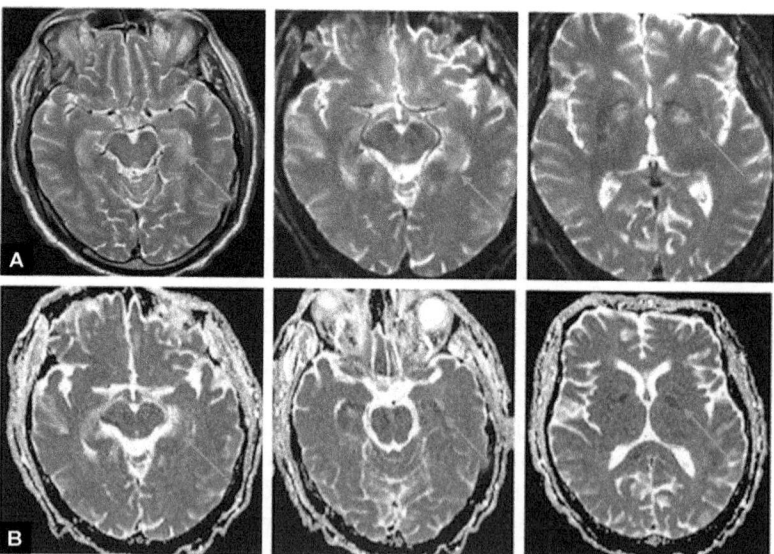

Figs. 2A and B: Magnetic resonance imaging showing focal hypoxic brain insult within subcortical regions of brain after HIBI (both sides) 7 days after ROSC. (A) Shows abnormal signaling in hippocampus and basal ganglia; (B) Diffusion weighted imaging reveals HIBI in Hippocampus and basal ganglia.

To sum up, the following changes in the computerized tomography done 24 hours post-ROSC may call for additional diagnostic interventions, neurology consultation, ICP monitoring or withdrawal of life sustaining treatment: localized or generalized cerebral edema, extra-axial or intraparenchymal hemorrhage, fracture skull or cerebral infarcts requires specialist consultation. Cerebral edema may be evident as reduction in gray-white ratio or effacement of sulci in post resuscitation period. Cerebral ischemic changes in MRI will be evident 2–5 days post resuscitation.

Biomarkers

Biomarkers are peptides and laboratory quantifiable agents used in prognostication of brain injury in comatose survivors of cardiac arrest. Prior to advent of therapeutic hypothermia, NSE (neuron serum-specific enolase) levels above 33 µg/L were considered strongly predictive of poor prognosis with FPR of less than 3%. The selective neuronal injury resulting in decreased NSE levels was discovered by Tiainen et al. making their reliability less accountable in patients not receiving Targeted Temperature Management (TTM).[24,27] Another serum biomarker of brain injury can potentially measure specific damage to astrocytes by S100 beta assays. They have a cut off value ranging from 0.2 to 1.5 mg/L and have been used in combination with NSE.[28]

The level of MAPK3, BCL2, and AKT1 as independent predictors of poor neurological outcome ($P < 0.05$) in early stages of post cardiac resuscitation were discovered by Eun and Yang in 2017.[29] High levels of anti-inflammatory cytokines (IL-1ra, sTNFr-I, and IL-10) had a direct correlation with elevated ICP and worse outcome in secondary injury following head trauma which led to conclusion that anti-inflammatory cytokine levels reflect the severity of neurological insult.[30]

Adrie et al discovered a direct correlation between elevated serum TNF levels, IL8 levels at 12 hours and mortality amongst survivors versus non-survivors post-cardiac arrest[31] (Table 1).

Near Infrared Spectroscopy (NIRS) and Regional Oxygen Saturation (rSVO$_2$)

The reduction in cardiac output, mean arterial blood pressure and deranged cerebral autoregulation after OHCA culminate in cerebral hypoperfusion. The resultant ischemia may be homogenous or heterogeneous and is difficult to quantify. A regional cerebral oxygen saturation monitor (rSVO$_2$) measured

Table 1: Serum levels of biomarkers at ROSC between the survivors and non-survivors			
Biomarker	Survivors (n = 45)	Non-survivors (n = 54)	P value
sCD40L (pg/mL)	7921.88 ± 8499.79	6069.07 ± 8134.92	0.001
IL-8 (pg/mL)	333.57 ± 640.56	1398.44 ± 3856.73	0.002
MDA-LDL (ng/mL)	492.70 ± 2943.99	2915.64 ± 12500.75	0.012
IL-10 (pg/mL)	705.93 ± 1749.59	1225.26 ± 2530.12	0.013
S100B (pg/mL)	607.08 ± 702.96	1128.31 ± 908.02	0.032
MPO (ng/mL)	1310.17 ± 2187.97	1398.88 ± 1607.37	0.053

with near infra-red spectroscopy (NIRS) (Fig. 3) with INVOS, Somantics, Troy, MI which was earlier used in cardiac surgery has its extended application in post ROSC patient. A saturation of 15% or below indicates 'no cerebral cortical perfusion' or level N.[32]

In a prospective study on 132 non-trauma OHCA patients admitted to emergency department none of the 33 patients survived to hospital discharge at 12 hours despite best treatment modalities. All 33 patients showed N value on $rSVO_2$ monitoring via bilateral electrodes placed on forehead within 3 min of admission to ER.[32] Thus, NIRS derived N value is a strong predictor of ultimate outcome in patients with cerebral injury. The advantages lie in it being noninvasive, simple and non-dependent on arterial pulsations and pressure and body temperature. Large trials are required to validate the use of $rSVO_2$ and NIRS in prognosticating OHCA patients.[32]

PROGNOSTICATION IN A TIMEWISE MANNER

Predicting Patient's Chances of Survival after ROSC Post-OHCA

To predict prognosis in the immediate ROSC period, Temple et al. developed two scoring systems namely the PAR (Prognosis after Resuscitation) and OHCA (Out of Hospital Cardiac Arrest Score).[33] While PAR score can be put into clinical practice; the OHCA score is complicated owing to its mathematical calculations. The time to commencement of CPR (no flow); poor quality CPR (low flow); metabolic derangements (lactate) and renal impairment (serum creatinine) are independent variables correlated with poor prognosis. Besides, these factors may be unknown at the time of circulatory arrest.

The PAR score is simple to calculate as tabulated in Table 2 and a cumulative score of 5 is associated with mortality. However, this should never be used to qualify or reject a patient for admission to critical care exclusively on its own merits. It comes handy as an objective assessment tool to help the clinician decide on admission when the clinical presentation is confusing.

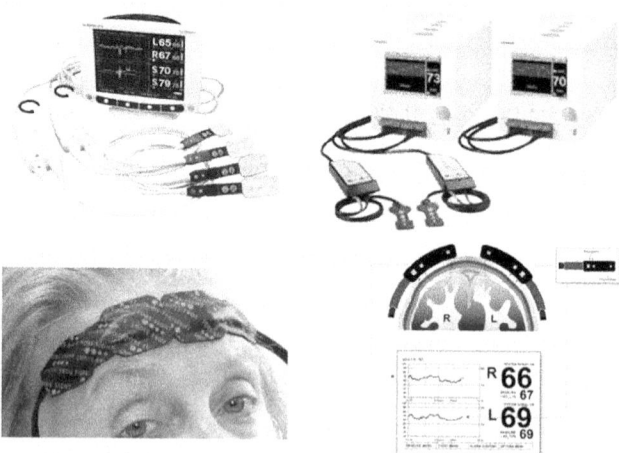

Fig. 3: Near infrared spectroscopy (NIRS) is used noninvasively to perform cerebral oximetry to assess site-specific adequacy of perfusion in the brain beneath its sensors. This enables you to obtain real-time data on regional oxygen saturation (rSO_2).

Table 2: Prognosis after resuscitation (PAR) score

Variables	Scores
Metastatic malignancy	10
Non-metastatic malignancy	3
Sepsis	5
Dependent functional status	5
Pneumonia	3
Creatinine >130 mmol liter−1	3
Age >70 year	2
Acute myocardial infarction	2

A score > 5 indicates non-survival.

Table 3: Independent predictors of a poor outcome at 6 months

Pre-hospital	After hospital admission
Older age	Bilateral absence of corneal and pupillary reflexes
Cardiac arrest occurring at home	
Initial rhythm as non-VF/non T	Glasgow coma scale motor response 1
Longer duration of no flow	Lower pH
Longer duration of low flow	$PaCO_2$ value < 4.5 kPa
Administration of adrenaline	

Predicting Patient's Chances of Survival after ROSC Post-OHCA

Louise Martinell in 2017 identified early factors to evaluate long-term prognosis following ROSC after out of hospital cardiac arrest.[34] The analysis described the state or quality of life of 933 unconscious patients after 6 months duration and classified them into CPC (Cerebral Performance Category Score) of 1–5, 5 being the worst outcome (Table 3). Simple and easy-to-use risk scoring system; patients at high risk for a poor outcome after OHCA may be identified early.

Another study was conducted to triage patients who would have a favorable chance of recovery after developing 'Post Cardiac Arrest Syndrome' but prior to induced hypothermia. A scoring system named PCAS (post-cardiac arrest syndrome) was developed which comprised of 8 factors to correlate with the ultimate neurological outcome.[35] These were initial rhythm (VF/asystole/PEA), whether arrest was witnessed, time to ROSC, pH, serum lactate and gray to white attenuation ratio on CT, hemoglobin and serum albumin. The scoring was both internally and externally validated. Ten independent variables of adverse outcome were identified at this stage. Six of these were linked to pre-hospital admission status and hence were not subject to modification. These were advanced age, Arrest occurring at home or out of hospital, initial rhythm other than VF or VT, long interval to commencement of CPR (No Flow), poor hemodynamic status (Low Flow), administration of epinephrine, presence or absence of pupillary and corneal reflexes, acidosis and low Glasgow coma scale. The CAST score evaluated the 30-day outcome of PCAS patients treated with hypothermia. The prognosis was bad in patients with CAST score of < 15.[36]

Predicting Patient's Chances of Survival in the Critical Care Unit

The CAHP Score helped to triage patients after admission to critical care. Neurological outcome was assessed in 819 patients admitted to ICU subsequent to OHCA.[37] The CAHP Score helps to identify and stratify patients with poor prognosis at an early stage of ICU admission. A scoring system was developed with 7 factors, each having a different weightage between 0 and 100. The seven factors are: age, non-shockable rhythm, time from collapse to basic life support, time from basic life support to return of spontaneous circulation, location of cardiac arrest, epinephrine dose and arterial pH.

Based on the score, three risks groups were identified:

Low-risk	≤ 150	39% chance of unfavorable outcome
Medium-risk	150–200	81% chance of unfavorable outcome
High-risk	≥ 200	100% chance of unfavorable outcome

Thus, the CAHP score represents a simple tool for early stratification of patients admitted in ICU after OHCA.

Long-term Rehabilitation

Heinz and Rollnik in 2015 conducted a study on a large sample size over a long duration.[38] The aim was to see the factors affecting the outcome of 93 patients who had hypoxic brain damage after OHCA but had been successfully resuscitated, managed in hospital and were now undergoing early rehabilitation. The mean length of stay was more than 80 days. On basis of clinical data, validated outcome scales or indexes were formed. There were BI (Barthel Index); ERI (Early remission Index); GCS (Glasgow Coma Scale); CRS (Coma Remission Scale) EEG Neuroimaging, VEP (Visual evoked potential) and SSEP.

The two most important variables affecting outcome from hypoxic brain injury were BI (Barthel Index) and duration of coma. Neuroradiological findings were predictive with direct correlation of bad outcome and hypodensities of basal ganglia. Thus, in line with other neuro-rehabilitation studies, activities of daily living (BI) was a strong predictor of ultimate outcome.

Neurological Prognostication Used in the Targeted Temperature Management Trial

Prognostication should be done on day 5 of cardiac arrest using 36°C core temperature. The protocol should be followed as per TTM Trial.[39] Cooling was done for all patients in TTM trial for minimal period of 72 hours. Prognostication was done upon rewarming for all unconscious patients thereafter. Neurological examination comprised of Glasgow Coma scoring; pupillary and corneal reflexes, SSEP and EEG. It is advisable to perform TTM at 36°C for cardiac arrest survivors. Prognosticate at day 5 post-cardiac arrest; Use the protocol as otherwise described in the TTM trial.

All patients should be actively treated until a minimum 72 hours after the intervention period, i.e. after rewarming, when neurological evaluation should be done on patients not regaining consciousness. Exceptions from this rule are given further.

1. Patients with myoclonus status in the first 24 hours after admission and a bilateral absence of N20-peak on median nerve somatosensory evoked potentials (SSEP).
2. Patients who are declared brain dead due to cerebral herniation.
3. Have advance directive or ethical reasons example for instance: previously unknown information about disseminated end-stage cancer or refractory shock with end-stage multiorgan failure.

At this point of time limitations in and withdrawal of active treatment could be instituted by the critical care physicians in conjunction with primary physician or the admitting physician. A multidisciplinary team discussion should be held along with next of kin and other members of staff and decision to discontinue or limit management be appropriately documented. In UK, it has become mandatory to fill in Withdrawal of Treatment Form/Do not escalate treatment Form/Do not Resuscitate Form as a part of medicolegal framework after such multidisciplinary team meetings. All forms need to be signed by two senior doctors preferably Consultants in presence of witnesses. Such improvisations have saved NHS from having to pay millions in judicial enquiries and future compensations to next of kin. A summarized approach ennumerating the poor prognostic indicators has been shown in Figure 4.

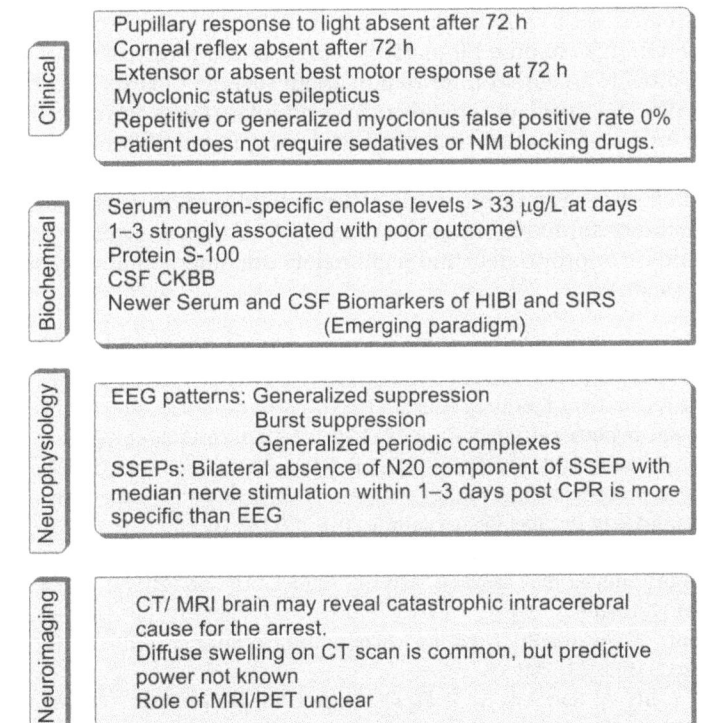

Fig. 4: Poor prognostic neurological features and indicators post-cardiac arrest.

Confounding Factors

- *Induced hypothermia*: Majority of studies have been carried out before induced hypothermia was widely used. There is evidence that cooling may alter interpretation of these results, but to what extent remains unclear.
- *Time of assessment:* Period of at least 72 hours post CPR is recommended. CT scan done too early may not show changes.
- *Use of sedatives and neuromuscular blockers.*
- *Metabolic derangements:* Presence of shock and organ failure are few of the important confounding factors.

CONCLUSION

Until 2015, advanced cardiac life support (ACLS) and European Resuscitation guidelines focused primarily to achieve ROSC in minimum possible time after OHCA. Thereafter in-depth advances in discovering heterogenic pathophysiological mechanisms due to 'no Flow' or 'low flow' state during cardiac arrest and release of Serum Biomarkers from brain to systemic circulation were made. These mechanisms were central to hypoxic ischemic brain injury (HIBI) and post arrest cardiac syndrome (PACS), the two main causes of mortality or unfavorable outcomes in survivors of cardiac arrest. The novel assay techniques of monitoring these biomarkers were also pivotal to prognosticate patients for their predicted outcome. Prognostication must commence very early on after ROSC (Return of spontaneous circulation), should be multimodal (Fig. 4) and be substantiated with various scoring systems during post resuscitation phase as discussed in this chapter. Biomarkers represent the future of prognostication since they provide an earlier information about severity of HIBI and other organ dysfunctions. The specialty is still in its primitive stages nevertheless seems promising for future. Cerebral oximetry has been validated on smaller scale and is awaiting large prospective trials and analysis, assessment and scoring must be done at all stages right from scene of arrest to long-term rehabilitation and a multidisciplinary approach should be made to withdraw or limit treatment. The latter should be appropriately and legitimately documented and signed by two senior physicians.

REFERENCES

1. Taccone F, Cronberg T, Friberg H, et al. How to assess prognosis after cardiac arrest and therapeutic hypothermia. Crit Care. 2014;18:202. DOI: 10.1186/cc13696.
2. Gräsner JT, Lefering R, Koster RW, et al. EuReCa ONE-27 Nations, ONE Europe, ONE Registry: A prospective one month analysis of out-of-hospital cardiac arrest outcomes in 27 countries in Europe. Resuscitation. 2016;105:188-95.
3. Sekhon MS, Ainslie PN, Griesdale DE. Clinical pathophysiology of hypoxic ischemic brain injury after cardiac arrest: a "two-hit" model. Crit Care. 2017;21:90 DOI: 10.1186/s13054-017-1670-9.
4. Sandroni C, Geocadin RG. Neurological prognostication after cardiac arrest. Curr Opin Crit Care. 2015;21(3):209-14.
5. Mosier J, Itty A, Sanders A, et al. Cardiocerebral resuscitation is associated with improved survival and neurologic outcome from out-of-hospital cardiac arrest in elders. Acad Emerg Med. 2010;17(3):269-75.

6. Ewy GA, Kern KB. Recent advances in cardiopulmonary resuscitation: cardiocerebral resuscitation. J Am Coll Cardiol. 2009;53(2):149-57.
7. Imberti R, Bellinzona G, Riccardi F, et al. Cerebral perfusion pressure and cerebral tissue oxygen tension in a patient during cardiopulmonary resuscitation. Intensive Care Med. 2003;29(6):1016-19.
8. Madathil RJ, Hira RS, Stoeckl M, et al. Ischemia reperfusion injury a modifiable therapeutic target for cardioprotection or neuroprotection in patients undergoing cardiopulmonary resuscitation. Resuscitation. 2016;105:85-91.
9. Bro-Jeppesen J, Johansson PI, Hassager C, et al. Endothelial activation/injury and associations with severity of post-cardiac arrest syndrome and mortality after out-of-hospital cardiac arrest. Resuscitation. 2016;107:71-9.
10. Nolan JP, Neumar RW, Adrie C, et al. Post-cardiac arrest syndrome: epidemiology, pathophysiology, treatment, and prognostication a scientific statement from the international liaison committee on resuscitation; the American Heart Association emergency cardiovascular care committee; the Council on Cardiovascular Surgery and Anesthesia; the Council on Cardiopulmonary, Prioperative, and Critical Care; the Council on Clinical Cardiology; the Council on Stroke. Resuscitation. 2008;79(1):350-79.
11. Sandroni C, Geocadin RG. Neurological prognostication after cardiac arrest. Curr Opin Crit Care. 2015;21(3):209-14.
12. Elmer J, Callaway CW. The brain after cardiac arrest. Semin Neurol. 2017;37(1): 019-024.
13. Raina K, Holm MB, Kim YJ, et al. Association between cerebral performance category, modified Rankin scale, and discharge disposition after cardiac arrest. Resuscitation. 2011;82:1036-40.
14. Fugate JE, Wijdicks EF, Mandrekar J, et al. Predictors of neurologic outcome in hypothermia after cardiac arrest. Ann Neurol. 2010;68:907-14.
15. Sandroni C, Geocadin RG. Neurological prognostication after cardiac arrest. Curr Opin Crit Care. 2015;21:209-14.
16. Greer DM. Unexpected good recovery in a comatose post-cardiac arrest patient with poor prognostic features. Resuscitation. 2013;84:e81-e82.
17. Golan E, Barrett K, Alali AS, et al. Predicting neurologic outcome after targeted temperature management for cardiac arrest: systematic review and meta-analysis. Crit Care Med. 2014;42:1919-30.
18. Couret D, Boumaza D, Grisotto C, et al. Reliability of standard pupillometry practice in neurocritical care: an observational, double-blinded study. Critical Care. 2016;20:99 DOI 10.1186/s13054-016-1239-z.
19. Matthews E, Bernstein JM. Prognostic value of the neurological exam in cardiac arrest patients treated with therapeutic hypothermia (S46.008). Neurology. 2016;86 (no. 16 Supplement) S 46.008.
20. Taccone FS, Cronberg T, Friberg H, et al. How to assess prognosis after cardiac arrest and therapeutic hypothermia Critical Care. 2014;18:202. http://ccforum.com/content/18/1/202.
21. Sandroni C, Cariou A, Cavallaro F, et al. Prognostication in comatose survivors of cardiac arrest: An advisory statement from the European Resuscitation Council and the European Society of Intensive Care Medicine. Intensive Care Medicine. 2014;40: 1816-31.
22. English WA, Giffin NJ, Nolan JP. Myoclonus after cardiac arrest: pitfalls in diagnosis and prognosis Anaesthesia. 2009;64:908-11.
23. Nolan J, Deakin C, Lockey A, et al. Resuscitation Council (UK) guidelines 2015: Post-resuscitation care. https://www.resus.org.uk/resuscitation-guidelines/.
24. Samaniego EA, Persoon S, Wijman CAC. Prognosis after cardiac arrest and hypothermia: a new paradigm. Curr Neurol Neurosci Rep. 2011;11:111-19.

25. Nolan JP, Soar J, et al. European Resuscitation Council and European Society of Intensive Care Medicine Guidelines for Post-resuscitation Care. 2015: Section 5 of the European Resuscitation Council Guidelines for Resuscitation 2015. Resuscitation. October 2015, pp. 202-22.
26. Taccone FS, Cronberg T, Friberg H, et al. How to assess prognosis after cardiac arrest and therapeutic hypothermia. Critical Care. 2014;18:202. DOI: 10.1186/cc13696.
27. Tiainen M, Roine RO, Pettilä V, et al. Serum neuron-specific enolase and s-100b protein in cardiac arrest patients treated with hypothermia. Stroke. 2003; 34:2881-2886.
28. Scolletta S, Donadello K, Santonocito C, et al. Biomarkers as predictors of outcome after cardiac arrest. Expert Rev Clin Pharmacol. 2012;5:687-99.
29. Jung Woo Eun, Hee Doo Yang, Sikyoung Jeong. Identification of novel biomarkers for prediction of neurological prognosis following cardiac arrest. Oncotarget. 2017; 8:16144-57.
30. Holly E, Hinson, Susan Rowell, Martin Schreiber. Clinical evidence of inflammation driving secondary brain injury: A systematic review. J Trauma Acute Care Surg. 2015;78:184-191.
31. Adrie, Adib-Conquy M, Laurent I, Monchi M, et al. Successful cardiopulmonary resuscitation after cardiac arrest as a "Sepsis-Like" syndrome Christophe. Circulation. 2002;106:562-8.
32. Ito N, Nishiyama K, Callaway CW, et al. Noninvasive regional cerebral oxygen saturation for neurological prognostication of patients with out-of-hospital cardiac arrest: a prospective multicenter observational study. Resuscitation. 2014;85:778-84.
33. Temple A, Porter R. Predicting neurological outcome and survival after cardiac arrest. Contin Educ Anaesth Crit Care Pain. 2012;12(6):283-7.
34. Martinell L, Nielsen N, Herlitz J, et al. Early predictors of poor outcome after out-of-hospital cardiac arrest. Critical Care. 2017;21:96 doi: 10.1186/s13054-017-1677-2.
35. Davies H, Loosely A, Dolling S, et al. Predicting survival in patients admitted to intensive care following out-of-hospital cardiac arrest using the prognosis after resuscitation score. Critical Care. 2014;18:491.
36. Nishikimi M, Matsuda N, Matsui K, et al. CAST: a new score for early prediction of neurological outcomes after cardiac arrest before therapeutic hypothermia with high accuracy. Intensive Care Med. 2016;42:2106-07.
37. Maupain C, Bougouin W, Lamhaut L, et al. The CAHP (Cardiac Arrest Hospital Prognosis) score: a tool for risk stratification after out-of-hospital cardiac arrest. Eur Heart J. 2016; 37:3222-28.
38. Heinz U, Rollnik JD. Outcome of hypoxic brain damage patients undergoing neurological early rehabilitation. BMC Res Notes. 2015;8:243. DOI 10.1186/s13104-015-1175-z.
39. Nielsen N, Wetterslev J, Cronberg T, et al. Targeted temperature management at 33°C versus 36°C after cardiac arrest. N Engl J Med. 2013;369:2197-2206.

CHAPTER 23

Anesthesia for Liver Transplantation

Vijay Vohra, Pooja Bhangui

KEY POINTS

- Liver transplant is now an established modality for end stage liver disease.
- Live donor liver transplant (LDLT) is more prevalent in the eastern countries whereas deceased donor liver transplants (DDLT) are common in the west.
- For LDLT, donor safety is most important and donor selection is very stringent.
- Comprehensive evaluation for Liver transplant recipient must include, cardiac, respiratory and renal work up.
- Invasive hemodynamic monitoring is essential and may require pulmonary artery catheter and pulse contour derived parameters.
- Intraoperative coagulation monitoring requires point of care monitor like TEG, TEM.
- Measures to reduce blood/blood product requirement should be initiated in all recipient surgeries.
- Prophylactic antifibrinolytics have a doubtful place in liver transplant surgery.
- Postoperative care emphasizes the need for complete asepsis.

INTRODUCTION

Thomas Starzl initiated liver transplant activity in its earnest in 1963 and he was able to perform the first successful human liver transplant in 1967. In 1983, the US FDA approved liver transplant as an acceptable therapeutic procedure for end stage liver disease.[1] Today, liver transplantation is widely accepted as the preferred treatment for adults and children with end stage liver disease and for selected patients of acute liver failure. This has been made possible because of progress and continuing refinement in surgical technique, immunosuppression and perioperative care of these patients. The anesthetic management for this procedure is quite challenging and involves managing complex issues of very dynamic changes in the coagulation and circulatory parameters through various phases of the surgery. The results of liver transplant surgery have improved significantly through the 1990s, but major bleeding, coagulopathy, electrolyte disturbances and cardiovascular instability still occur more frequently than in any other routine surgical procedure.

Deceased donor liver transplants (DDLT) are predominant in the western world including United States and Europe. In India and in some of the eastern countries like India, South Korea, and Japan; the availability of deceased donors is limited due to lack of education and religious beliefs, which prevent donation after brain death is declared. Therefore, both deceased as well as live donor liver programs are in use in these countries. DDLT becomes more of an emergency procedure as the transplant is carried out as and when an organ becomes available. Live donor liver transplant (LDLT) on the other hand can be planned; recipient can be optimized and has the potential of good organ matching. There is no waiting time in LDLT program and this minimizes the risk of further decompensation in the recipient. The organs procured during LDLT are good quality as they are taken from a healthy donor after thorough investigation. So, in the living donor setting, you have a healthy graft but the volume of the graft could be an issue, and a minimal of 0.8% of the body weight is considered to be an acceptable graft size for the recipient. Further, the surgical procedure for LDLT is technically more difficult and requires a good understanding of the hepatobiliary anatomy. Donor safety has a major importance in living donor transplants and only donors who have no significant co morbid condition are taken up for organ donation.

LIVER TRANSPLANT INDICATIONS

Transplantation is indicated when liver disease progresses to a stage where recovery is not possible. This could be both chronic liver disease (cirrhosis), as well as acute liver failure and the decision to list a patient is based more on the severity of liver dysfunction than the actual cause. The timing of liver transplantation is important, it should not be done too early or left it too late which may affect overall patient outcome. The indications for liver transplant are listed in Table 1.

OBJECTIVE ASSESSMENT OF LIVER DISEASE SEVERITY

Criteria for End Stage Liver Disease

Various disease severity scoring system are in use and more scoring systems are being tried in different parts of the world. The commonest one is **Child-Pugh classification**, which was modified to **Child-Turcotte-Pugh (CTP)**, and this is based on two clinical and three laboratory parameters (Table 2). This classification initially included another important clinical parameter that is nutrition, which was later dropped to make a more objective scoring system.

The scores are also used to allocate organs whereby sicker patients get priority in organ allocation.

Model for End Stage Liver Disease score (MELD Score) was first introduced in United States in 2002 for allocation of organs. It has been validated as a good predictor of mortality while the patients are on waiting list for transplantation.[2,3] It is a mathematical score taking into consideration serum bilirubin, prothrombin time (PT-INR), and serum creatinine with different weightage of all three components. A patient requiring hemodialysis pretransplant affects the calculation of MELD score and the patient acquires maximum points for serum creatinine. The mathematical calculation is as follows:

MELD = 3.78 [Ln serum bilirubin (mg/dL)] + 11.2 [Ln INR] + 9.57 [Ln serum creatinine (mg/dL)] + 6.43
Where Ln is a natural algorithm.

Higher MELD score indicates greater severity of the liver disease and need for early transplantation. MELD the score is valid for adults and children more

Table 1: Indications for liver transplant

Acute liver failure
Hepatitis A, acetaminophen, autoimmune hepatitis
Hepatitis B
Hepatitis C, cryptogenic
Drugs, hepatitis D
Wilson's disease, Budd-Chiari syndrome
Fatty infiltration—acute fatty liver of pregnancy, Reye's syndrome

Cirrhosis from chronic liver disease
Chronic hepatitis B virus infection
Chronic hepatitis C virus infection
Alcoholic liver disease
Autoimmune hepatitis
Cryptogenic liver disease
Nonalcoholic fatty liver disease

Malignant diseases of the liver
Hepatocellular carcinoma
Carcinoid tumor
Islet cell tumor
Epithelioid hemangioendothelioma
Cholangiocarcinoma

Metabolic liver disease
Wilson's disease
Hereditary hemochromatosis
Alpha-1 antitrypsin deficiency
Glycogen storage disease

Cystic fibrosis
Glycogen storage disease I and IV
Crigler-Najjar syndrome
Galactosemia
Type 1 hyperoxaluria
Familial homozygous hypercholesterolemia
Hemophilia A and B

Vascular diseases of the liver
Budd-Chiari syndrome
Veno-occlusive disease

Cholestatic liver diseases
Primary biliary cirrhosis
Primary sclerosing cholangitis
Secondary biliary cirrhosis
Biliary atresia
Alagille syndrome
Byler's disease

Miscellaneous
Adult polycystic liver disease
Nodular regenerative hyperplasia
Caroli's disease
Severe graft-versus-host disease
Amyloidosis
Sarcoidosis
Hepatic trauma

Table 2: Child-Turcotte-Pugh (CTP) score

	1	2	3
Encephalopathy	None	1 and 2	3 and 4
Ascites	Absent/slight	Moderate	Not controlled by diuretics
Bilirubin (mg%)	1–2	2–3	>3
Albumin (gm%)	>3.5	2.8–3.5	<2.8
PT (INR)	<1.7	1.7–2.3	>2.3

CTP: Class A: 5–6; Class B: 7–9; Class C: 10–15

than 12 years old. The main advantage of MELD is that it is a continuous system of rating disease severity.

MELD score allocation changes in case of hepatocellular carcinoma; the minimum score automatically becomes 24 irrespective of other parameters.

Similarly, extra MELD points are also given to patients with hepatopulmonary syndrome, which is limited to patients with PO_2 less than 60 mm Hg. Other conditions that get prioritized are hyperoxaluria and portopulmonary hypertension (POPH).

Generally, patients with late Childs B or C cirrhosis (score 9-15) or with a MELD >14 are listed for liver transplantation.

Children under the age of 12 years have different criteria for listing them for liver transplantation. ***PELD Score*** used for children takes into consideration serum albumin, prothrombin time (INR), weight and bilirubin. The mathematical calculation is as follows:

PELD = 4.80 [Ln serum bilirubin (mg/dL)] + 18.57 [Ln INR] - 6.87 [Ln albumin (g/dL)] + 4.36 (<1 year old) + 6.67 (growth failure)

Where Ln is a natural algorithm.

Children less than one year of age and growth failure get consideration in calculating PELD score as these groups do poorly on the waiting list.

There have been continuous attempts to further refine these criteria incorporating other parameters for assessing disease severity. Serum sodium is incorporated in the recently adopted score in United Kingdom called **UKELD**. Organ allocation using UKELD was started from 1st April 2013 and has been in use since. Patients with a score of 49 or more can be listed for transplantation. Organ allocation by this score would lead to reduced waiting list mortality but its effect on post-transplant survival is too complex to predict.[4]

UKELD = (5.395 × INR) + (1.485 × S Creatinine) + (3.13 × S Bilirubin) - (81.565 × S Sodium) + 435][4]

Criteria for Acute Liver Failure

The patients with acute liver disease cannot be rated according to CTP or MELD. The most accepted criteria for transplanting in acute liver failure is the ***King's College Criteria***[5] which has separate distinguishing parameters for those having acetaminophen toxicity and others as follows:

- Criteria for Acetaminophen toxicity patients
  pH < 7.3 or INR > 6.5 and serum creatinine level > 3.4 mg/dL
- Criteria for other patients
  INR >6.5 (PT >100 sec), or any 3 of the following:
  a. Age <10 or >40 years
  b. Aetiology non-A, non-B hepatitis, or idiosyncratic drug reaction
  c. Duration of jaundice before hepatic encephalopathy >7 days
  d. INR >3.5
  e. Serum bilirubin >17.6 mg/dL.

Clichy's Criteria

Clichy's Criteria was developed based on a French prospective study, which identified patients having lowest survival rate without liver transplant. These patients had hepatic encephalopathy accompanied with low levels of factor V. The criteria are as follows:

- Factor V level < 20%, Age < 30 years + hepatic encephalopathy
- Factor V level < 30%, Age > 30 years + hepatic encephalopathy.

In this cohort, they showed a positive predictive value of 80% and negative predictive value of 98%.[6] Further studies did not replicate these predictive values and the score was found to be inferior to the widely used King's College Criteria.

PREOPERATIVE EVALUATION

The recipient is assessed independently by the surgeon, hepatologist and the anesthesiologist and then a formal multidisciplinary team meeting (also including radiologists and transplant coordinators) is held in which all recipient and donor (in case of LDLT) details are presented and discussed, before final medical approval for transplantation.

The anesthetic assessment is carried out early during the recipient evaluation process so that pertinent issues (or sometimes prohibitive risks) are picked up at the initial stages itself, and detailed evaluation for the same may be done. Some of the prohibitive risks include gross hyponatremia, portopulmonary hypertension, severe cardiomyopathy, etc. Various organ systems are assessed as for any major surgery with emphasis on issues/complications seen in end stage liver disease. Cardiovascular system is assessed as these patients can have wide fluctuations in cardiac output intraoperatively and cirrhotic cardiomyopathy may be unmasked in the perioperative period. Infections need be ruled out before planning transplant, as these are often immunocompromised and therefore at risk of acquiring infections.

Hemodynamic profile of end stage liver disease is one of overall hyperdynamic state with low systemic vascular resistance and high cardiac output. All patients undergo 12 lead electrocardiography and stress echocardiography. As these patients of chronic liver disease can easily develop fluid overload, functional tricuspid regurgitation might be visible on echocardiography. Cardiomyopathy is known to exist in cirrhotic liver disease, which is revealed on stress testing. End stage liver disease is associated with low systemic vascular resistance and high cardiac output and may precipitate ischemic event in patients with compromised coronary vasculature. It may not be possible to perform a stress test in all liver transplant patients, due to the use of beta-blockers which prevent achieving predicted heart rate during stress. Such patients can be screened by CT angiography or withdrawing beta-blockers for a few days before attempting stress test. Coronary calcium score is another modality used to determine the presence of coronary artery disease, which has a good negative predictive value. Patients with coronary artery disease may need to undergo CT coronary angiography or conventional angiography.

Assessment of renal function is critical in the perioperative management of these patients. Poor preoperative renal function is a predictor of poor prognosis and these patients are at a higher risk for intraoperative blood loss, postoperative need for dialysis, perioperative morbidity and mortality.[7] As serum creatinine is not a sensitive index of renal function, creatinine clearance is the more preferred indicator for renal dysfunction. These tests should be interpreted with caution keeping in mind the use of diuretics and volume expansion measures like use of terlipressin and albumin infusion. Hepato renal syndrome should always be suspected as the cause of renal failure and treated aggressively. Terlipressin, an analogue of vasopressin, started in the dose of 0.5–1 mg three times a day has been shown to improve renal function with improvement of serum creatinine levels and creatinine clearance by increasing the central blood volume.[7]

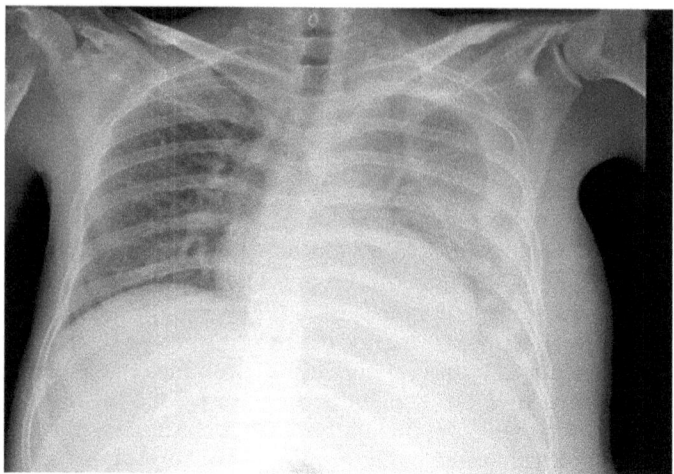

Fig. 1: Chest X-ray showing hydrothorax.

In chronic liver disease ascites develops due to portal hypertension and is sometimes accompanied by hydrothorax. This can cause respiratory distress and may require therapeutic drainage. The hydrothorax (Fig. 1) should be left alone in spite of the size of hydrothorax, if it is not producing any respiratory symptoms. In the event of long standing hydrothorax, CT chest should be done, to know the expansibility and state of the underlying lung after therapeutic drainage of the hydrothorax. In the context of Indian patients, pulmonary tuberculosis should be ruled out by doing ADA or Quantiferon TB Gold Test. None of these tests are confirmatory but tissue diagnosis is not always possible. Left sided hydrothorax must be viewed with high suspicion of tuberculosis and high level of ADA (> 40 U/L) in the pleural fluid point towards tubercular pathology.[8]

ANESTHESIA PREPARATION AND PREMEDICATION

Preoperative preparation includes re-evaluation of the patient especially, if the patient has been admitted from home. All patients must undergo screening process to rule out any infective issues and culture of blood, urine and ascitic fluid is done. X-ray chest is done close to the surgery to see any change in the size of hydrothorax. Gross ascites, if present can affect ventilation and cause basal atelectasis and collapse. Arterial blood gases are done to see the metabolic state and oxygenation. Metabolic acidosis can develop, if there is progression of portal vein thrombosis. Poor oxygenation is seen, if there is evidence of hepatopulmonary syndrome. These patients have a prolonged intensive care stay, and may need tracheostomy early in the postoperative period. Early tracheostomy may not have mortality benefit but is associated with lower incidence of pneumonia.[9] Other causes of hypoxia should be investigated. All patients should be started on incentive spirometry at the time of initial assessment. This helps prevent development of microatelectasis especially in those with large ascites. A transthoracic echocardiograph should be done within a week of the transplant to ascertain cardiac function, pulmonary artery pressure, volume status and presence of pericardial effusion.

Premedication is generally not required except in children or younger patients. Prophylactic antibiotics are an integral part of the perioperative protocol and should cover both gram positive and gram-negative organisms. These patients are immunocompromised, are susceptible to infections and translocation of bacteria from the intestines is a distinct possibility. The antibiotics are given at the time of induction of anesthesia unless the patient is already on antibiotics for other infective issues like spontaneous bacterial peritonitis (SBP).

ANESTHETIC TECHNIQUE

The recipients are anesthetized in the operating room only and the patient is placed on a gel mattress with a warm water under blanket which has circulating water with thermostatic control kept at 39–42°C. Forced air blanket is used for upper and lower body warming. An ECG monitor, pulse oxymeter and automatic blood pressure monitor are attached to the patient before induction.

After preoxygenation, anesthesia is usually induced with midazolam 1–2 mg, fentanyl 1–1.5 μg/kg and propofol 1–2 mg/kg. If the patient has gross ascites or is full stomach, rapid sequence intubation is facilitated by rocuronium or suxamethonium otherwise conventional anesthesia is practiced for induction. Anesthesia is maintained with fentanyl 1–2 μg/kg/hour with air/oxygen/desflurane or isoflurane. Desflurane has the advantage of quick recovery and very low hepatic metabolism, but isoflurane is known to better preserve the hepatic artery buffer response and the splanchnic blood flow.[10] Nitrous oxide is avoided as it causes distension of intestines on prolonged use and is also known to cause cardiovascular depression.

Any of the relaxants can be used viz; cisatracurium, rocuronium or vecuronium. Cisatracurium is 3-times more potent than atracurium without releasing histamine or cardiovascular depressing profile. Cisatracurium undergoes spontaneous degradation, which makes it ideal for ESLD patients who have renal dysfunction. Rocuronium is probably better than vecuronium because it has no active metabolites, whereas break down products of vecuronium have some skeletal muscle relaxant properties.

Venous Access

Liver transplant surgery is associated with massive blood loss especially, if there is a history of previous upper abdominal surgery, or the patient is highly coagulopathic and has significant portal hypertension to start with. Peripheral venous access may be difficult, if the patient has had previous hospital admissions before the transplant.

Large-bore intravenous infusions are set up in the arms, if peripheral access is available. After induction of anesthesia, ultrasound guided central venous cannulation is established with two central venous catheters, one large bore for rapid infusion and another triple/four lumen for infusion of drugs and blood products. Pulmonary artery catheter (PAC) is floated to monitor pulmonary artery pressures. Right internal jugular vein is preferred because of its straighter course. At our center, the practice is to use *Advance Venous Access catheter 9F*, which has three lumens and a port for floating PAC, if required. If venovenous bypass is planned, then a 10F re-enforced catheter is used in the axillary vein or the internal jugular vein. If axillary vein is to be used for inflow, open access is usually obtained surgically and for this left side vein is used. Venovenous bypass entails cannulation of the femoral vein along with portal vein (after explanting the native liver), which constitute outflow from the patient and inflow to the bypass. This blood is then returned to the patient in the upper half of the body via axillary vein or internal jugular vein.

Coagulation Monitoring

A full coagulation screen, including platelet count, PT/INR, fibrinogen levels and thromboelastography (TEG) are routinely done preoperatively, and at regular intervals in the operation theatre to monitor coagulation.[11] Another point of care monitor for coagulation monitoring available which has more automation is thromboelastometry (TEM).[12] At our center, it is a practice to have on site coagulation monitoring in operating theatre or close by, and reliance is on thromboelastography (TEG) rather than PT for intraoperative coagulation status. On an average 6–8 TEGs are done during the surgical procedure. The first TEG is done at the start of the operation, once or twice during dissection phase, hourly during anhepatic phase, an hour after reperfusion, at any time if there is inexplicable bleeding and before sending the recipient to the ICU at the completion of surgery. Associated electrolyte abnormalities, hyponatremia and hypomagnesemia, require guarded correction and sodium should not be corrected by more than 12 mmol/L over 24 hours as rapid correction can cause osmotic demyelination.[13]

Blood and Blood Products

Routinely 10 units of blood and 10 units of Fresh Frozen Plasma and 3 Units of Platelets Apheresis are arranged and kept ready in the blood bank fridge kept in the OT complex for all adult recipients. Routine correction of coagulation prior to insertion of ultrasound guided central venous catheterization seems unnecessary, as the complication rate is negligible.

Intraoperatively, FFP and/or platelets are infused based on the coagulation parameters, PT and/or TEG. Absolute platelet count does not reflect the state of coagulation in patients of chronic liver disease with portal hypertension and hypersplenism. TEG is a better modality and prolonged reaction time along with maximum amplitude (mA) less than 40 mm justifies platelet supplementation. High-risk patients (those with portal hypertension, history of upper abdominal surgery or bacterial peritonitis) may require prophylactic antifibrinolytic therapy. Subclinical fibrinolysis is present in most patients with chronic liver disease and some centers advocate the use of antifibrinolytic therapy in all patients for liver transplant as this is known to reduce overall blood and blood product requirement.

Antifibrinolytic therapy is used in the form of tranexamic acid, epsilon amino caproic acid and aprotinin. Our preference is to use tranexamic acid 10 mg/kg bolus followed by 5 mg/kg/hr till the new liver is reperfused. There is wide variation in the dose of this drug and up to 40 mg/kg has been used.[14] More described drug for this purpose in the literature is aprotinin 50,000 unit test dose, and after 15 mins, 2 million units over 30 minutes, followed by 500,000 units per hour till the end of surgery. Patients with Budd-Chiari syndrome, hepatocellular carcinoma or those with a history of deep vein thrombosis or other thrombotic tendency, acute liver failure patients and pediatric age group patients are excluded from antifibrinolytic therapy.

The risk of thrombotic complications with the antifibrinolytic therapy must be weighed before giving these drugs prophylactically. There is literature support for its use in selected liver transplant recipients with good patient outcome in terms of reduced blood transfusion requirement. Case reports of intravascular thrombosis and thromboembolism during liver transplantation have been reported with the use of antifibrinolytic therapy.[15]

PHASES OF TRANSPLANTATION

Dissection Phase

This phase begins with start of the surgical procedure and ends when the liver is explanted, i.e. beginning of the anhepatic phase. During this phase, there are large hemodynamic changes due to blood loss, manipulation of liver and handling of the inferior vena cava (IVC). The blood loss could be massive and the most important consideration is to maintain intravascular volume by infusion of blood, blood products and colloids, depending on the hematocrit and coagulation status. Calcium chloride/gluconate must be added in adequate dose to avoid hypotension.

Once dissection of the liver is done and all the vessels and bile duct have been isolated (sometimes in the anhepatic phase), trial clamping of IVC is performed for at least one minute to see the hemodynamic effects and assess adequacy of the patient's ability to withstand caval clamping when new liver is being revascularized. There is an expected drop in cardiac output and it is to be assessed whether this period of inferior vena cava clamping can be managed with vasopressors and volume adjustments. If the systolic pressure falls to less than 70% of its previous value (SAP < 80–90 mm Hg or MAP < 60 mm Hg), in the presence of adequate blood replacement, or if ECG changes occur, bypass support may be needed. In our center, we rarely resort to venovenous bypass during inferior vena cava clamping probably because the patients who are accepted for transplants normally do not have significant heart disease.

Anhepatic Phase

Hemodynamic changes during this period are related to IVC clamping and to physiological changes caused by the removal of the liver. Quite often patients start stabilizing during anhepatic phase because the liver, which was producing various vasoactive substances, is now out of circulation. IVC clamping results in a decrease in venous return and thereby cardiac output is reduced. These changes are more marked in the absence of extensive collaterals from the portal circulation. Partial clamping for the implantation is done, if the patient does not tolerate cross clamping. Similarly, if there is preoperative renal dysfunction, complete clamping of the IVC is avoided during anhepatic phase. Absence of liver function results in inability to metabolize citrate leading to citrate intoxication and lowering of ionized calcium. This can cause significant myocardial depression. Hypocalcemia must be corrected before reperfusion, the aim being to have ionized serum calcium level closer to 1.2 mmol/L before the vascular clamps are removed and the new liver comes into circulation. Serum calcium is built up to counter high level of K^+ in the effluent from the new liver, which gets into circulation on reperfusion.

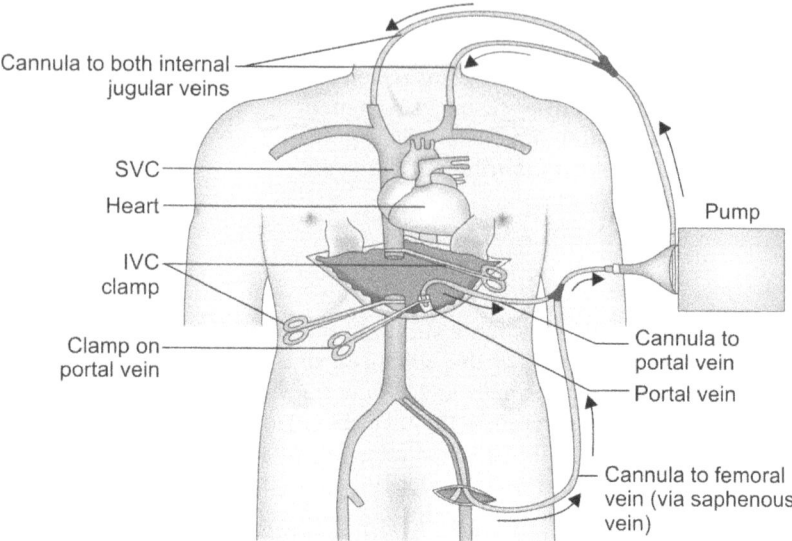

Fig. 2: Venovenous bypass (diagramatic representation).
(SVC: Superior vena cava; IVC: Inferior vena cava).

Portal vein clamping heralds the beginning of anhepatic phase which causes further rise in portal pressures and may increase surgical bleeding and congestion of the bowel.[16,17] If anhepatic phase is likely to be prolonged, portacaval shunt is established and which will prevent bowel congestion. Using venovenous bypass (VVB) can obviate this, but it has its own inherent side effects of air embolism, etc. that requires monitoring.[18] Piggyback technique decreases the need for VVB.[19] Attempts to increase filling pressures by blood and fluid replacement must be cautious at this stage, because of the danger of fluid overload at the time of liver revascularization, when normal venous return and central blood volume are restored.

Venovenous Bypass

Venovenous bypass (Fig. 2) is a standard procedure in DDLT where liver along with vena cava are dissected out and replaced with two caval ends with liver attached to it. Other reasons for using VVB during liver transplant are to maintain hemodynamic stability, to preserve cardiac, pulmonary, cerebral, renal and intestinal blood flow and function, to reduce the need for blood transfusion and to provide a longer anhepatic phase for better surgical performance especially when surgery is complicated. Veroli et al. advised the use of VVB in patients with 30% drop in mean arterial pressure and 50% decrease in cardiac index during a 5 min test clamping of inferior vena cava.[20] However, several studies have failed to show any effect on morbidity or mortality in these patients with or without the use of VVB.[21,22] Administration of vasopressors and strict volume adjustment can help to maintain preload and hemodynamic stability without an increased risk of volume overload and pulmonary edema following reperfusion of the liver.[23] In LDLT, there is preservation of recipient vena cava and therefore one can even do partial caval clamping and do the venous anastomosis.

Reperfusion Phase

The ultimate test is when the new liver comes into circulation after hepatic vein and portal vein clamps are released. Ischemia reperfusion injury can occur at this stage and the extent of this injury depends upon cold ischemia time, quality of the donor graft and size of the graft. Giving prednisolone before reperfusion can minimize the extent of this injury. Variable prednisolone doses up to 1 gm have been used in different studies, but our practice is to give 10 mg/kg once patient becomes anhepatic.

Reperfusion can cause dramatic cardiovascular changes, which may or may not last for a long time.[24] There may be a sudden increase in serum potassium levels, which can be offset by giving calcium bolus. There could be sudden decrease in heart rate, mean arterial pressure and systemic vascular resistance due to release of vasoactive substances from ischemic liver graft and from static blood from the gut getting back into circulation.[25] It is important to ensure that ionized calcium levels before reperfusion are normal. Treatment of hypotension is with vasopressors like phenylephrine, or noradrenaline. It is common practice to use one of these prophylactically, along with calcium on unclamping of the portal vein. Normally there is no more blood loss after this stage but at times fibrinolysis continues and may require continued antifibrinolytic therapy and blood or blood products.

Post-reperfusion Syndrome

This is defined as a drop in blood pressure of more than 30% from baseline, lasting for 1 minute or more, and occurring within 5 minutes of reperfusion. This occurs due to release of vasodilatory substances and metabolites from the graft and congested intestines. The treatment is with vasopressors as well as sodium bicarbonate. The effluent from the hepatic vein may have very high potassium levels and may require treatment with calcium chloride intravenously. Post-reperfusion syndrome is seen more often with deceased donor transplant than with living donor liver transplant.

SPECIFIC COMPLICATIONS OF TRANSPLANT PROCEDURE

Major Bleeding

This procedure has the potential for rapid and sudden blood loss and it is essential to transfuse at a rate sufficient to maintain hemodynamic parameters in the near normal range. Some form of rapid infusion device should be available to correct rapidly changing hemodynamic status. It should be remembered that concentrated and washed cells must be supplemented with colloids and that rapid blood replacement will lead to citrate intoxication leading to hypocalcemia, and even hyperkalemia.

Metabolic Acidosis

During dissection and anhepatic phase, metabolic acidosis can develop due to tissue hypoperfusion resulting from shunting associated with liver disease. Treatment should be aimed at correcting the underlying problem, ascertaining that there is no respiratory component and by mild hyperventilation. Sodium bicarbonate should be used cautiously as this adds to sodium load.

After reperfusion of the liver, metabolic acidosis typically worsens as a result of sudden release into the circulation of acidotic material from the ischemic liver and obstructed splanchnic bed. This is generally self-limited and resolves over a few hours without specific treatment.

Dyselectrolytemia

Electrolyte disturbances are common in ESLD patients. Transfusion of blood and blood products lower ionized serum calcium levels which may fall further during anhepatic phase, when citrate metabolism ceases completely. If blood loss is not substantial, values return to normal after reperfusion without the need for further treatment. The aim should be to keep serum calcium within the normal range (1.1-1.3 mmol/L) at all times, especially during the period preceding reperfusion.

Hyponatremia maybe pre-existing in some ESLD patients presenting for liver transplant and indicates severity of liver disease. The condition is associated with higher incidence of hepatorenal syndrome, hepatopulmonary syndrome and spontaneous bacterial peritonitis.[26] Rapid correction of hyponatremia is known to cause neurological complications including osmotic demyelination syndrome.[27,28] Sodium level should be maintained closer to the preoperative levels and certainly not increase by more than 12 mmol/L in 24 hours, which can lead to cerebro pontine myelinolysis (CPM). Hyperkalemia can occur on release of the clamps and though it lasts for a short time the effect can be catastrophic. Prophylactic calcium chloride is given and measures to prevent a further marked increase are essential to reduce the risk of hyperkalemic arrest at reperfusion. This may require washing of bank blood (use cell saver), glucose/insulin neutralizing infusion and use of calcium gluconate/calcium chloride. Flushing of the new graft with ringer lactate or gelatin solution before reperfusion helps minimize this complication.

Fluid Balance and Renal Function

Brief period of oliguria or anuria may occur during IVC clamping. Dextrose 5% infusion is started along with another crystalloid from the beginning of the surgery. Preferred crystalloid solution is plasmalyte A which has pH corrected to 7.4. Intravascular volume is maintained with albumin, 6% hydroxyl ethyl starch (HES), blood and blood products as indicated by measurements of hematocrit and TEG. Mannitol is given as free radical scavenger and as osmotic diuretic in a dose of 0.5-1.0 g/kg before inferior vena caval clamping, when an abrupt fall or temporary cessation of urine output is usual. Vasopressors may be required at this stage, noradrenaline, adrenaline, phenylephrine have all been used. There may be a need to give intravenous fluids, if there is inadequate response to vasopressors. The maintenance of urine output is desirable although the efficacy of low-dose dopamine for this reason is unproven.[29]

Hypothermia

The body temperature invariably decreases during induction of anesthesia, during preparation of surgery, evaporative loss from large exposed peritoneal surface, use of venovenous bypass and infusion of cold fluids. The hypothermia will get further aggravated, when the donor liver is placed in the abdomen. Lower body temperature affects the coagulation, drug metabolism and myocardial contractility. It is therefore imperative to use protective measures like use of heated mattress, warm and humidified gases and warming of all intra venous fluids. The exposed areas can be covered and draped with cotton to prevent losing heat from the surface. Insulating the bypass circuit can also prevent heat loss. The temperature should be kept above 36°C. A gradual recovery from hypothermia takes place once the operation is completed and the patient is covered in insulated blankets.

Marked increase in the amount of blood in splanchnic circulation is seen in the end stage liver disease leading to increase in portal venous pressure. Portal hypertension also translates into development of porto-systemic shunts as the disease progresses.[30,31] Surgical dissection in these circumstances does lead to blood loss.

INTRAOPERATIVE TRANSFUSION OF BLOOD AND BLOOD PRODUCTS

Intraoperatively blood and blood products are given on clinical basis, laboratory testing and on the evidence of thromboelastography done at regular intervals with the target hemoglobin of 9 g%. Packed cell infused are preferred to be leucodepleted. Routine use of TEG reduces transfusion of blood components, especially fresh frozen plasma and platelets. Alternative method of rationalizing the use of blood products is by using the algorithm described for reduction of blood loss is the use of recombinant activated factor VII (rFVIIa). Two recent retrospective studies obtained favorable results with reduced transfusion of packed red blood cells and fresh frozen plasma in patients treated with (rFVIIa).[32,33] As a policy we at our center use recombinant factor VIIa as a rescue therapy for uncontrolled bleeding. One of the algorithms for blood product use is shown in Flowchart 1.

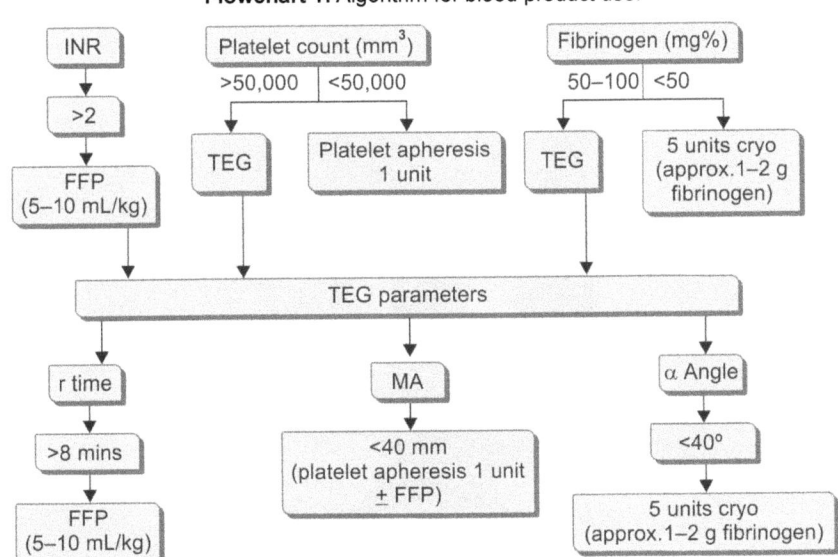

Flowchart 1: Algorithm for blood product use.

Blood Conservation Strategies

Liver transplantation has a potential of massive blood losses and various conservation strategies are adopted to minimize blood/blood product requirement. Correction of coagulation defects with plasma transfusion does not necessarily decrease blood loss during liver transplantation. It may lead to a hypervolemic state, which can even increase blood loss during surgery.

- **Low CVP**

  Lowering of central venous pressure is used to reduce blood losses during liver dissection before the anhepatic phase without any deleterious results.[34] CVP can be lowered by fluid restriction, phlebotomy and by avoiding plasma transfusion in order to diminish the transfusion of blood products.

- **Cell Saver**

  The use of intraoperative cell saver (Fig. 3) has the potential to reduce the need for heterologous transfusion, thereby reducing the risks of disease transmission. In a prospective study, the use of cell saver was shown not only to reduce transfusion but also to be cost effective.[35] One aspect that needs to be kept in mind is that with cell saver, blood comes from the abdominal cavity into collection bags, is washed, collected into other bags and then reinfused. During this travel from the abdominal cavity to reinfusion, there is possibility of contamination and infection. Cell saver is to be avoided in malignancy. Cell saver processing also reduces ammonia, lactate as well as potassium levels in the blood (Table 3).[36]

- **Antifibrinolytic Agents**

  Antifibrinolytic agents have been used to reduce intraoperative bleeding, as there is ongoing fibrinolysis in most patients with chronic liver disease. This is due to presence of circulating tissue plasminogen activator (t-PA) during the anhepatic phase and the burst release of t-PA associated with the reperfusion of the liver graft. Diseased liver is not able to clear t-PA from circulation but once new liver starts functioning, fibrinolysis may not be seen on TEG.

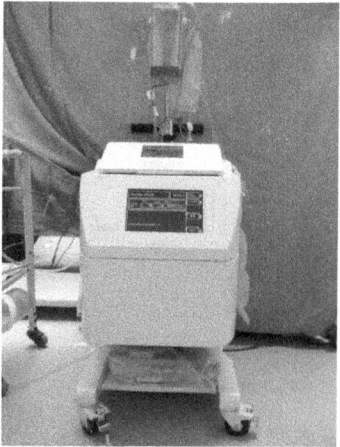

Fig. 3: Cell-saver.

Table 3: Electrolyte changes with cell-saver

Serum values (Normal)	In vivo pre-CSP	Patient' blood in vitro post-CSP	In vivo post-CSP	Banked PRBCs Pre-CSP	Banked PRBCs Post-CSP
Ammonia (15–40 µmol/L)	85	40	43	693	92
Lactate (0.5–2.2 mmol/L)	16.4	5.1	5.9	24.8	10.6
Potassium (3.5–5.0 mEq/L)	4.2	1.1	3.6	>30	1.3

(CSP: Cell-saver processing; PRBC: Packed red blood cells).

Aprotinin has been shown to reduce transfusion requirements in surgeries with significant blood loss and has been used for liver transplant as well as cardiac surgery.[37]

Tranexamic acid, which is a synthetic derivative of lysine exerts its antifibrinolytic effect by reversibly blocking plasminogen. It has been used in a dose of 2 mg/kg to 40 mg/kg body weight with good effect on transfusion reduction.[38]

Prothrombin complex concentrate is a concentrated form of coagulation factors (factor II, VII, IX, and X). It has a utility in the management of coagulopathy of transplant recipients especially, if intravascular fluid volume is an issue and is currently undergoing trial (PROTON – trial).[39]

PRIMARY NONFUNCTION/INITIAL POOR FUNCTIONING GRAFT

Persistence of metabolic acidosis after reperfusion and hemodynamic instability points towards a suboptimal liver graft. Congested or greyish appearance of the liver, coagulopathy, inadequate urine output, and high inotropic requirement are signs of poor graft function. Supportive management includes use of N-acetylcysteine (NAC) 150–300 mg/kg over 24 hours, which acts as a free radical scavenger. Noradrenaline and vasopressin can be used at this juncture to preserve hemodynamics and support till the graft shows signs of improvement. NAC infusion can be continued postoperatively also for up to 5 days.

Poor graft function is seen, if the quality of the liver graft is marginal, which happens largely in the organs retrieved from deceased donors. Marginal donors are being accepted for transplantation due to a shortage of donor organs and growing waiting lists of patients requiring liver transplantation. These organs are more prone for ischemia reperfusion injury compared to normal grafts.

POSTOPERATIVE CARE

Monitoring continues in the postoperative period from where it was left in the operating theater in terms of hemodynamic status, coagulation status and the graft functioning. Pulmonary artery pressure (PAP) monitoring may be discontinued in the intensive care unit, if the pressures are stable and near normal. High venous pressure will prevent venous drainage from the new graft. Positive end expiratory pressure and Intermittent Positive Pressure should be minimized to enable better outflow from the new liver.

Most patients are ventilated for a variable period, depending on their preoperative status and the intraoperative course. Select patients can be extubated early on transfer to the intensive care unit. There has been an attempt to fast track some of these patients from the intensive care unit. To successfully fast track it is important to use short-acting drugs and appropriate use of narcotics and benzodiazepines to allow early return of spontaneous breathing and awakening at the end of surgery. Patients with encephalopathy, large blood and blood product requirement, obesity, high Child's Pugh Score are not good candidates for fast tracking. Furthermore, obesity (BMI >32) and preoperative encephalopathy are likely to result in failed attempts at immediate extubation. It is not certain that endotracheal extubation at the end of surgery will result in shorter intensive-care-unit stay or in significant cost savings.

Doppler studies are done daily to assess the vascular integrity of the graft and trends in the blood flow of hepatic artery, portal vein and hepatic vein are recorded at least once a day. In children, it may be carried out twice a day as they have a high risk of vascular complications. These studies are more relevant in the living donor liver transplant surgery as there is possibility of mismatch of the size of artery or vein. Hepatic artery thrombosis (HAT) is a serious complication and must watch out for in all recipients. HAT requires urgent re-exploration and if not correctable, will eventually lead to retransplantation.[40]

Aggressive chest physiotherapy supplemented with incentive spirometry is prescribed for all recipients. It helps, if all patients are counseled preoperatively about the need to do incentive spirometry. Postoperative infection is a major hazard in these patients and over 80% mortality in liver transplant is related to infective issues. Barrier nursing, hand hygiene and appropriate antibiotic therapy should be used in these immunocompromised patients.

CONCLUSION

Liver transplantation has come to be accepted as a life saving procedure for end stage liver disease. Liver transplant programs requires multidisciplinary approach with involvement of transplant surgery, anesthesiology, hepatology, blood transfusion services, intensivists, physiotherapist and intensive care nursing staff. The care of liver transplant patient presents a unique challenge, not seen with any other surgical procedure. A good understanding of the pathophysiology of the disease and of the surgical procedure is essential to sustain a successful liver transplant program.

REFERENCES

1. Yu S, Keeffe EB. Liver transplantation. In: Zakim D, Boyer TD (Eds). Hepatology: A Textbook of Liver Disease (4th ed). Elsevier, Philadelphia, Pa, USA. 2003. pp. 1617-56.
2. Kamath PS, Wiesner RH, Malinchoc M, et al. A model to predict survival in patients with end-stage liver disease. Hepatology. 2001;33:464-70.
3. Wiesner R, Edwards E, Wiesner R, et al. Model for end stage liver disease (MELD) and allocation of donor livers. Gastroenterology. 2003;124:91-6.
4. Barber K, Madden S, Allen J, et al. Elective liver transplant list mortality: development of a united kingdom end stage liver disease score. Transplantation. 2011;92:469-76.

5. O'Grady JG, Alexander GJM, Hayllar KM, et al. Early indicators of prognosis in fulminant hepatic failure. Gastroenterology. 1989;97(2):439-45.
6. Bernuau J, Samuel D, Durand F, et al. Criteria for emergency liver transplantation in patients with acute viral hepatitis and factor V below 50% of normal: a prospective study. Hepatology. 1991;14:49A.
7. Allegretti AS, Israelsen M, Krag A, et al. Terlipressin versus placebo or no intervention for people with cirrhosis and hepatorenal syndrome. Cochrane Database of Systematic Reviews 2017, Issue 6. Art.No.: CD005162. DOI: 10.1002/14651858.CD005162.pub4.
8. Vorster MJ, Allwood BW, Diacon AH, et al. Tuberculous pleural effusion: advances and controversies. J Thorac Dis. 2015;7(6):981-91.
9. Siempos LL, Ntaidou TK, Filippidis FT, et al. Effect of early versus late or no tracheostomy on mortality and pneumonia of critically ill patients receiving mechani-cal ventilation: a systematic review and meta-analysis. Lancet Respir Med. 2015;3(2):150-8.
10. O'Riordan J, O'Beirne HA, Young Y, et al. Effects of desflurane and isoflurane on splanchnic microcirculation during major surgery. Br J Anaesth. 1997;78:95-6.
11. Ozier Y, Pessione F, Samain E, et al. Institutional variability in transfusion practice for liver transplantation. Anesth Analg. 2003;97:671-9.
12. Fayed N, Mourad W, Yassen K, et al. Preoperative thromboelastometry as a predictor of transfusion requirements during adult living donor liver transplantation. Transfus Med Hemother. 2015;42:99-108.
13. Sterns RH, Riggs JE, Schochet SS. Osmotic demyelination syndrome following correction of hyponatremia. N Eng J Med. 1986;314:1535-42.
14. Boylan JF, Klinck JR, Sandler AN, et al. Tranexamic acid reduces blood loss, transfusion requirements, and coagulation factor use in primary orthotopic liver transplantation. Anesthesiology. 1996;85:1043-8.
15. Ramsay MAE, Randall HB, Burton EC. Intravascular thrombosis and thromboembolism during liver transplantation: antifibrinolytic therapy implicate? Liver Transplantation. 2004;10(2):310-4.
16. Haagsma EB, Gips CH, Wesenhagen H, et al. Liver disease and its effect on haemostasis during liver transplantation. Liver International. 1985;5(3):123-8.
17. Bechstein WO, Neuhaus P. Bleeding problems in liver surgery and liver transplantation. Chirurg. 2000;71(4):363-8.
18. Budd JM, Isaac JL, Bennett J, et al. Morbidity and mortality associated with large-bore percutaneous venovenous bypass cannulation for 312 orthotopic liver transplantations. Liver Transplant. 2001;7(4):359-62.
19. Tzakis A, Todo S, Starzl TE. Orthotopic liver transplantation with preservation of the inferior vena cava. Ann Surg. 1989;210:649-52.
20. Veroli P, Hage C, Ecoffey C. Does adult liver transplantation without venovenous bypass result in renal failure? Anesth Analg. 1992;75:489-94.
21. Schwarz B, Pomaroli A, Hoermann C, et al. Liver transplantation without venovenous bypass: morbidity and mortality in patients with greater than 50% reduction in cardiac output after vena cava clamping. J Cardiothorac Vasc Anesth 2001;15(4):460-2.
22. Wall WJ, Grant DR, Duff JH, et al. Liver transplantation without venous bypass. Transplantation. 1987;43:56-61.
23. Wu Y, Oyos TL, Chenhsu RY, et al. Vasopressor agents without volume expansion as a safe alternative to venovenous bypass during cavaplasty liver transplantation. Transplantation. 2003;76(12):1724-8.
24. Blanot S, Gillon MC, Ecoffey C, et al. Circulating endotoxins during orthotopic liver transplantation and post-reperfusion syndrome (letter). Lancet. 1993;342:859-60.
25. Estrin JA, Beiani KG, Ascher ML, et al. Hemodynamic changes on clamping and unclamping of major vessels during liver transplantation. Transplant Proc. 1989;21:3500-05.

26. Angeli P, Wong F, Watson H, et al. Hyponatremia in cirrhosis: results of a patient population survey. Hepatology. 2006;44(6):1535-42.
27. Abbasoglu O, Goldstein RM, Vodapally MS, et al. Liver transplantation in hyponatremic patients with emphasis on central pontine myelinolysis. Clin Transplant. 1998;12(3): 263-9.
28. Wszolek ZK, McComb RD, Pfeiffer RF, et al. Pontine and extrapontine myelinolysis following liver transplantation: relationship to serum sodium. Transplantation. 1989;48:1006-12.
29. Swygert TH, Roberts LC, Valek TR, et al. Effect of intraoperative low-dose dopamine on renal function in liver transplant recipients. Anesthesiology. 1991;75:571-6.
30. Wagener G, Gubitosa G, Renz J, et al. Vasopressin decreases portal vein pressure and flow in the native liver during liver transplantation. Liver Transplantation. 2008;14(11):1664-70.
31. Mukhtar A, Salah M, Aboulfetouh F, et al. The use of terlipressin during living donor liver transplantation: effects on systemic and splanchnic hemodynamics and renal function. Crit Care Med. 2011;39(6):1329-34.
32. Kalicinski P, Markiewicz M, Kaminski A, et al. Single pretransplant bolus of recombinant activated factor VII ameliorates influence of risk factors for blood loss during orthotopic liver transplantation. Ped Transpl. 2005;9(3): 299-304.
33. Niemann CU, Behrends M, Quan D, et al. Recombinant factor VIIa reduces transfusion requirements in liver transplant patients with high MELD scores. Transf Med. 2006;16(2):93-100.
34. Massicotte L, Lenis S, Thibeault L, et al. Effect of low central venous pressure and phlebotomy on blood product transfusion requirements during liver transplantations. Liver Transplantation. 2006;12(1):117-23.
35. Phillips SD, Maguire D, Deshpande R, et al. A prospective study investigating the cost effectiveness of intraoperative blood salvage during liver transplantation. Transplantation. 2006;81(4):536-40.
36. Brown MR, Ramsay MAE, Swygert TH. Exchange autotransfusion using the Cell saver during liver transplantation. Anesthesiology. 1989;70:168-9.
37. Lentschener C, Roche K, Ozier Y. A review of aprotinin in orthotopic liver transplantation: can its harmful effects offset its beneficial effects? Anesth Analg. 2005;100(5): 1248-55.
38. Dalmau A, Sabate A, Acosta F, et al. Tranexamic acid reduces red cell transfusion better than epsilon-aminocaproic acid or placebo in liver transplantation. Anesth Analg. 2000;91:29-34.
39. Arshad F, Lckx B, Beem RTV, et al. Prothrombin complex concentrate in the reduction of blood loss during orthotopic liver transplantation: Proton-trial. BMC Surgery. 2013;13:22.
40. Mourad MM, Liosis C, Gunson BK, et al. Etiology and management of hepatic artery thrombosis after adult liver transplantation. Liver Transplantation. 2014;20(6):713-23.

CHAPTER 24

Myocardial Protection during Cardiac Surgery: An Overview of Cardioplegia

Deepak K Tempe, Deepti Saigal

KEY POINTS

- Administration of cardioplegia solution after aortic cross clamping leads to instantaneous cardiac arrest thereby decreasing energy consumption and preserving energy stores.
- Potassium is the most common agent for inducing cardiac arrest, now used in a concentration of 10–30 mEq/L. Other important constituents of cardioplegia solution include buffering agents to maintain pH, agents to maintain hyperosmolarity and prevent myocardial edema, ATP regenerators and agents to improve myocardial protection.
- Blood has several advantages when used as a cardioplegia vehicle. These include enhanced oxygen carrying capacity, good rheological properties, ideal oncotic pressure, presence of endogenous buffers and free radical scavengers.
- Cardioplegia can be delivered to the myocardium in an antegrade (via aorta or coronary artery) or retrograde (coronary sinus or right atrium) fashion. While antegrade delivery helps achieve instant cardiac arrest, retrograde delivery is a more reliable route in coronary artery stenosis and aortic regurgitation. The combined route employing antegrade induction and retrograde route for continuous or repeat delivery has become an accepted practice.
- Continuous warm blood cardioplegia ensures a continuous supply of oxygen and energy substrates to the heart thus producing "aerobic arrest". However, it poses the risk of hyperkalemia, hyperglycemia, increased bleeding risks and increased risk for cerebral complications. Any discontinuation for surgical or other purposes lets to periods of warm ischemia which are unsafe.
- Terminal hot shots before unclamping of aorta provide oxygenated and enriched blood to the myocardium and also wash out the accumulated toxins.

INTRODUCTION

The most important difficulty perceived during the early period of cardiac surgery was the fact that the heart is an organ that moves (beats) while it works, and that it is always full of blood. To overcome these difficulties, cardioplegia was introduced and over the years has been refined and is a standard practice nowadays. The word cardioplegia derives its meaning from the Greek word *kardia* meaning heart and *plege* meaning stroke. Hence, literally cardioplegia means paralysis of the heart. Aortic cross clamping followed by administration of cardioplegia solution to achieve pharmacologically induced electromechanical cessation of the cardiac activity is an accepted practice during cardiac surgeries. This not only provides an immobile and bloodless surgical field, but also yields myocardial protection by quiscencing the myocardium. Although there is little role of cardioplegia in beating heart coronary artery bypass graft (CABG) surgery; the evolution of cardioplegia solutions continues as its use is indispensable in all on-pump procedures namely cardiac valve surgery, pediatric cardiac surgery and other complex cardiac surgical procedures including minimally invasive cardiac surgery.

WHY CARDIOPLEGIA?

The initial measures for providing intraoperative myocardial protection included the use of hypothermia. However, it went into disrepute with increased incidence of myocardial damage (stone heart) with prolonged periods of combined hypothermia and ischemia. It was subsequently postulated that chemically arresting the heart would preserve high energy phosphate stores and provide myocardial protection.

Arrested heart is the demand for any intracardiac procedure. The immobile heart hastens the work of the surgeon and also prevents lethal air embolism that may occur upon the opening up of a beating cardiac chamber. It also provides a bloodless field to the surgeon by preventing refilling from the pulmonary artery and coronary sinus. However, application of aortic cross clamp and administration of cardioplegia does not lead to immediate cessation of cardiac electromechanical activity. The mechanical arrest is preceded by fibrillation and contractions which deplete the myocardium of its high energy phosphate stores[1] leading to genesis of anaerobic milleu and potentiation of reperfusion injury. The institution of immediate cardioplegic arrest ensures that myocardial oxygen consumption (MVO_2) and consequent depletion of high energy phosphates (adenosine triphosphate ATP, adenosine diphosphate ADP) is significantly reduced.[2]

Hence, one of the major aims of using cardioplegia is the myocardial protection. Major advances have taken place in cardiac surgery with increase in the nature, complexity and length of procedures being performed; these have also been paralleled by advances in molecular biology and pharmacology. Evolution and assessment of new cardioplegia techniques for their composition, delivery vehicles, ideal temperature and administration methods thus continue so as to provide immediate arrest, a good surgical field (bloodless and relaxed heart), optimum myocardial protection along with easy reversibility of the arrest. However, the safe time limit of aortic cross clamping even with the use of cardioplegia protection cannot be defined. It will depend on the vulnerability of the myocardium to ischemic damage and needs to be individualized. So, it will also depend on the extent of the pre-existing myocardial disease that the patient has. It was generally agreed that the outcome is adversely affected when the cross-clamp time exceeds 120 min. The current thinking is that the postoperative myocardial damage is determined more by how the heart is protected, than how long the aorta is clamped.[3,4]

PHYSIOLOGICAL BASIS

The knowledge of cardiac electrophysiology is the key for understanding the functioning of cardioplegia solutions. The resting membrane potential (RMP) of cardiac myocytes is maintained around –91 mV by an active (energy or ATP dependent) 3Na$^+$(sodium)/2K$^+$(potassium) ion exchange pump. The initial rapid depolarization (phase 0) of the action potential (AP) is caused via rapid intracellular movement of Na$^+$ ions via fast Na$^+$ channels (get activated when RMP reaches –65 mV to –70 mV), which depolarizes the cell membrane up to +50 mV. This is followed by the phase of early rapid repolarization (phase 1) which occurs due to the inactivation of the fast Na$^+$ channels and activation of transient outward current of K$^+$. Thereafter, the opening up of long-type calcium (Ca^{2+}) channels leads to influx of cations into the cardiomyocyte, this balances with opening of the outward K$^+$ channels, thereby generating the plateau phase (phase 2). This intracellular influx of Ca^{2+} causes cytosolic release of Ca^{2+} from cytoplasmic reticulum and consequent contraction (electro-mechanical coupling). Phase 3 is the phase of final rapid repolarization occurring due to the activation of Ca^{2+} channels and the delayed K$^+$ rectifier channels. The normal pacemaker activity is maintained by activation of pacemaker channels I_f or the fast sodium current. I_f along with a decreasing permeability to K$^+$, causes spontaneous diastolic depolarization (phase 4).

COMPOSITION OF CARDIOPLEGIA SOLUTION

Agents to Induce Pharmacological Arrest

Potassium

Potassium is the most common agent used for cardioplegic arrest. The ability of potassium to cause diastolic arrest was reported by Ringer way back in 1883.[5] In the normal physiologic state with a K$^+$ concentration of 3.5–5.0 mEq/L, the RMP of cardiac myocyte cellular membrane is –85 mV. An increase in the extracellular K$^+$ decreases the membrane permeability to K$^+$ and brings the RMP to about –50 mV which is well beyond the Na$^+$ channel threshold. Therefore, these fast Na$^+$ channels remain closed, preventing any further depolarization and propagation of the AP at the sinoatrial (SA) node. Since there is no further repolarization also, hyperkalemia thus leads to a state of depolarized arrest. In 1929, Hooker introduced the concept of pharmacological arrest of heart. One ml of 2.5% potassium chloride (KCl) was injected into the coronary artery of a dog heart producing rapid cardiac arrest, which was reversed to sinus rhythm after wash out of potassium.[6] In 1954–55, Lam et al.[7] used intraventricular KCl injection for arresting the heart in hypothermic dogs. They reversed the effect of KCl by manual massage. However due to persistent ventricular fibrillation and difficulty in resumption of cardiac activity; further investigations were not performed. Instead, Lam and colleagues investigated the use of acetylcholine as a cardioplegic agent.[8] Acetylcholine 10 mg/kg was administered for rapid cardiac arrest, this was associated with sporadic beats and contractions of the atria and ventricles upon stimulation by the touch of surgical instruments. Reversal of acetylcholine happened by its wash out during reperfusion. It was suggested by Melrose that the difficulties encountered by Lam's KCl solution were because of the use of chloride salt. Melrose described the use of potassium citrate solution for inducing cardiac arrest in 1955.[9] Melrose solution contained very high concentrations of potassium (245–980 mg/L). However, it soon went into disrepute for almost 20 years due to reports on poor postoperative myocardial contractility and left ventricular failure.[10,11]

During this nidus of 20 years, several other techniques to provide myocardial protection were used and investigated. These included topical hypothermia, normothermic arrest, intermittent aortic occlusion, coronary perfusion and induced ventricular fibrillation.[12,13] But none was associated with improved clinical outcomes;[14] mortality rates were not reduced. Finding an optimum method of myocardial protection became the need of the hour as it was imperative for the success of any cardiac surgical procedure and the growth of the surgical field. Hence, there was renewed interest in chemical cardioplegia techniques; these were further investigated in various centers. It was also demonstrated that it was not the toxic effect of high K^+ concentration, but the chelation of intracellular Ca^{2+} and magnesium (Mg^{2+}) ions by citrate that was responsible for the deleterious myocardial effects of the Melrose's solution.[15] With further studies, it was established that lower concentrations of K^+ (10–30 mmol/L) were enough to produce diastolic arrest and also provided optimum functional recovery simultaneously.[16,17] This led to the revival of potassium based cardioplegia solutions for inducing cardiac arrest during cardiopulmonary bypass (CPB). Various solutions were developed with lower concentrations of potassium by Gay and Eberts et al., Bretschinder et al., Sondergard et al., Buckberg et al., Bainbridge et al., and others (Table 1). The solutions were broadly of two types: those based on extracellular matrix like Gay's and STH (St. Thomas Hospital) solution, and those based on intracellular matrix like Bretschneider's solution.[18-20]

Myocardial exposure even to the lower potassium levels in the above formulated solutions has been associated with several myocardial functional and morphological changes in post-cardioplegia period. Potassium causes depolarized arrest with the RMP of cellular membranes maintained at around −50 mV. There is a volley of currents that not only causes a detrimental increase in Na^+ and Ca^{2+} concentration in cells, but also causes energy utilization. ATP depletion causes intracellular acidosis with consequent activation of Na^+/H^+ ion exchanger, which further activates Na^+/Ca^{2+} ion exchanger. The resultant increases in intracellular Na^+ and Ca^{2+} ion concentrations cause mitochondrial damage, contractures, cellular edema, apoptosis and cell death. Restoration of ionic imbalances to attain electroneutrality is also an active process that consumes ATP at the time of reperfusion and potentiates damages.[21,22] Potassium also causes microvascular injury and the concentration of potassium in cardioplegia solutions determines the extent of endothelial damage.[23] It has also been associated with coronary vasospasm causing impaired myocardial perfusion in the post-cardioplegia period.[24] The key seems to be to determine the optimum concentration of various ions in the cardioplegia solution.

Magnesium

Initial reports of the use of magnesium sulfate ($MgSO_4$) for the purpose of cardioplegia date back to 1958.[25] Magnesium aspartate was introduced for cardioplegia by Kirsch et al. in 1969.[26] It augments the arrest produced by potassium by virtue of its effect on transmembrane ion movements. Blockade of intracellular metabolism yields additional margin of safety. Use of Mg aspartate also accelerates the regeneration of ATP from inosine phosphate. Latest evidence concludes the undoubted role of inclusion of Mg in cardioplegia solutions for augmenting myocardial protection.[27]

Table 1: Composition of various cardioplegia solutions

	Melrose solution	Kirsch's solution	Bretschneider's solution 1	Bretschneider's solution 2	Bretschneider's solution 3	Buckberg's solution	St Thomas Hospital Solution 1	St Thomas Hospital Solution 2 (Plegisol)	Gay and Eberts	Hamburg	Tyers
KCl	25% K citrate	0.3%	1.5–2 mmol/L	5 mmol/L	0.75 g/L	30 mmol/L	16 mmol/L	16 mmol/L	25 mEq/L	5 mmol/L	20 mmol/L KHCO$_3$ 10 mmol/L
Magnesium		2.5% (as-partate)	0.5–2.5 mmol/L	1 mmol/L	0.2 g/L (MgCl$_2$)		MgCl$_2$ 16 mmol/L	16 mmol/L		Aspartate 2 mmol/L	MgCl$_2$ 1.5 mmol/L
Procaine hydrochloride			0.2%	0.2%	2 g/L		1 mmol/mL	2 mmol/L		4 mmol/L	
Sodium chloride			50–60 mmol/L	10 mmol/L	0.7 g/L	91 mmol/L	147 mmol/L	110 mmol/L	200 mEq/L	25 mmol/L	88 mmol/L
Calcium chloride						2 mmol/L	2 mmol/L	1.2 mmol/L		0.5 mmol/L	0.5 mmol/L
Sorbitol		4.5%									
Mannitol			320 mosm/L	320 mosm/L	43.5 g/L					200 mmol/L	
Glucose			0.5–1 mmol/L			50% 40 mL (with 40 units insulin)			2 g/L	10 mmol/L	
Plasmanate						850 mL					
Salt poor albumen						50 mL				Haes 6%	
Others										Na acetate 27 mmol/L Na gluconate 23 mmol/L Oxygen Methylprednisolone	Heparin

Contd...

Contd...

	Melrose solution	Kirsch's solution	Bretschneider's solution 1	Bretschneider's solution 2	Bretschneider's solution 3	Buckberg's solution	St Thomas Hospital Solution 1	St Thomas Hospital Solution 2 (Plegisol)	Gay and Eberts	Hamburg	Tyers
Buffer						THAME 20 ml			$NaHCO_3$ 1 g/L	$NaHCO_3$ 25 mmol/L	
pH			7.4	7.4			5.5–7	7.8			
Osmolarity							300–320 mosm/L	285–300 mosm/L		320 mosm/L	275 mosm/L
Dose	Diluted in a ratio of 1:9 with oxygenated blood	50 mL	1 L	1 L		250 mL loading over one minute followed by 150 mL/min for two min	1 L				

Procaine

It is a Na⁺ channel blocker and hence augments the action of potassium. It also offers the advantage of being a membrane stabilizer. It was introduced by Bretschneider in his cardioplegia formulations.[19]

Adenosine

Although the return of potassium based cardioplegia solutions have revolutionized the progress of cardiac surgery; with the above known adverse effects of potassium and inclusion of elderly and sicker patients in the surgical population; more agents were introduced to induce cardiac arrest. The toxic effects of myocardial exposure to high potassium concentrations used in cardioplegia solutions and documented cardioprotective effects[28] of adenosine have paved the way towards growing use of adenosine as an adjunct to potassium for inducing cardiac arrest in cardioplegia solutions.[29,30] It is postulated to be useful especially in patients who are at risk of low cardiac output syndromes (LCOS). Adenosine has been used in conjunction with lower doses of potassium solutions as well as with lignocaine.[22] However, its use as a sole agent in replacement of supranormal potassium is limited because of rapid catabolism and short half-life of adenosine (0.6 seconds).

Four subtypes of adenosine receptors have been identified; namely A_1 A_2, A_3, and A_4. Stimulation of A_1 receptors enhances the outward K⁺ current causing persistent hyperpolarization thereby inhibiting SA and AV node depolarization leading to rapid cardiac arrest. The cardioprotective effects are also mediated by A_1 activation. However, since the cardioprotective effects outweigh the A_1 receptor activation; additional mechanisms have been suggested. This additional cardioprotective effect can be explained by its role as a substrate for resynthesis of high energy phosphates. Also, unlike potassium; it prevents an increase of intracellular calcium.[31] Adenosine also protects the mitochondrial integrity and function; this is mediated via mito KATP channels, and is reflected as a better mechanoenergetic efficiency or a better utilization of oxygen for ATP formation. Adenosine has a suppressive effect on the inflammatory component of reperfusion injury by three mechanisms. There is direct inhibition of neutrophils leading to reduced superoxide anion generation and reduced expression of adhesion molecules, A_2 receptor mediated inhibition of endothelial activation and finally A_3 receptor mediated inhibition of neutrophil adherence to the endothelium.[32,33]

Agents to Maintain Hyperosmolarity

Various agents such as mannitol, sorbitol, glucose-insulin and plasma proteins are added so as to maintain hyperosmolarity of the solution so as to prevent myocardial edema.[34]

Buffers

The cellular metabolic processes (e.g. membrane pump) are pH dependent. Bicarbonate, inorganic phosphates and THAM (trometamol; tris-hydroxymethyl aminomethane) have been used as buffering agents to maintain the pH and minimize the ischemic injury.[35] Advantages of using THAM include its ability to act as an intracellular buffer, appropriate pKa which changes in parallel with change in physiological pH as temperature varies, and most importantly unlike bicarbonate; it is a closed buffer system. It has a superior buffering capacity to histidine. However, higher doses (>12 mmol/L) can cause myocardial depression and systemic toxic effects.[36] The histidine/histidine chloride buffer pair possesses an ideal temperature profile and also acts as a free radical scavenger. It is the buffer used in the Bretschneider histidine-tryptophane-a-ketoglutarate (HTK) solution (CustodiolTM, Dr. F. Kö hler Chemie, Alsbach-Ha"hnlein, Germany).[37]

ATP Regenerators

These include xanthine, ribose, adenosine, alpha ketoglutarate.

Adjuncts for Myocardial Protection

The role of various agents such as calcium channel blockers, potassium channel openers (diazoxide) and sodium hydrogen exchanger inhibitors (eniporide) has been studied to minimize ischemic and reperfusion injuries and improve myocardial protection. However, none is being used routinely because of insufficient data to support the beneficial effects.[38-40]

HTK Solution

It is based on the original Bretschneider's solution. Histidine is the buffering agent. Alpha ketoglutarate serves as an energy substrate as it is an intermediate metabolite of Kreb's cycle and a precursor of nicotinamide dinucleotide. Tryptophan functions as a membrane stabilizer. Osmolarity is maintained using mannitol. Many studies have proved the beneficial effects of this solution for myocardial protection. Because of its long duration of action; it has been propagated as the cardioplegia solution of choice for minimally invasive mitral valve surgery. Cases of hemodilution and subsequent hyponatremia because of absorption in CPB circuit have been reported.[37,41]

CARDIOPLEGIA VEHICLE

Blood versus Crystalloid Cardioplegia

Various strategies have been developed to improvise the cardioplegia solutions so as to maximize myocardial protection. Use of blood as a vehicle for delivery of cardioplegia solution was one of them, definitely this was a turning point in the practice of cardioplegia technique.

Blood has several qualities which support its use as a cardioplegia delivery medium. First of all, it has a greater oxygen carrying capacity due to presence of hemoglobin. The rheological properties of blood enhance microcirculation. It has an ideal oncotic pressure that prevents myocardial edema. Natural buffering capacity due to presence of endogenous buffers such as carbonic anhydrase and histidine containing molecules along with the presence of antioxidants such as glutathione, peroxidase and catalase are additional benefits. Blood provides ideal metabolic substrates to heart for anaerobic (glucose) as well as aerobic (free fatty acids) metabolism. Buckberg, who pioneered the concept of blood cardioplegia had quoted that blood provides several benefits to the surgeon "that cannot be measured". He postulated that blood being the natural fluid for organ perfusion should be preferred over crystalloid as a cardioplegia medium.[42,43]

At the same time, there are certain disadvantages with the use of blood cardioplegia. These include impairment of vision while performance of distal coronary anastomosis. Also presence of white blood cells and cytokines act as propagators to the inflammatory responses and reperfusion injury. Leuko-reduced blood cardioplegia could be used as an alternative to blood cardioplegia to offset the inflammatory damages, this area needs further exploration. Depletion of at least 90% leucocytes in blood cardioplegia is recommended along with initial five minutes of reperfusion with the leuko-reduced blood so as to attenuate the reperfusion injury.[44,45]

Hemodiluted blood cardioplegia came into use because it preserved the advantages offered by blood, reduced the crystalloid load; and a lowered hematocrit decreased rouleaux formation that caused sludging and probably impaired the uniform distribution of the blood cardioplegia solution at the microcirculatory level. A 4:1 ratio of blood to crystalloid was used. This also made it easy to accommodate the other ingredients such as glucose, bicarbonate and THAM. Hemodilution, however can pose the risk of myocardial edema.

Microplegia is the use of low volume of blood cardioplegia without any hemodilution. Thus, it possesses all the qualities of blood cardioplegia and lowers the risk of myocardial edema.[43]

There is no clear cut clinical evidence whether hemodiluted blood cardioplegia or microplegia is superior to crystalloid cardioplegia. Many randomized controlled trials (RCTs) and their meta-analysis have been performed with inconclusive results regarding return of cardiac activity, incidence of LCOS, incidence of postoperative myocardial infarction (MI) and length of hospital stay.[46-49]

Perfluorocarbon-based Cardioplegia

Perfluorocarbon-based cardioplegia instead of blood or crystalloid-based cardioplegia solutions have also been studied by certain investigators. It was associated with better oxygen delivery to myocardium during the ischemic phase as compared to blood cardioplegia that translates into oxidative metabolism and preservation of high energy phosphate stores, prevention of intracellular acidosis and inorganic phosphate accumulation; thereby leading to better post-ischemic functional recovery and lesser reperfusion related morphological damages.[50,51] However, certain investigators stated that although perfluorocarbons do preserve high energy phosphates and aerobic metabolism during the ischemic phase; there is no metabolic or functional advantage concurred in the reperfusion phase.[52] The role of perfluorocarbons as a cardioplegia vehicle is not well defined and requires further validation in the form of large RCTs and meta-analysis.

ADMINISTRATION: APPROACHES AND METHODS

Proper administration of cardioplegia and its uniform distribution in myocardium is the precursor to its ability to offer optimum myocardial protection. The commonly used administration approaches are: antegrade cardioplegia, retrograde cardioplegia and combined anterograde- retrograde cardioplegia.

Antegrade Cardioplegia

This is one of the commonest approaches for cardioplegia delivery used by cardiac surgeons world over because of its ease and simplicity. It has been stated as the preferred approach in minimally invasive mitral valve surgery. It involves the delivery of cardioplegia solution via a cardioplegia cannula inserted in the root of aorta (Figs. 1A and B). After the commencement of CPB, the cardioplegia line is flushed. The aortic pressure is lowered to around 50–60 mm Hg and the aorta is cross clamped. The perfusionist is then asked to deliver cardioplegia solution at a rate of 300 mL/min so as to achieve full closure of aortic valve followed by a rate of 200 mL/min. Use of intraoperative transesophageal echocardiography (TOE) to rule out aortic regurgitation (AR), or direct holding of the left ventricle (LV) in the surgeons hand to rule out LV spillage can reassure about the proper delivery of cardioplegia solution. Antegrade cardioplegia produces immediate diastolic arrest, but has the following disadvantages:

❑ It requires a competent aortic valve to prevent leakage into the LV. It is thus an ineffective method in patients with AR. However, the surgeon can administer the cardioplegia directly via the coronary ostia by using a coronary ostial cannula (Fig. 2). This poses the potential risk of damage to the ostia, coronary

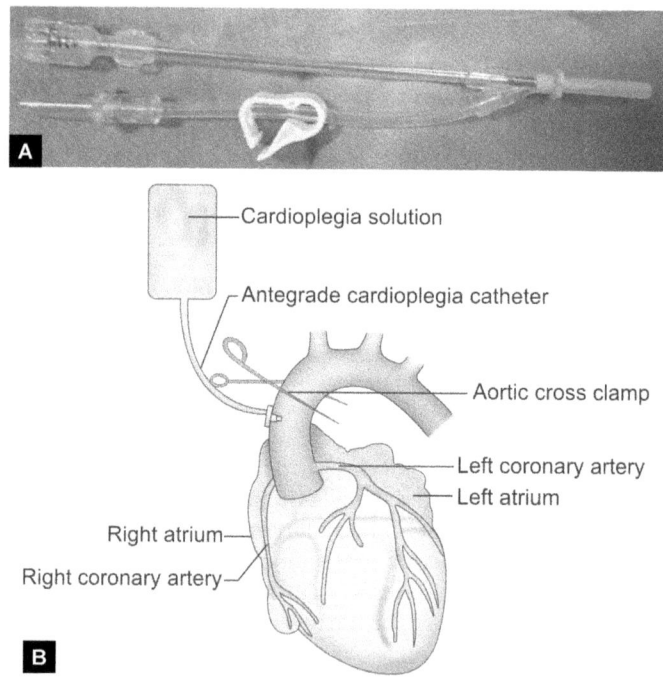

Figs. 1A and B: (A) Antegrade cardioplegia–aortic root cannula; (B) Schematic diagram showing administration of the antegrade cardioplegia.

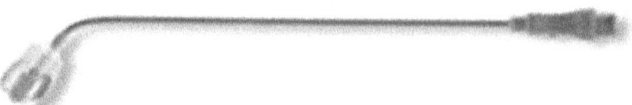

Fig. 2: Antegrade cardioplegia—coronary ostial cannula.

artery dissection and delayed onset ostial coronary artery stenosis [post 1-6 months of aortic valve replacement (AVR), incidence up to 5%, more common in left coronary artery].[53] Infact, coronary artery stenosis should be suspected in all patients who complain of angina after AVR. TOE can be a useful tool to diagnose acute coronary ostial stenosis in patients with intra-operative LV dysfunction due to acute ostial stenosis.[54] The incidence of complications is independent of intermittent or continuous dosage of cardioplegia as well as intermittent withdrawal or continuous coronary arterial presence of the catheter. The ostial injury and subsequent healing fibrotic process causing stenosis may be related to the infusion pressure of the cardioplegic fluid and overdilatation of the vessel by the catheter tip.[53] With the development of better quality cardioplegia cannula, this problem has been largely overcome.

❑ A uniform distribution of the cardioplegia solution requires an unobstructed arterial system. In patients with coronary artery disease (CAD), there is an inadequate supply of cardioplegia to the ill-perfused myocardial areas, thereby causing suboptimal myocardial protection.

Retrograde Cardioplegia

After being introduced in 1950s,[55] retrograde cardioplegia delivery became popular by 1970s mainly to overcome the demerits of the conventional antegrade approach. A retrograde delivery of cardioplegia is performed via a cannula inserted in the coronary sinus (Fig. 3). The cannula can be placed under direct vision by atriotomy which mandates dual venous cannulation. This need can be circumvented by blind insertion of a stylet based coronary sinus catheter after making a small puncture in the right atrium. It should be positioned correctly to ensure retroperfusion in all tributaries of the coronary sinus. TOE guidance can aid coronary sinus cannulation by assessing adequate depth of insertion, decreasing the time required for placement and reducing associated trauma.[56,57] After its insertion, the balloon of the catheter should be gently inflated so as to seal the coronary sinus opening to prevent the spillage. The maximum infusion pressure should not exceed 40 mm Hg and delivery rate should be around 100 mL/min to prevent jet induced lesions. The cardioplegia returns to the root of aorta and it must be vented by aortic root vent. In patients undergoing aortic valve replacement (AVR), aortic root vent is not necessary, as the aorta is already opened for replacing the valve. The cannula stays in place once the balloon is inflated, additionally it may be secured using an anchoring suture. Retrograde cardioplegia can also be administered directly inside the right atrium, this is known as atrial cardioplegia. This was introduced with the hypothesis of improved right ventricle (RV) protection over coronary sinus retroplegia by enhancement of the delivery to the RV directly by way of the Thebesian veins. However, atrial cardioplegia requires occlusion of the two venae cavae and the main pulmonary artery to prevent leakage. The RV distension secondary to this technique poses a doubt on the efficacy of RV preservation. Also, there may be inadequate delivery of cardioplegia to the LV with right atrial injection of the cardioplegia making LV protection also inadequate.[58,59] The present practice is to use specially designed retrograde cardioplegia cannula with self inflating balloon tips that inflate with infusion of cardioplegia, which are inserted blindly or under TOE guidance into the coronary sinus.

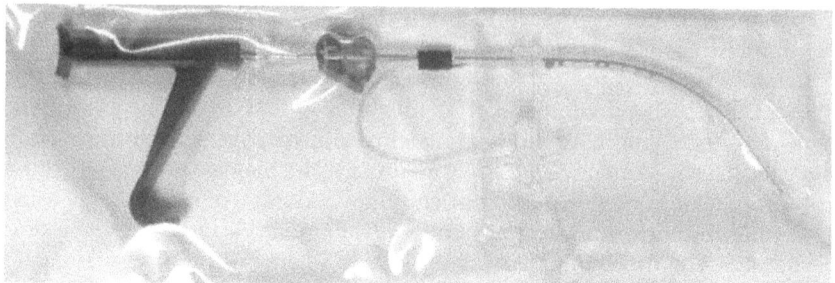

Fig. 3: Retrograde cardioplegia—coronary sinus catheter.

Retrograde cardioplegia has the following advantages:
1. It provides an effective means for cardioplegia delivery in AR.[60] Direct coronary ostial cannulation and its associated complications can be avoided.
2. It can be used in patients with calcification of the aortic walls and narrow aortic lumens.
3. In complex and lengthy procedures such as multiple valve replacements or aortic aneurysm repairs or certain pediatric corrections that require a longer cross clamp times and thus a re-administration of cardioplegia, a retrograde technique provides uninterrupted surgery and eliminates the need for aortic re-exposure.
4. There is a lower incidence of supraventricular arrhythmias due to the hypothermic and protective effect bestowed on right heart by direct spillage of the retroperfusate.
5. Myocardial protection is also improved because of a more uniform distribution of the cardioplegia in the myocardium, especially relevant for hypertrophic LVs as in aortic stenosis.
6. It is an effective method for myocardial protection in the presence of CAD wherein the diseased myocardium cannot be perfused antegradely.[61] The venous system on the other hand is an unobstructed system, free of atherosclerosis and can be a more reliable route for distribution of the cardioplegia solution to the entire myocardium.

Disadvantages of retrograde cardioplegia include:
1. Coronary sinus injury:
    ➤ Rupture of the coronary sinus may result from sudden over-inflation of the balloon. To prevent this, the balloon should be gently inflated until it just occludes the lumen of the coronary sinus, not aiming for a tight seal. This is not necessary if cannula with a self inflating balloon tip is used.
2. Delay in cardiac arrest:
    ➤ Rapid occurrence of cardiac arrest is the principle of myocardial protection offered by cardioplegia administration. Although a delayed onset of cardiac arrest (due to slow administration) has been reported and theoretically this should be associated with depletion of the high energy stores, there is no evidence of a cause-effect relationship. That means, a delayed cardiac arrest with retrograde cardioplegia has not led to poor postoperative outcomes.[62]

3. Inadequate RV preservation:[63]
   ➢ Initial animal anatomical studies had shown that the RV and right side of the interventricular septum is not drained by coronary sinus.[64] This was speculated as a reason for probable inadequate RV protection by retrograde cardioplegia. However, firstly, there was no further clinical evidence of inadequate RV protection even in studies carried on dogs, probably due to the presence of effective veno-venous channels. Secondly, because of the differences in dog and human cardiac venous anatomy, the above findings cannot entirely be extrapolated to human subjects. In fact, the drainage pattern of human RV is also favorable for RV protection with the use of retrograde cardioplegia. Thebasian veins draining directly into the RV allow for topical hypothermic and cardioplegic protection to the ventricle as well as right side of interventricular septum. Also, the anterior cardiac vein from the RV anastomoses with the tributaries of coronary sinus before emptying into the right atrium. Hence, it gets retroperfused with retroplegia injected into coronary sinus. Finally, the posterior interventricular vein that drains the diaphragmatic wall of RV and the veins draining the posterior part of the interventricular septum enter the coronary sinus just at the opening of the sinus into right atrium. If the retroplegia cannula is properly positioned and not over inserted thereby not obscuring the opening of the posterior interventricular vein in the coronary sinus, this vein will be adequately retroperfused too. Equally good preservation of both the ventricles has been shown in some studies.[65]
4. Prolonged delivery times:
   ➢ Since the rate of administration is 100 mL/min versus 300 mL/min for antegrade route; it takes a longer duration to deliver the same amount of cardioplegia solution. In patients with CAD, delivery time may go up to 30 min. However; this very feature offers the advantage of delaying the wash out of cardioplegia by the non- coronary collateral blood flow. A prolonged and continuous flow helps maintain delivery of substrates and buffering agents, causes removal of toxic metabolites and improves the overall oxygen delivery when blood or oxygenated crystalloid cardioplegia is used.

Combined Antegrade and Retrograde Cardioplegia

A combined technique of antegrade and retrograde cardioplegia has gained popularity in the last few decades. The combined mode of delivery provides immediate cardiac arrest after antegrade cardioplegia; and also preserves the benefits of subsequent retrograde cardioplegia.[66-68] Although this has been found to be useful for best myocardial protection in CAD patients,[69-71] its role in patients with normal LV function and in the absence of CAD is debatable.[72,73] The combined technique is also useful in patients undergoing complex procedures requiring longer cross clamp times, as the cardioplegia can be repeated using the retrograde route without interruption of the surgery.[74]

TEMPERATURE: COLD, WARM, TEPID

It is a known fact that hypothermia decreases the metabolic rate and decreases myocardial oxygen requirements thus decreasing the ischemic damage.

Hence, "warm ischemia" is believed to be more damaging than "cold ischemia". The role of hypothermia for myocardial protection is probably as old as cardiac surgery itself. It was found that electromechanical arrest decreased MVO_2 by 90% in the working heart at normothermia, this was reduced by an extra 20–30% with hypothermia. Initially hypothermia was used as the sole method or in conjunction with aortic cross clamping for arrest and preservation of the cardiac function. However with the rebirth of chemical cardioplegia in 1970s, hypothermia was incorporated in the form of topical hypothermia, and more importantly as cold crystalloid cardioplegia. Cold crystalloid cardioplegia causes myocardial hypothermia and decreases the ischemic injury until delivery of the next cardioplegia dose. Cold crystalloid cardioplegia with a temperature up to 10°C to 12°C was the main component of myocardial protection in the earlier decades.[75,76] The need for profound hypothermia was questioned due to following reasons:[77]

1. The oxygen demand of the arrested heart being as low as 0.3 mL/100 g/minute at 20°C, further hypothermia was not considered beneficial.
2. Since asanguineous crystalloid cardioplegia was increasingly being replaced with blood cardioplegia solutions, there was a risk of decreased oxygen uptake by myocardial tissue due to leftwards shift of the oxygen-hemoglobin dissociation curve. It was found that at 20°C, only 50% of the total oxygen content was available for uptake, this further decreased by additional 30% at 10°C. Tissue hypercarbia and acidosis may offset the hypothermia related prevention of oxygen unloading.
3. Hypothermia also caused increased rouleaux formation, sludging and activation of cold agglutinins; thus affecting the flow and distribution of blood cardioplegia.
4. Hypothermia can only decrease the metabolism and does not stop it completely; the anaerobic metabolism continues; it was found that energy needs of anaerobic metabolism were not met during hypothermia; and hence cold ischemia is not free of ischemic damages. In fact, it was demonstrated that hypothermia caused greater suppression of the glycolytic pathway for ATP production than the oxygen consumption (demand more than supply) which could potentiate the ischemic damages.
5. It also caused membrane destabilization, intracellular Ca^{2+} sequestration, inhibition of important enzymes like Na^+-K^+ ATPase leading to myocardial cellular edema.
6. Profound hypothermia necessitated prolonged reperfusion periods for return to normothermic levels, increasing the risk of reperfusion injury.
   Above factors, combined with the advent of blood cardioplegia that ensured delivery of oxygen and substrates to the arrested myocardium gave birth to the idea of continuous normothermic or warm blood cardioplegia that constituted warm aerobic arrest.[77,78]

Antegrade tepid blood cardioplegia (27°C–32°C) was introduced to combine the advantages of warm and cold blood cardioplegia and to minimize the detrimental effects (increased incidence of cerebral complications, increased bleeding risk) of warm blood cardioplegia.[4,79-81]

REPEAT DOSES (INTERMITTENT/REPEAT), CONTINUOUS INFUSIONS

Apart from popularizing blood cardioplegia, Buckberg and colleagues, in 1976, also postulated the importance of intermittent reinfusion of cardioplegic solution to replace the losses due to the washout of cardioplegia solution from non-coronary collateral perfusion. Replenishment by intermittent infusions maintains the heart in an arrested state, maintains hypothermia (if cold cardioplegia is used), decreases myocardial edema and also provides for delivery of energy substrates and wash out of the accumulated toxic metabolites. Studies in normal hearts show that up to four hours of safe aortic clamping can be achieved by intermittent doses of cold blood cardioplegia. Reinfusion may not be necessary in cases where cross clamp times are not long. Intermittent dosings are preferable when continuous cardioplegia flow may impede the surgical vision and impair technical precision.[82]

CURRENT CARDIOPLEGIA STRATEGIES

Combined Warm Antegrade and Intermittent Cold Retrograde Cardioplegia

Conceptualized by Buckberg and colleagues, this technique combines the advantages of the two routes of delivery as well as warm induction followed by cold intermittent protection, offsetting the shortcomings of individual techniques. A warm induction is useful in resuscitation of diseased hearts with poor function like in patients with acute MI, low ejection fractions or cardiogenic shock. Delivery of substrate (aspartate, glutamate, etc.) enriched normothermic blood cardioplegia helps in recovery of these ischemically damaged and substrate depleted hearts, and cold intermittent doses decrease the ischemic damage especially when interruptions in surgery are not desirable.[83-86]

Continuous Warm Blood Cardioplegia

The concept that "there is no reperfusion injury without ischemia" and the well established use of blood as a cardioplegia vehicle were the major principles for the birth and survival of continuous blood cardioplegia. This strategy aims to prevent any duration of myocardial ischemia during aortic cross-clamping by continuous retrograde delivery of blood cardioplegia. Due to a continuous provision of metabolic substrates and oxygen (mimicking a "perfused" state) even though the heart is arrested, it leads to a situation of "aerobic arrest". Hence, aortic clamping does not lead to anaerobiasis and consequent reperfusion injury. The need for hypothermic protection is also obviated because of uninterrupted perfusion of the heart.[87,88] As the heart is normothermic, systemic hypothermia can also be deferred.

After antegrade induction of hyperkalemic normothermic blood cardioplegia, continuous retrograde infusion of normothermic cardioplegia is continued throughout the surgical procedure. The potassium concentration in this second phase of cardioplegia can be titrated down (6 mEq/L) or up (if there is resumption of electrical activity). Also, continuous perfusion may be provided by the antegrade or retrograde route at a rate of 50–150 mL/min, which may have to be increased to 150–250 mL/min for hypertrophic hearts and redo surgeries.[77]

Ikonomidis et al.[89] have suggested that maintenance of aerobic metabolism requires flow rates of at least 200 mL/min, these are detrimental if given by the coronary sinus. The same has been performed along with coronary sinus pressure monitoring, and have shown to decrease the lactate production and maintain coronary venous pH within normal limits.

Lichtenstein et al. have concluded several benefits with continuous warm blood cardioplegia including earlier spontaneous return of normal sinus rhythm, shorter reperfusion times (time interval between aortic unclamping and withdrawal of CPB) and a lower incidence of postoperative LCOS and MI. Hence, they emphasized that continuous warm blood cardioplegia may provide optimum myocardial protection in patients with poor cardiac reserves.[90] Many trials have proved the beneficial effects of continuous warm blood cardioplegia.[91-93] Nevertheless, continuous warm blood cardioplegia has the following drawbacks. Most surgeons discontinue the cardioplegic flow for some time, especially while performance of distal anastomosis. This leads to a period of unwanted warm ischemia. To prevent damages during these periods; cardioplegia should have a hemoglobin of at least 8 g% and flow rates of at least 100 mL/min when being perfused.[94] Continuous cardioplegia can also cause systemic hyperglycemia and hyperkalemia.[4]

Intermittent Antegrade Warm Blood Cardioplegia

This was introduced by Calafiore in 1995 with the aim of providing a bloodless field to the surgeon that was not possible with continuous warm blood cardioplegia. Doses were repeated at 15 minutes intervals. Hypothermia is completely avoided. However, use of antegrade route limits spread of cardioplegia distal to the critically stenosed coronary arterial segments. This inadequate delivery along with periods of interruption (warm ischemic periods) may contribute to inadequate myocardial protection.[95]

Warm Terminal Reperfusion ('Hot-Shot')

This is based on the same principle as antegrade warm cardioplegic induction of the diseased hearts. A terminal infusion of normothermic, oxygenated, substrate enriched blood cardioplegia to the arrested heart just before the removal of aortic cross clamp provides oxygen and energy substrates, counters acidosis and hypothermia, chelates calcium and also limits myocardial edema.[96] The oxygen is utilized towards cellular repair rather than electromechanical activity. The hot-shot cardioplegia can also be administered via retrograde route in patients with left ventricular hypertrophy undergoing AVR.

Controlled Reperfusion

Controlled reperfusion is a strategy to reduce reperfusion injury during coronary revascularization after acute coronary occlusion.[45,97] After completion of the final distal anastomosis and release of the aortic clamp, the controlled blood cardioplegic solution is administered at a flow rate of up to 50 mL/min per graft with a perfusion pressure not exceeding 50 mm Hg for 20 min into the grafts only.

CONCLUSION

With the expanding horizon of different components, vehicles, routes and dosing strategies of cardioplegia available in the armamentarium of the cardiac anesthesiologist and surgeon; there will exist institutional and personal preferences based on evidence as well as experience. However, the technique should be tailored according to the condition of the heart and the demand of the surgery. Combining various approaches to compensate individual shortcomings may aid to provide optimum myocardial protection. Inadequate myocardial protection can lead to increased morbidity thereby increasing the length and cost of hospital stay.

REFERENCES

1. Schaff HV, Dombroff R, Flaherty JT, et al. Effect of potassium cardioplegia on myocardial ischemia and post arrest ventricular function. Circulation. 1978;58:240-9.
2. Goldstein SM, Nelson RL, McConnell DH, et al. Effects of conventional hypothermic ischemic arrest and pharmacological arrest on myocardial supply/demand balance during aortic cross clamping. Ann Thorac Surg. 1977;23:520-8.
3. Tempe DK. Myocardial protection during cardiopulmonary bypass. In: Clinical Practice of Cardiac Anaesthesia, 3rd edition; CBS Publishers, Delhi. pp. 342-64.
4. Buckberg GD. Warm versus cold blood cardioplegia: A self- imposed and counterproductive dilemma. Ann Thorac Surg. 1993;56:1007-15.
5. Ringers S. A further contribution regarding the influence of the different constituents of the blood on the contraction of the heart. J Physiol. 1883;4:29-42.
6. Hooker DR. On recovery of the heart in electric shock. Am J Physiol. 1930;91:305-28.
7. Lam CR, Geoghegan T, Sergeant CH, et al. Clinical experiences with induced cardiac arrest during intracardiac surgical procedures. Ann Surg. 1957;146:439-49.
8. Sergeant CK, Geoghegan T, Lam CR. Further studies in induced cardiac arrest using the agent acetylcholine. Forum of American College of Surgeons. 1956;7:254-7.
9. Melrose DG, Dreoer B, Bentall HH, et al. Elective cardiac arrest. Lancet 1955;2:21-2.
10. Helmsworth JA, Kaplan S, Clark LC, et al. Myocardial injury associated with asytole induced with potassium citrate. Ann Surg. 1959;149:200-6.
11. McFarland DG, Dreyer B, Bentall HH, et al. Myocardial necrosis following elective cardiac arrest induced with potassium citrate. J Thorac Cardiovasc Surg. 1960;40:200-8.
12. Griepp RB, Stinson EB, Shumway NE. Profound local hypothermia for myocardial protection during open-heart surgery. J Thorac Cardiovasc Surg. 1973;66:731-41.
13. Kay EB, Head LR, Nogueira C. Direct coronary artery perfusion for aortic valve surgery. Report of technique. JAMA. 1953;168:1767-8.
14. Cooley DA, Reul GJ, Wukasch DC. Ischemic contracture of the heart: "stone heart". Am J Cardiol. 1972;29:575-7.
15. Hoelscher B. Studies by electron microscopy on the effects of magnesium chloride-procaine amide or potassium citrate on the myocardium in induced cardiac arrest. J Cardiovasc Surg (Torino). 1967;8:163-6.
16. Gharagozloo F, Bulkley BH, Hutchins GM, et al. Potassium-induced cardioplegia during normothermic cardiac arrest. Morphologic study of the effect of varying concentrations of potassium on myocardial anoxic injury. J Thorac Cardiovasc Surg. 1979;77:602-7.
17. Gay WA, Ebert PA. Functional metabolic and morphological effects of potassium-induced cardioplegia. Surgery. 1973;74:283-90.
18. Braimbridge MV, Chayen J, Bitensky L, et al. Cold cardioplegia or continuous coronary perfusion? J Thorac Cardiovasc Surg. 1977;74:900-6.
19. Sondergaard T, Senn A. Clinical experience with cardioplegia according to Bretschneider. Langenbecks Arch Chir. 1967;319:661-5.

20. Tyers GFO, Manley NJ, Williams GH, et al. Preliminary clinical experience with isotonic hypothermic potassium induced arrest. J Thorac Cardiovasc Surg. 1977;74:674-81.
21. Chambers DJ, Hearse DJ. Developments in cardioprotection: 'polarized' arrest as an alternative to 'depolarized' arrest. Ann Thorac Surg. 1999;68:1960-6.
22. Dobson GP, Jones MW. Adenosine and lidocaine: a new concept in nondepolarizing surgical myocardial arrest, protection, and preservation. J Thorac Cardiovasc Surg. 2004;127:794-805.
23. Mankad PS, Chester AH, Yacoub MH. Role of potassium concentration in cardioplegic solutions in mediating endothelial damage. Ann Thorac Surg. 1991;51:89-93.
24. Sellke FW, Shafique T, Schoen FJ, Weintraub RM. Impaired endothelium-dependent coronary microvascular relaxation after cold potassium cardioplegia and reperfusion. J Thorac Cardiovas Surg. 1993;105:52-8.
25. Sealy WC, Young WG, Brown IW, et al. Potassium, magnesium, and neostigmine for controlled cardioplegia. Studies on the dog using extracorporeal circulation and hypothermia. Arch Surg. 1958;77:33-8.
26. Kirsch U, Rodewald G, Kalmar P. Induced ischemic arrest and clinical experience with cardioplegia in open heart surgery. J Thorac Cardiovasc Surg. 1972;63:121-30.
27. Duan L, Zhang CF, Luo WJ, et al. Does magnesium-supplemented cardioplegia reduce cardiac injury? A meta-analysis of randomized controlled trials. J Card Surg. 2015;30:338-45.
28. Ely SW, Berne RM. Protective effects of adenosine in myocardial ischemia. Circulation. 1992;85:893-904.
29. Fremes SE, Levy SL, Christakis GT, et al. Phase 1 human trial of adenosine-potassium cardioplegia. Circulation. 1996;94:370-5.
30. Hudspeth DA, Nakanishi K, Johansen JV, et al. Adenosine in blood cardioplegia prevents postischemic dysfunction in ischemically injured hearts. Ann Thorac Surg. 1994;58:1637-44.
31. Jovanovic A, Alekseev AE, Lopez JR, et al. Adenosine prevents hyperkalemia induced calcium loading in cardiac cells: relevance for cardioplegia. Ann Thorac Surg. 1997;63:153-61.
32. Johansen JV, Thourani VH, Ronson RS, et al. Pathophysiology of ischemic reperfusion injury. Broadspectrum cardioprotection with adenosine. Ann Thorac Surg. 1999;68:1942-48.
33. Jakobsen O, Muller S, Aarsaether E, et al. Adenosine instead of supranormal potassium in cardioplegic solution improves cardioprotection. Eur J Cardio-thorac Surg. 2007;32:493-500.
34. Foglia RP, Steed DL, Follette DM. Iatrogenic myocardial edema with potassium cardioplegia. J Thorac Cardiovasc Surg. 1979;78:217-22.
35. Follette N, Fly K, Mulder N, et al. Prolonged safe aortic clamping by combining membrane stabilization: Multidose cardioplegia and appropriate pH perfusion. J Thorac Cardiovasc Surg. 1977;74:682-9.
36. Nahas GG, Sutin KM, Fermon C, et al. Guidelines for the treatment of acidaemia with THAM. Drugs. 1998;55:191-224.
37. Garbade J, Davierwala P, Seeburger J, et al. Myocardial protection during minimally invasive mitral valve surgery: strategies and cardioplegic solutions. Ann Cardiothorac Surg. 2013;2:803-8.
38. Klass O, Fischer UM, Perez E, et al. Effect of the Na^+/H^+ exchange inhibitor eniporide on cardiac performance and myocardial high energy phosphates in pigs subjected to cardioplegic arrest. Ann Thorac Surg. 2004;77:658-63.
39. Ducko CT, Stephenson ER, Jayawant AM, et al. Potassium channel openers: are they effective as pretreatment or additives to cardioplegia? Ann Thorac Surg. 2000;69:1363-8.

40. De Jong JW. Cardioplegia and calcium antagonists: A review. Ann Thorac Surg. 1986;42:593-8.
41. Braathen B, Jeppsson A, Scherstén H, et al. One single dose of histidine-tryptophan-ketoglutarate solution gives equally good myocardial protection in elective mitral valve surgery as repetitive cold blood cardioplegia: a prospective randomized study. J Thorac Cardiovasc Surg. 2011;141:995-1001.
42. Follette DM, Mulder DG, Maloney JV, et al. Advantages of blood cardioplegia over continuous coronary perfusion or intermittent ischemia. Experimental and clinical study. J Thorac Cardiovasc Surg. 1978;76:604-19.
43. Jakob VJ. Whole blood cardioplegia: Do we still need to dilute? JECT. 2016;48:9-14.
44. Hayashi Y, Sawa Y, Nishimura M, et al. Clinical evaluation of leukocyte depleted blood cardioplegia for pediatric open heart operation. Ann Thorac Surg. 2000;69:1914-9.
45. Martin J, Benk C. Blood cardioplegia. Multimedia Manual of Cardiothoracic Surgery. Obtained from www.area-c54.it/public/blood%20cardioplegia.pdf. Last visited on 15-05-2017.
46. Ovrum E, Tangen G, Tollofsrud S, et al. Cold blood versus cold crystalloid cardioplegia: a prospective randomised study of 345 aortic valve patients. Eur J Cardio-thorac Surg. 2010;38:745-9.
47. Gong B, Ji B, Sun Y, et al. Is microplegia really superior to standard blood cardioplegia? The results from a meta-analysis. Perfusion. 2015;30:375-82.
48. Algarni KD, Weisel RD, Caldarone CA, et al. Microplegia during coronary artery bypass grafting was associated with less low cardiac output syndrome: a propensity-matched comparison. Ann Thorac Surg. 2013;95:1532-8.
49. Zeng J, He W, Qu Z, et al. Cold blood versus crystalloid cardioplegia for myocardial protection in adult cardiac surgery: a meta-analysis of randomized controlled studies. J Cardiothorac Vasc Anesth. 2014;28:674-81.
50. Novick RJ, Stefaniszyn HJ, Michel RP, et al. Protection of the hypertrophied pig myocardium. A comparison of crystalloid, blood, and Fluosol-DA cardioplegia during prolonged aortic clamping. J Thorac Cardiovasc Surg. 1985;89:547-66.
51. Flaherty JT, Jaffin JH, Magovern GJ, et al. Maintenance of aerobic metabolism during global ischemia with perfluorocarbon cardioplegia improves myocardial preservation. Circulation. 1984;69:585-92.
52. Rousou JH, Dobbs WA, Engelman RM. Fluosol cardioplegia—a method of optimizing aerobic metabolism during arrest. Circulation. 1982;66:155-9.
53. Funada A, Mizuno S, Ohsato K, et al. Three cases of iatrogenic coronary ostial stenosis after aortic valve replacement. Circ J. 2006;70:1312-7.
54. Ono N, Sawai T, Hisanari Ishii JA. Coronary ostial stenosis detected by transesophageal echocardiography after aortic valve replacement: A case report. Clinical Reports. 2017;3:14.
55. Blanco G, Adam A, Fernandes A. A direct experimental approach to the aortic valve II. Acute retroperfusion of the coronary sinus. J Thorac Surg. 1956;82:171-6.
56. Aldea GS, Connelly G, Fonger JD, et al. Directed atraumatic coronary sinus cannulation for retrograde cardioplegia administration. Ann Thorac Surg. 1992;54:789-90.
57. Gundry SR, Sequiera A, Razzouk AM, et al. Facile retrograde cardioplegia: transatrial cannulation of the coronary sinus. Ann Thorac Surg. 1990;50:882-7.
58. Crooke GA, Harris LH, Grossi EA, et al. Biventricular distribution of cold blood cardioplegic solution administered by different retrograde techniques. J Thorac Cardiovasc Surg. 1991;102:631-7.
59. Philippe M, Iwnica AP. Cardioplegia by way of the coronary sinus for valvular and coronary surgery. JACC. 1991;18:628-6.
60. Moisa RB, Zeldis SM, Alper SA, et al. Aortic regurgitation in coronary artery bypass grafting: Implications for cardioplegia administration. Ann Thorac Surg. 1995;60:665-8.

61. Noyez L, Van Son JA, Van der Werf T, et al. Retrograde versus antegrade delivery of cardioplegic solution in myocardial revascularization. A clinical trial in patients with three vessel coronary artery disease who underwent myocardial revascularization with extensive use of the internal mammary artery. J Thorac Cardiovasc Surg. 1993;105: 854-63.
62. Fiore AC, Naunheim KS, Kaiser GC, et al. Coronary sinus versus aortic root perfusion with blood cardioplegia in elective myocardial revascularization. Ann Thorac Surg. 1989;47:684-8.
63. Kaukoranta PK, Lepojarvi MVK, Kiviluoma KT, et al. Myocardial protection during antegrade versus retrograde cardioplegia. Ann Thorac Surg. 1998;66:755-61.
64. Caldarone CA, Krukenkamp IB, Misare BD, et al. Perfusion deficits with retrograde warm blood cardioplegia. Ann Thorac Surg. 1994;57:403-6.
65. Rangaraj AT, Ghanta RK, Umakanthan R, et al. Real-time visualization and quantification of retrograde cardioplegia delivery using near infrared fluorescent imaging. J Card Surg. 2008;23:701-8.
66. Radmehr H, Soleimani A, Tatari H, et al. Combined antegrade-retrograde cardioplegia have any superiority over antegrade cardioplegia? Heart, Lung and Circulation. 2008;17:475-7.
67. Buckberg GD, Drinkwater DC, Laks H. A new technique for delivering antegrade/retrograde blood cardioplegia without right heart isolation. Eur J Cardiothorac Surg. 1990;4:163-7.
68. Hoffenberg EF, Ye J, Sun J, et al. Antegrade and retrograde continuous warm blood cardioplegia: A 31P magnetic resonance study. Ann Thorac Surg. 1995;60:1203-9.
69. Onorati F, Renzulli A, Feo MD, et al. Does antegrade blood cardioplegia alone provide adequate myocardial protection in patients with left main stem disease? J Thorac Cardiovasc Surg. 2003;126:1345-51.
70. Candilio L, Malik A, Ariti C, et al. A retrospective analysis of myocardial preservation techniques during coronary artery bypass graft surgery: are we protecting the heart? J Cardiothorac Surg. 2014;9:184-96.
71. Chocron S, Alwan K, Toubin G, et al. Crystalloid cardioplegia route of delivery and cardiac troponin I release. Ann Thorac Surg. 1996;62:481-5.
72. Savunen T, Kuttila K, Rajalin A, et al. Combined cardioplegia delivery offers no advantage over antegrade cardioplegia administration in coronary surgical patients with a preserved left ventricular function. Eur J Cardio-thorac Surg. 1994;8:640-4.
73. Aldea GS, Hou D, Fonger JD, et al. Inhomogeneous and complementary antegrade and retrograde delivery of cardioplegic solution in the absence of coronary artery obstruction. Thorac Cardiovasc Surg. 1994;107:499-504.
74. Pelletier LC, Carrier M. Antegrade/retrograde cardioplegia for valve replacement: A prospective study. Ann Thorac Surg. 1999;68:1681-5.
75. Hearse OJ, Stewart DA, Braimbridge MV. Hypothermic arrest and potassium arrest: metabolic and myocardial protection during elective cardiac arrest. Circ Res. 1975;36:481-9.
76. Louagie YAG, Jamart J, Gonzalez M, et al. Continuous cold blood cardioplegia improves myocardial protection: a prospective randomized study. Ann Thorac Surg. 2004;77:664-71.
77. Mauney MC, Kron IL. The physiologic basis of warm cardioplegia. Ann Thorac Surg. 1995;60:819-23.
78. Caputo M, Ascione R, Angelini GD, et al. The end of the cold era: from intermittent cold to intermittent warm blood cardioplegia. Eur J Cardiothorac Surg. 1998;14:467-75.
79. Yeh CH, Wang YC, Wu YC, et al. Continuous tepid blood cardioplegia can reserve coronary endothelium and ameliorate the occurrence of cardiomyocyte apoptosis. Chest. 2003;123:1647-54.

80. Abah U, Roberts PG, Ishaq M, et al. Is cold or warm blood cardioplegia superior for myocardial protection? Interact CardioVasc Thorac Surg. 2012;14:848-55.
81. Trescher K, Gleiss A, Boxleitner M, et al. Short term clinical outcomes for intermittent cold versus intermittent warm blood cardioplegia in 2200 adult cardiac surgery patients. J Cardiovasc Surg (Torino). 2017;58:105-12.
82. Yves D Durandy. Is there a rationale for short cardioplegia re-dosing intervals? World J Cardiol. 2015;7:658-64.
83. Rosenkranz ER, Johansen VJ, Buckberg GD, et al. Benefits of normothermic induction of cardioplegia in energy-depleted hearts, with maintenance of arrest by multidose cold blood cardioplegic infusions. J Thorac Cardiovasc Surg. 1982;84:667-76.
84. Rosenkranz ER, Okamoto F, Buckberg GD, et al. Safety of prolonged aortic clamping with blood cardioplegia. Aspartate enrichment of glutamate-blood cardioplegia in energy-depleted hearts after ischemic and reperfusion injury. J Thorac Cardiovasc Surg. 1986;9:428-35.
85. Drinkwater DC, Laks H, Buckberg GD. Antegrade retrograde blood cardioplegia without right heart isolation: a new simplified method of optimizing cardioplegic delivery. J Thorac Cardiovasc Surg. 1990;100:56-64.
86. Bhayana JN, Kalmbach T, Booth FV, et al. Combined antegrade retrograde cardioplegia for myocardial protection: a clinical trial. J Thorac Cardiovasc Surg. 1989;98:956-60.
87. Lichtenstein SV, Ashe KA, El Dalati H, et al. Warm heart surgery. J Thorac Cardiovasc Surg. 1991;101:269-74.
88. Lichtenstein SV, Abel JG, Panos A, et al. Warm heart surgery: experience with long cross-clamp times. Ann Thorac Surg. 1991;52:1009-13.
89. Ikonomidis JS, Yau TM, Weisel RD, et al. Optimal flow rates for retrograde warm cardioplegia. J Thorac Cardiovasc Surg. 1994;107:510-9.
90. Lichtenstein SV, Abel JG, Salerno TA. Warm heart surgery and results of operation for recent myocardial infarction. Ann Thorac Surg. 1991;52:455-60.
91. Morishige N, Tashiro T, Yamada T, et al. Retrograde continuous warm blood cardioplegia reduces oxidative stress during coronary artery bypass grafting. Ann Thorac Cardiovasc Surg. 2002;8:31-7.
92. Grech ED, Baines M, Steyn R, et al. Evidence that continuous normothermic blood cardioplegia offers better myocardial protection than intermittent hypothermic cardioplegia. Br Heart J. 1995;74:517-21.
93. Rashid A, Jackson M, Page RD, et al. Continuous warm versus intermittent cold blood cardioplegia for coronary bypass surgery in patients with left ventricular dysfunction. Eur J Cardiothorac Surg. 1995;9:405-8.
94. Yau TM, Weisel RD, Mickle DAG, et al. Optimal delivery of blood cardioplegia. Circulation. 1991;84:380-8.
95. Calafiore AM, Teodori G, Bosco G, et al. Intermittent antegrade warm blood cardioplegia in aortic valve replacement. J Card Surg. 1996;11:348-54.
96. Teoh KH, Christakis GT, Weisel RD, et al. Accelerated myocardial metabolic recovery with terminal warm blood cardioplegia (hot shot). J Thorac Cardiovasc Surg. 1986;91:888-95.
97. Beyersdorf F. The use of controlled reperfusion strategies in cardiac surgery to minimize ischaemia/reperfusion damage. Cardiovascular Research. 2009;83:262-8.

Journal Scans

Sanjeev Aneja, Ashok Jadon, Yatin Mehta, Monish Nakra, Ashok Kumar Saxena

Journal Scan 1—Sanjeev Aneja

Increased Early Systemic Inflammation in ICU-Acquired Weakness; A Prospective Observational Cohort Study

Witteveen E, Wieske L, van der Poll T, et al. On behalf of the Molecular Diagnosis and Risk Stratification of Sepsis (MARS) Consortium. Crit Care Med. 2017;45(6):972-9.

BACKGROUND

Intensive Care Unit acquired weakness (ICU-AW) refers to generalized muscle weakness in critically ill patients for which no other etiology can be identified other than critical illness itself. It is an important complication of critical illness.[1] It is present in approximately 11–67% of cases requiring mechanical ventilation. ICU-AW involves nerves (critical illness polyneuropathy CIP) or muscles (critical illness myopathy CIM) but most often involves both nerves and muscles.[1-3] The main risk factors, sepsis and the systemic inflammatory response syndrome suggest an inflammatory pathogenesis.[1,2] It is suggested that exaggerated inflammatory response in sepsis and systemic inflammatory response syndrome damages the nerves and muscles. This can present as infiltration of muscles and nerves by systemic inflammatory markers and increased levels in plasma.[4] Studies on increased level of inflammatory mediators in plasma of patients developing ICU-AW are limited and have methodological limitations.[5,6] In this present prospective observational study authors included 204 consecutive patients requiring mechanical ventilation for more than 48h and compared the inflammatory markers in patients who developed ICU-AW with those who did not.

ABSTRACT

ICU-acquired weakness is a serious complication in patients who are mechanically ventilated in the intensive care unit. Increased systemic inflammatory response has long been thought to be associated with ICU-acquired weakness. In this prospective observational cohort study involving 204 patients admitted in mixed ICU and requiring ventilation for 48 hours or more, authors have compared the pattern of rise in systemic inflammatory markers in the patients who develop ICU-acquired weakness to those who do not develop weakness. ICU-acquired weakness was diagnosed based on manual muscle strength testing by trained physiotherapists. A Panel of systemic inflammatory markers and soluble vascular adhesion molecules were measured in plasma samples on day 0, 2, and 4 after ICU admission. Of 204 patients, 99 developed ICU-acquired weakness. There was 1.5 to 2 fold increase in the levels of interleukin-6, interleukin-8, interleukin-10, and fractalkine in these patients after adjusting for confounders. The authors concluded that systemic inflammatory markers interleukin-6, interleukin-8, interleukin-10, and fractalkine are the most important discriminative markers in patients who develop ICU-acquired weakness in the first four days after admission.

COMMENTARY

In the present study Witteveen et al. have determined whether patients who develop ICU acquired weakness have different pattern of systemic inflammatory markers as compared to patients who do not develop ICU-AW. Authors have been working on the muscle and nerve inflammation in ICU-AW for quite some time, and have published informative articles on this topic before also.[4] But probably this is the first study where they have investigated patterns of systemic inflammatory markers in ICU-AW. Number of patients included in the present study are large as compared to previous studies on ICU acquired weakness. Of the 204 patients, 99 patients (48%) developed ICU acquired weakness as diagnosed by manual muscle strength testing (MMT), using the medical research council scale (MRC). These tests were performed as soon the patients became attentive and awake as it is mandatory for the patient to be cooperative before conducting these tests. MRC scale is used to grade the muscle strength testing of 6 different groups of muscle bilaterally. Each muscle group is scored from 0 to 5, with higher scores indicating greater strength. It is inexpensive and easy to use. Other inexpensive and easy to use test to diagnose ICU acquired weakness is Handgrip Dynamometry. Many authors have preferred Handgrip Dynamometry over MRC and found it to be associated with better functional outcome of the ICU patients. Full nerve conduction study with electromyography and muscle biopsy constitute the gold standard for the diagnosis of ICU acquired weakness. But they are time intensive, costly, painful, moderately invasive and commonly refused by patients. As a result, these gold standard tests are not much used in human studies. MRC score used for diagnosis of ICU acquired weakness by the present authors has high sensitivity, specificity and negative predictivity. Mean MRC score of less than 4 for the diagnosis of ICU acquired weakness is in accordance with international consensus statement.[7]

Authors tried to find the pattern of early inflammatory response. They collected samples on the day of admission (day 0), day 2 and 4 after ICU admission, which makes it a unique study. This is probably the first study to know the pattern of early inflammatory response in ICU acquired weakness. Large panel of inflammatory markers consisting of pro and anti-inflammatory cytokines, chemokine and soluble vascular adhesion molecule were used. Estimating the values of all inflammatory markers in large number of patients makes statistical analysis and any inference very difficult. It is more difficult in the present case as inflammatory response is the cascade of activated markers and they all are highly correlated. Secondly there are lot of cofounders for ICU-acquired weakness which also needs to be taken care. Authors used multiple statistical methods to determine pattern of inflammatory markers and their association with ICU-acquired weakness.

To know the pattern of inflammatory markers, authors created heat map with hierarchical clustering of columns. A heat map is a graphical way of displaying a table of numbers by using colors to represent numerical values. The clustering algorithm groups related rows and/or columns together by similarity. This resulted in identification of three clusters. Markers in cluster 1 (including IL-6, IL-8, IL-10, IFNγ, and fractalkine) were higher in ICU-acquired weakness.

There are various cofounders for ICU-acquired weakness in the literature, e.g. age, gender, presence of sepsis, use of corticosteroid, APACHE score or sequential organ failure assessment (SOFA) score. Most of the studies have included APACHE score, but the present author included SOFA score to decrease the number of variables and assuming the correlation between two scores. Which is an understandable step. To overcome the problem of multicollinearity and to exclude low variance principal components, authors applied Principal Component (PC) regression analysis. This concluded that IL-6, IL-8, IL-10, and fractalkine to be the most important discriminative markers. The raised levels of these markers were found at the time of admission in ICU also which suggests that these markers may cause ICU-AW and are not because of ICU-AW. This suggestion of author is not surprising as these inflammatory markers play an important role in the disbalanced inflammatory response seen in sepsis.[8] High level of IL-6 as an early indicator of muscle dysfunction has been reported earlier in a prospective observational study.[9] They are also used as biomarkers to distinguish between survivors and nonsurvivors in ICU.

Over all this is a well-planned study on large number of patients with and without sepsis. This showed that association was not limited to patients with sepsis. By using better method to diagnose ICU-AW and selection of statistical tests especially principal component regression analysis is the main strength of this study. This observational study can show the association of inflammatory markers and ICU-AW, but no causal relationship can be deduced. ICU-AW has high morbidity and mortality because of respiratory muscle weakness, pharyngeal dysfunction and symptomatic aspiration. ICU-AW may be important contributor to postintensive care syndrome. Therapeutic options to prevent or treat ICU-AW are limited and may include intensive insulin therapy, nutritional management, neuromuscular electrical stimulation and mobilization and physical therapy. Therefore, there is need to predict the development of ICU-AW in the clinical ICU setting. This study does not help in the prediction of development of ICU-acquired weakness.

There is need to develop biomarkers to predict the development and severity of ICU-AW, as the present available biomarkers are not validated. Further research in to bedside evaluation tool like bedside ultrasound to evaluate muscle atrophy and muscle structural damage will be helpful.

REFERENCES

1. Jolley SE, Bunnell AE, Hough CL. ICU-acquired weakness. Chest. 2016;150(5):1129-40.
2. Zorowitz RD. ICU-acquired weakness: a rehabilitation perspective of diagnosis, treatment, and functional management. Chest. 2016;150(4):966-71.
3. Kress JP, Hall JB. ICU-acquired weakness and recovery from critical illness. N Engl J Med. 2014;370(17):1626-35.

4. Witteveen E, Wieske L, Verhamme C, et al. Muscle and nerve inflammation in intensive care unit—acquired weakness: a systematic translational review. J Neurol Sci 2014;345:15-25.
5. Winkelman C, Johnson KD, Gordon N. Associations between muscle-related cytokines and selected patient outcomes in the ICU. Biol Res Nurs. 2015;17:125-34.
6. Verheul GA, de Jongh-Leuvenink J, Op de Coul AA, et al. Tumor necrosis factor and interleukin-6 in critical illness polyneuromyopathy. Clin Neurol Neurosurg. 1994; 96:300-4.
7. Stevens RD, Marshall SA, Cornblath DR, et al. A framework for diagnosing and classifying intensive care unit-acquired weakness. Crit Care Med. 2009;37(10 Suppl): S299-S308.
8. Aziz M, Jacob A, Yang WL, et al. Current trends in inflammatory and immunomodulatory mediators in sepsis. J Leukoc Biol. 2013;93:329-42.
9. Weber-Carstens S, Deja M, Koch S, et al. Risk factors in critical illness myopathy during the early course of critical illness: a prospective observational study. Crit Care. 2010;14:R119.

Journal Scan 2—Ashok Jadon

Occupational Stress of Anesthesia: Effects on Aging

Zanaty OM, El Metainy S, Abdelmaksoud R. J Clin Anesth. 2017;39:159-64.

BACKGROUND

Aging is a normal physiological process. Many intrinsic and extrinsic factors can facilitate the process of aging and stress is one of them. Stress in moderation provides the driving force which enables mankind to function optimally. Excessive stress however, is detrimental and results in mental or physical disintegration.[1] Although, more research is needed on the exact mechanisms by which psychological stress contributes to biological aging, it is suggested that, chronic stress creates a fight-or-flight reaction and as a result, stress chemicals are released into the body and which creates accelerated biological aging.[2] Among medical professionals, anesthesiologists are known to suffer from excessive stress due to nature of their work and environment in which they work. This stress when become chronic results in increased biological aging which can be measured by aging related changes in skin, increased level of stress hormones and free radicals along with decrease in telomere length.[3]

ABSTRACT

Psychological stress is known to facilitate the biological aging and aging of skin in human beings. Biomarkers like decreased telomere length, increased free radicle levels and changes in the skin of face have been studied and shown a reliable correlation with aging. A prospective observational study was done to evaluate the stress related aging in anesthesiologists with the presumption that their work is more stressful than their colleagues working in laboratory and academic specialties. Total 366 ASA I–II physicians of 30–50 years of age were categorized in two equal groups. Anesthesiologists Group A (n = 183), and physicians of laboratory and academic specialties Group B (n = 183). Assessment of Physical health, emotional well-being, skin aging analysis, telomere length and measurement of markers of oxidative stress were done. Physical health score and emotional health score showed higher values in Group A than Group B. Markers of oxidative stress were also significantly higher in Group A than Group B. Upper and lower face esthetic unit summary score showed higher values in Group A than Group B. Telomere (TTAGGG) repeats for terminal restriction fragments (TRF) of Group A individuals revealed a significant decrease of TRF compared to Group B (p = 0.001). It was concluded that anesthesiologists who are chronically exposed to occupational stress showed evidence of biological and skin aging with higher face scores and free radical with obvious shorter telomere length.

COMMENTARY

According to the nature and functionality of the occupation, there are risk and high-risk occupations. Anesthesiology is classified as high-risk specialty that promotes high levels of stress. Lack of control over work situations, administrative responsibilities, work overload, professional relationships and work-home conflict are significant factors for stress in anesthesiologists. All these factors cumulatively lead to "Burnout".[4] Burnout is a concept that consists of three dimensions: emotional exhaustion, depersonalization and lack of personal accomplishment.[5] More than 40% of anesthesiologists suffer from high emotional exhaustion or burnout which is actually responsible for all the deleterious effects of stress including the accelerated biological aging.

Initial studies have focused their research on either finding out the prevalence of stress among various work situations (including anesthesiologists) or factors causing the stress and burnout (physical, psychosocial or other environmental factors). The assessment of outcomes was done through interviews or question based inventory. These assessments although helpful to generate an information about severity of stress related issues, often have variable results and inherent limitations of subjective bias. Furthermore, the use of a self-administered questionnaire can generate differences in interpretation of the questions. For an example, in a study by Larsson et al.[6] when anesthesiologists were interviewed, they maintained that they enjoyed work and could see no external obstacles to doing a good job. Therefore, new research incorporated more objective measures to assess the effect of stress.

The levels of stress were assessed by measurement of levels of stress hormones and free radicals. The effect of stress on skin aging have been done by various validated tools through face photography, and the biological aging have been measured by measuring the length of telomere.[3,7] Telomeres are the oligomeric DNA-protein complexes that cap chromosomal ends in cells. The length of telomeres serves as a biomarker of a cell's biological age. When cells divide, the telomere is not fully replicated because of the limitations of the DNA polymerase in completing the replication of the ends of the linear molecule, leading to telomere shortening with every replication. Finally, after numerous shortenings, the cell is arrested into senescence.[8] The results of these studies have consistently shown that high level of constant stress resulted in increased level of stress hormone and free radicals, changes in facial skin of aging and decreased length of telomere which indicates the cellular aging.[3,9,10]

The present study[7] is unique in a sense that, it has used multiple tools to assess the effect of prolonged stress on skin aging and biological aging in anesthesiologists. Question based inventory were used to measure physical health and emotional well-being among anesthesiologists. Upper face and lower face photographs were used to determine the skin aging through validated scoring systems. The markers of oxidative stress were assessed by measuring increased levels of thiobarbituric acid reactive substance (TBARS), decreased levels of SOD (antioxidant enzyme) and DNA analysis of cells was done to assess telomere length in the mononuclear cells (PBMCs) of peripheral blood. The data were compared with nonanesthesiologist physicians from laboratory and academic specialties.

Health and Stress Profile used to assess the level of stress showed significantly high scores (high stress) among anesthesiologists. It was observed that the level of stress increased with increasing work load. Results also showed that this difference persisted even after age based subgroup comparison (e.g. 30-40 years and 40-50 years). Secondary outcomes which included skin aging analysis, levels of stress hormones and telomere shortening (all are stress related effects) also showed positive correlation in anesthesiologists.

The strength of this study was an objective and evidence-based approach to verify the prevalence of high stress in anesthesiologists through validated tools and quantitative measurement of various stress biomarkers responsible for skin and biological aging. This study further strengthens the viewpoint of previous studies about excessive stress and burnout in anesthesiologists and its detrimental effects like skin aging and biological aging. However, this study also had some limitations. To avoid potential confounding variables which might have affected telomere length, physicians who had any known systemic illness such as hypertension, coronary artery disease, diabetes mellitus, or affective disorders were not enrolled in this study. Also, few other important cofounding factors (number of children in female participants and childhood adverse life events) which were not excluded could have affected the results. These factors also affect the length of telomeres.[11]

Like other studies this study also focused on environmental correlates, but it is likely that personality factors also play an important part in the development of burnout. It is known that personality is consistently related to burnout, and it is recommended that, personality variables be included as predictors in future research on burnout.[12] Two more limitation of the present study as accepted by author were the small sample size and not taking the effect of ultra violet rays' exposure on skin aging in to consideration. It is well-known that large sample size helps in minimizing the various inherent statistical errors and biases which may influence the outcomes and thus conclusions. The effect of ultraviolet rays on skin aging is a known fact and cannot be undermined.[13]

The authors in the present study have concluded that biological and skin aging is evident in anesthesiologists who are chronically exposed to occupational stress, with obvious shorter telomere length, higher lower and upper face scores, and higher free radicals. This study is strongly suggestive of the fact that, we are on the right path (which emphasized that anesthesiologists suffer with burnout and its deleterious effects in form of skin and biological aging) however, we have not yet reached the destination, e.g. prevention. Therefore, question is, can it be prevented? Studies have suggested that with lifestyle modification (through diet, exercises, yoga and other relaxation measures) the intensity of side effects can be reduced and thus speed of aging. A study by Babizhayev et al.[14] supports a therapeutic concept of using nonhydrolyzed forms of naturally occurring imidazole-dipeptide based compounds carnosine and carnitine, making it clinically possible that slowing down the rate of telomere shortening could slow down the human aging process in specific tissues where proliferative senescence is known to occur with the demonstrated evidence of telomere shortening appeared to be a hallmark of oxidative stress and disease.

REFERENCES

1. Cohen S, Janicki-Deverts D, Miller GE. Psychological stress and disease. JAMA. 2007;298(14):1685-7.
2. Epel ES. Psychological and metabolic stress: a recipe for accelerated cellular aging? Hormones. 2009;8(1):7-22.
3. Ahola K, Siren I, Kivimaki M, et al. Work-related exhaustion and telomere length: a population-based study. PLoS One [Internet]. 2012;7(7):e40186.

4. Shanafelt T. Burnout in anesthesiology — a call to action. Anesthesiology. 2011;114:1-2.
5. Maslach C. Burnout. The Cost of Caring. Englewoods Cliffs, NJ: Prentice-Hall, 1982.
6. Larsson J, Rosenqvist I, Holmstrom I. Enjoying work or burdened by it? How anaesthetists experience and handle difficulties at work: A qualitative study. Br J Anaesth. 2007;99:493-9.
7. Zanaty OM, Metainy SE, Abdelmaksoud R, et al. Occupational stress of anesthesia: effects on aging. J Clin Anes. 2017;39:159-64.
8. Chan SRWL, Blackburn EH. Telomeres and telomerase. Philosophical transactions of the Royal Society B: Biological Sciences. 2004;359(1441):109-21.
9. Chen Y, Lyga J. Brain-skin connection: Stress, inflammation and skin aging. Inflammation & Allergy Drug Targets. 2014;13(3):177-90.
10. Epel ES, Blackburn EH, Lin J, et al. Accelerated telomere shortening in response to life stress. Proceedings of the National Academy of Sciences of the United States of America. 2004;101(49):17312-315.
11. Kananen L, Surakka I, Pirkola S, et al. Childhood adversities are associated with shorter telomere length at adult age both in individuals with an anxiety disorder and controls. PLos ONE 2010;5: e10826. Available at: http://journals.plos.org/plosone/article?id=10.1371/journal.pone.0040186.
12. Alarcon G, Eschleman KJ, Bowling NA. Relationships between personality variables and burnout: a meta-analysis. Work and Stress. 2009;23(3):244-63.
13. Pillai S, Oresajo C, Hayward J. Ultraviolet radiation and skin aging: roles of reactive oxygen species, inflammation and protease activation, and strategies for prevention of inflammation → induced matrix degradation–a review. Int J Cosme Sci 2005;27(1):17-34.
14. Babizhayev MA, Kasus-Jacobi A, Vishnyakova KS, et al. Novel neuroendocrine and metabolic mechanism provides the patented platform for important rejuvenation therapies: targeted therapy of telomere attrition and lifestyle changes of telomerase activity with the timing of neuron-specific imidazole-containing dipeptide-dominant pharmaconutrition provision. Recent Pat Endocr Metab Immune Drug Discov. 2014;8(3):153-79.

Journal Scan 3—Yatin Mehta

The SLUScore: A Novel Method for Detecting Hazardous Hypotension in Adult Patients Undergoing Noncardiac Surgical Procedures

Stapelfeldt WH, Yuan H, Dryden JK, et al. Anesth Analg. 2017;124(4):1135-52.

BACKGROUND

Maintaining a stable intraoperative hemodynamics is a priority in anesthesia practice. Intraoperative hypotension is one of the very few modifiable risk factors which can have adverse perioperative outcome, if not corrected on time. Although severe Intraoperative hypotension is attended to promptly, mild to moderate hypotension is not always aggressively managed in our clinical practice. The brevity of the duration of such hypotension along with occasional surgical demands of a bloodless surgical field are some of the causes of delayed intervention. Various authors have shown that the long-term patient outcomes are affected by extended periods of less severe hypotension.[1-6] However, not much data is available as to what is the safe lower limit of hypotension, both as a number and duration of exposure that patients can tolerate without any long term sequelae. Modern electronic anesthesia information management systems (AIMS) along with integrated clinical decision support (DSS) functionality can record and store patient data and inform about the severity and the duration of patients' deviation from certain vital sign ranges. Working on the hypothesis that the postoperative outcome is associated with not only the severity of hypotension, but also on the duration of time spent below a range of mean arterial pressure (MAP) thresholds, the researchers at Saint Louis University School of Medicine, St. Louis, Missouri conceived "The SLUScore™" as a hemodynamic assessment and postoperative risk stratification tool. The authors predicted that an elevated SLUScore™ is associated with an increased risk of cardiac morbidity and all-cause mortality within 30 days of surgery.

ABSTRACT

Data were retrieved from AIMS for 152,445 adult patients undergoing noncardiac surgery including; patient demographics, Charlson comorbidity score, type of anesthetic used, anesthesia duration, blood loss, minute-to-minute MAP values, and all cause mortality within 30 days of surgery. The patients were divided into two population cohorts: a developmental cohort of 35,904 patients from Cleveland Clinic's main campus and a validation cohort of 116,541 patients from Cleveland Clinic, the Vanderbilt Medical Center, and the Saint Louis University Medical Center. The data collected from the developmental cohort included the periods of time accumulated below each one of the 31 thresholds between 75 and 45 mm Hg (hypotensive exposure times), the number of minutes for each of the 31 MAP thresholds and the 30 day mortality. This particular hypotensive time duration with the corresponding MAP threshold was labeled as "smart exposure limit sets". Within each of the "smart exposure limit sets" information about fraction of patients exceeding one or more of these exposure limits, number of exposure limits exceeded, observed mortality of patients exceeding none of the limits, observed mortality of patients exceeding one or more of these limits, the adjusted increase in the odds of mortality per exposure time limit that had been exceeded was obtained and a novel risk score, the SLUScore™ (range 0–31) was conceived. The validity of this score was tested in the validation cohort. It was observed that progressively greater hypotensive exposures were associated with greater 30-day mortality. In the developmental cohort, a SLUScore > 0 (average 13.8) was found in 40% of patients who had twice the mortality, adjusted odds increasing by 5% per limit exceeded. When tested in the validation cohort, a SLUScore > 0 (average 14.1) identified 35% of patients who had twice the mortality, each incremental limit exceeded portending a 5% compounding increase in adjusted odds of mortality, independent of age and Charlson score (C = 0.73, 0.72–0.74, $P < .05$). Thus, the SLUScore represented a novel method for identifying nearly 1 in every 3 patients experiencing greater 30-day mortality related to more severe intraoperative hypotensive exposures.

COMMENTARY

Ever since Sessler et al. demonstrated that "triple low" of low minimum alveolar concentration (MAC) of inhalational anesthetic, low bispectral index (BIS) and low MAP can adversely affect the postoperative outcome,[3] many researchers have proved the deleterious effects of intraoperative severe hypotension. However, long-term postsurgical outcome may be adversely affected by less than severe hypotension often encountered in anesthesia. The reference study was designed to develop a method for identifying patients at increased risk of death within 30 days in association with the severity and duration of intraoperative hypotension (MAP between 75 and 45 mm Hg). The working hypothesis was that the postoperative outcome is associated with not only the severity of hypotension, but also on the duration of time spent below a range of MAP thresholds.

Patient optimization is a dynamic process. It involves preoperative as well as intraoperative optimization for the best possible outcome. As anesthesiologists, it is our primary duty to keep the patient oxygenated during the surgery and as perioperative physicians we should not only look at the immediate postoperative period for the successful conduct of anesthesia, but also the long-term well-being of the patient as a whole. Most of the times, even elevation of troponin levels are asymptomatic. After a seemingly uneventful noncardiac surgery, a modestly elevated non-high-sensitivity troponin T levels during the first 3 postoperative days were associated independently with excessive 30-day mortality.[7] Cardiac dysfunction, renal dysfunction, sepsis, deep wound infection, gastrointestinal ischemic complications due to compromise of splanchnic circulation following Intraoperative hypotensive episodes are the leading causes of postoperative death within first 30 days.[8] Use of vasopressors further aggravates the resistance to splanchnic circulation already compromised by the physiological sympathetic stimulation.

The reference study was brilliantly designed to develop a method for identifying patients who were at increased risk of death within 30 days in association with a serious yet modifiable risk factor, i.e. the severity and duration of intraoperative hypotension. Rather than deriving a predictive model for 30-day mortality, the study objective was to create a logarithmic ratio scale. Such quantification might allow certain fractions of patients to be identified who may be at some increased postoperative mortality risk alerted by intraoperative hypotensive exposures.

The observations were made after adjustment for those main confounding factors that are principally unalterable at the time of surgery like patient age and comorbidity. For universal reproducibility and acceptability, the authors solely depended on routinely captured clinical data, with all its associated limitations including the latency due to intermittent cycling at 3-5 minutes.

The researchers have introduced the SLUScore™, a novel scoring system with values ranging from 0 (no hypotensive exposure) to 31 (the maximal number of exposures exceeded beyond the "smart exposure limit sets"), with each increment of the SLUScore reflecting in an equivalent 5% increase in 30-day postoperative mortality. In the 116,541 patients studied as part of the validation cohort, it is alarming to note that 1 in every 3 patients exceeded some or all of these "smart exposure limit sets" and experienced approximately twice the 30-day all-cause mortality in association with a SLUScore™ of > 0 versus a SLUScore™ of 0. This finding was independent of the patients' comorbidity. While nearly all patients crossed the 75 mm Hg threshold and so achieved a SLUScore > 0, the 30-day mortality increased compoundly in patients crossing progressively lower MAP thresholds. One additional finding was the impact of extent of hypotension on the necessary time of exposure to achieve the "smart exposure limit" or vice versa. Even just a few minutes accumulated below an MAP of 50 projected a sharp increase in 30-day mortality. Major confounding factors in the final analysis that remain, are the procedural risk and duration of surgery. In my opinion, this bias may have been nullified to a great extent by the power of the study. The researchers of the article went on to propose SLUScore™ as a real time hemodynamic assessment and postoperative risk stratification tool in the operating room. The reference study has the much needed power (a total of 152,445 adult patients) and if simplified further would create the impact it deserves in our clinical practice. However, it seems unlikely to be applicable in the near future as the present monitors in most of the centers do not have electronic AIMS or DSS functionality. One other limitation of using SLUScore as an intervention tool is that the final SLUScore of a particular patient is available only at the end of the surgery. However, the authors have done a commendable job in taking up from where Sessler et al. (the "triple low" state) had left by defining the exact level of hypotension and the particular duration that need to be accumulated at that point to predict risk of 30-day mortality. It would be interesting to see when developed as an intervention tool, if the SLUScore in an ongoing surgery can guide intraoperative management to reduce the 30-day all cause mortality.

REFERENCES

1. Bijker JB, van Klei WA, Vergouwe Y, et al. Intraoperative hypotension and 1-year mortality after noncardiac surgery. Anesthesiology. 2009;111:1217-26.
2. Stapelfeldt WH, Dalton J, Bromley P, et al. Risk-based decision support thresholds for hypotension in adult patients undergoing noncardiac surgery. Anesth Analg. 2013;116:S-291.
3. Sessler DI, Sigl JC, Kelley SD, et al. Hospital stay and mortality are increased in patients having a "triple low" of low blood pressure, low bispectral index, and low minimum alveolar concentration of volatile anesthesia. Anesthesiology. 2012;116:1195-203.
4. Walsh M, Devereaux PJ, Garg AX, et al. Relationship between intraoperative mean arterial pressure and clinical outcomes after noncardiac surgery: toward an empirical definition of hypotension. Anesthesiology. 2013;119:507-15.

5. Stapelfeldt WH. Duration of hypotension (still) matters. Anesthesiology. 2015;122:470.
6. Kertai MD, White WD, Gan TJ. Cumulative duration of "triple low" state of low blood pressure, low bispectral index, and low minimum alveolar concentration of volatile anesthesia is not associated with increased mortality. Anesthesiology. 2014;121:18-28.
7. Botto F, Alonso-Coello P, Chan MT, et al. Myocardial injury after noncardiac surgery: a large, international, prospective cohort study establishing diagnostic criteria, characteristics, predictors, and 30-day outcomes. Anesthesiology. 2014;120:564.
8. Reilly PM, Wilkins KB, Fuh KC, et al. The mesenteric hemodynamic response to circulatory shock: an overview. Shock. 2001;15:329-43.

Journal Scan 4—Monish Nakra

Generalizable Biomarkers in Critical Care: Toward Precision Medicine

Sweeney TE, Khatri P. Crit Care Med. 2017;45(6):934-9.

BACKGROUND

Biomarkers has been in vogue since long; humans have been in search of that elusive molecule which proves or disproves presence of a disease or a syndrome. It is an oversimplified statement as very few biomarkers have actually been demonstrated to have association with syndromic diseases in ICU. The process is so dynamic that research of these molecules have persistently fallen short of expectations. Dr Sweeney and Dr Khatri dwells on why these studies do not succeed and what requires to be corrected, so that medical science and humanity benefits.

ABSTRACT

The authors noted with concern that due to the dynamic nature of disease and syndrome in ICU patients, the discovery of biomarkers have lagged behind and no biomarker has been associated with a disease consistently. There are various reasons for failure of studies researching these metabolites. Disease definition, etiology, severity, management, outcome, etc. are different for each patient. The number of variables in these studies are numerous and their sample size is less. Miniscule number of studies share their data and hence meta-analysis is not consistent. Search of a biomarker passes through stages of discovery, early validation, late validation and post market studies and most of the studies do not cross the first stage. The authors put forward futuristic ideas to help investigators with biomarkers in their quest.

COMMENTARY

Metabolomics is a study of small molecules called metabolites, within cells, biofluids, tissue and organisms. It started getting crystallized in scientific manner at the turn of the last century and in the year 2001, Biomarkers Definitions Working Group[1] defined biomarker as "a characteristic that is objectively measured and evaluated as an indicator of normal biological processes, pathogenic processes, or pharmacologic responses to a therapeutic intervention". In this guideline by Atkinson et al. a basic framework of biomarker identification and validation was proposed. They indicated that the road to discovery is not easy. The analytical process should have three steps which were (a) Analytical validation: analyses of available evidence of an assay, (b) Qualification: assessment of associations between the biomarker and disease states, including data showing effects of interventions on both biomarkers and clinical outcomes; and (c) Utilization: specific use proposed and the applicability of available evidence to this use. The present article has widened the search path and suggested four steps for life cycle (a) discovery (b) early validation (c) late validation and (d) post market studies.

Big issue in discovery of biomarkers is reproducibility and generalizability. After the human genome project, there was hope that most critical illnesses can be identified by specific biomarkers, but it could not be achieved. In critical care medicine, the illnesses which were studied most were acute kidney injury (AKI), acute respiratory distress syndrome (ARDS), sepsis, TBI (traumatic brain injury) and delirium. The most acceptable reason was that cluster of diseases lead to a common syndrome in critical care which cannot be associated with a single reproducible biomarker. The patients of ICU are heterogeneous and the etiology of the common syndrome is varied. As a result, any single biomarker is not associated with a syndrome. This lead to clinicians with a view that each time a syndrome is investigated, it would require many tests. In addition, it may not be possible for a biomarker to deliver similar performance in seemingly similar conditions and the treatment could get compromised. Hence, research should first clearly define a disease, classify it into sub-types and then find presence or absence of a biomarker for the same. Perez-Gracia et al.[2] in their interesting article guide metabolomics and mention that few reliable biomarkers have been identified in retrospective studies in patients who were under standard treatment outside study protocols. They suggest that the best strategy would be to collect samples prospectively from patients both in study protocol and on standard treatment and study them retrospectively to boost sample size and hypothesis. However, even this study could not find answers on how to improve sample size related issues. They suggested that though randomized trials are gold standard, even nonrandomized and retrospective studies could be acceptable. Buyse[3] et al. in their article in 2011 classified biomarkers as either clinical biomarker or pharmacokinetic/pharmacodynamic biomarker. Clinical biomarkers are further classified as prognostic or predictive biomarkers. They suggest retrospective analysis of prospective patients as the best case scenario for biomarker validation. In contrast, the present study does not explore this possibility. They suggest that, if public sharing of data is the norm, meta-analysis and hypotheses generation will be easier and each study will not have to 'invent the wheel' again and again. Without this step, these studies will lead to nowhere in times to come, until there is a massive improvement in our knowledge of the disease process, which itself is hampered due to privatization of data.

Literature is flushed with studies on markers for Sepsis, AKI, ARDS, delirium, TBI and many other critical illnesses. Out of plethora of biomarkers studied very few hold clinical significance like serum procalcitonin, KIM, NGAL, etc. However, in spite of poor advances in metabolomics, the outcome of sepsis has been regularly improving.[4] This is certainly due to holistic approach to the patient and concentrating on organ support rather than focusing on biomarkers. Perhaps these studies are early in their times and more knowledge of disease process is required before reliable biomarkers are available. Way forward could be a statement declaration by medical fraternity worldwide to share raw data and retrospective analysis of patients in and out of study protocols to help metabolomics succeed. May be the clinical trials registry can have a clause ensuring the same.

REFERENCES

1. Atkinson AJJ, Colburn WA, DeGruttola VG, et. al. Biomarkers and surrogate endpoints: preferred definitions and conceptual framework. Clinical Pharmacology and Therapeutics. 2001;69(3):89-95.
2. Perez-Gracia JL, Sanmamed MF, Bosch Campos AL, et al. Strategies to design clinical studies to identify predictive biomarkers in cancer research. Cancer Treatment Reviews. 2017;53:79-97.
3. Buyse M, Michiels S, Sargent DJ, et al. Integrating biomarkers in clinical trials. Expert Review of Molecular Diagnostics. 2011;11(2):171-82.
4. Kaukonen KM, Bailey M, Suzuki S, et al. Mortality related to severe sepsis and septic shock among critically ill patients in Australia and New Zealand, 2000-12. JAMA. 2014;311(13):1308-16.

Journal Scan 5—Ashok Kumar Saxena

Physical Activity Behavior Predicts Endogenous Pain Modulation in Older Adults

Naugle KM, Ohlman T, Naugle KE, et al. PAIN. 2017;158(3):383-90.

BACKGROUND

A large number of older adults are at risk for chronic pain compared with the young adults. This is largely due to age-related changes in endogenous pain processes with decreased pain inhibition and increased pain facilitation. There is some evidence that increased physical activity may improve pain inhibition and facilitation though it has not been objectively evaluated. The aim of this study was to evaluate whether objective measures of physical activity behavior predicted pain inhibitory function on the conditioned pain modulation (CPM) test and pain facilitation on the temporal summation (TS) test in healthy older adults.

ABSTRACT

A total of fifty-one healthy older adults (60 to 77 yrs; 21 males/30 females; 46 Caucasians, 4 African Americans, 1 Hispanic) were enrolled and they wore an accelerometer (Actigraph GT3X+) on the hip to measure physical activity levels for 7 days. Temporal summation (TS) which refers to increased perception of pain in response to repetitive, noxious stimulus delivered at frequencies above 0.3 Hz and conditioned pain modulation (CPM) which refers to the reduction of pain produced by a test stimulus by a second noxious conditioning stimulus in a remote body site (pain inhibition by pain), were measured. The details of sedentary time period, light physical activity (LPA), and moderate-to-vigorous physical activity (MVPA) were retrieved from the accelerometer.

In the statistical analysis, spearman bivariate correlation between TS and CPM scores and psychological and physical activity variables were conducted. Also, hierarchical linear regressions were done to evaluate the relationship between physical activity and TS and CPM, while controlling the factors known to affect experimental pain testing. The results revealed that LPA and sedentary time, significantly predicted the pain inhibitory function on the CPM test, with minimal sedentary time and greater LPA per day linked with greater pain inhibitory capacity. Also, MVPA predicted pain facilitation on the TS test, with enhanced MVPA, linked with less TS of pain. It was concluded that sedentary time and LPA could be linked to pain inhibitory capacity in older healthy adults, whereas MVPA is linked to pain facilitatory process.

COMMENTARY

It is for certain and it is for sure that physical therapy is an essential and integral part of the multimodal approach in the management of chronic pain. This interesting study by Naugle et al.[1] is a great initiative to explore that to what extent the physical activity behavior can predict the effect on temporal summation (TS) of pain and inhibition of pain on conditioned pain modulation (CPM) test. Recently, Arendt-Nielsen et al. attempted to evaluate the experimental and clinical applications of quantitative sensory testing when applied to skin, muscles and viscera, and concluded that TS of pain is the human behavioral correlate of ascending facilitatory limb and CPM is the human behavioral correlate of descending inhibitory limb of central pain modulation.[2] With this background, the recent substantial body of evidence provided by Ellingson et al., Naugle et al., and Umeda et al., proves the relationship between physical activity behavior and endogenous pain modulatory function with an effective pain modulation seen in more active patients.[3-5] They also suggested that minimum physical activity results in reduction of endogenous pain inhibitory and facilitatory systems seen in elderly population.

It has been opined that the individuals who are highly active physically, have a reduced risk for predisposition to chronic pain.[6,7] Now from this study by Naugle et al., it is not clear whether this relationship of physical activity with pain happens in patients with pain, and whether level of physical activity modulates the excitability and inhibition or is it the other way round in that differences in pain excitability and inhibition modulates the activity levels.

In this study, the participants were 51 healthy adults in the age group of 60 to 77 years, with majority of Caucasians (46 adults) and only 4 African Americans and one Hispanic. All participants were motivated to wear an accelerometer on the hip to measure physical activity levels. Greater temporal summation to heat was linked with lower moderate-to-vigorous physical activity, and also lower levels of light physical activity was linked with less conditioned pain modulation (CPM) to heat, but not to pressure after a cold water conditioning. Hence it was concluded that physical activity levels may modulate central excitability and central inhibition.

It has been observed that prior voluntary wheel running attenuates neuropathic pain by preventing development of hyperalgesia, development of chronic pain and activation of central neurons.[8,9] Furthermore, it has been observed that regular physical activity minimizes excitability of central neurons as evident by phosphorylation of the NRI unit of NMDA receptor, altered neuroimmune signaling in the CNS, and enhanced release of endogenous opioids and serotonin, in the brainstem pain inhibitory pathways.[9-11]

The responses to deep tissue pressure or heat can depict variable responses. Few individuals can be more sensitive to noxious heat, and few sensitive to ischemia, and few sensitive to heat temporal summation. Hence in this particular study, association between physical activity and CPM, were inconsistent in older adults. This study also observes that incidence of chronic pain goes up in the older adult population and that older adults are less physically active than younger adults. The study analyzed that physical activity may be a significant factor in influencing pain sensitivity. In simple language, higher enhanced levels of activity are associated with reduced pain facilitation and enhanced pain inhibition. As evident in this study's power analysis, the study was adequately powered to conduct a linear regression model with 2 covariates. As this study contained more than 2 covariates, it is possible that with a larger sample size, the model with MVPA (moderate-to- vigorous physical activity) predicting CPM-heat would have been significant.

In essence, the higher levels of physical activity are linked with reduced pain facilitation and enhanced pain inhibition. The older adults should be encouraged to be active throughout the day with light physical activity, while minimizing prolonged sedentary time.

REFERENCES

1. Naugle KM, Naugle KM, Ohlman T, et al. Physical activity behavior predicts endogenous pain modulation in older adults. PAIN. 2017;158:383-90.
2. Arendt-Nielsen L, Yarnitsky D. Experimental and clinical applications of quantitative sensory testing applied to skin, muscles and viscera. J Pain. 2009;10:556-72.
3. Ellingson LD, Shields MR, Stegner AJ, et al. Physical activity, sustained sedentary behavior and pain modulation in women with fibromyalgia. J Pain. 2012;13:195-206.
4. Naugle KM, Riley JL. Self-reported physical activity predicts experimental models of pain facilitation and inhibition. Med Sci Sports Exerc. 2014;46:622-9.
5. Umeda M, Lee W, Marino CA, et al. Influence of moderate intensity physical activity levels and gender on conditioned pain modulation. J Sports Sci. 2016;34:467-76.
6. Landmark T, Romundstad P, Borchgrevink PC, et al. Associations between recreational exercise and chronic pain in the general population: evidence from the HUNT3 study. PAIN. 2011;152:2241-7.
7. Zhang R, Chomistek AK, Dimitrakoff JD, et al. Physical activity and chronic prostatitis/Chronic pelvic pain syndrome. Med Sci Sports Exerc. 2015;47:757-64.
8. Grace PM, Fabisiak TJ, Green-Fulgham SM, et al. Prior voluntary wheel running attenuates neuropathic pain. PAIN. 2016;157:2012-23.
9. Sluka KA, O'Donnell JM, Danielson J, et al. Regular physical activity prevents development of chronic pain and activation of central neurons. J Appl Physiol. 2013;114:725-33.
10. Bobinski F, Ferreira TA, Cordova MM, et al. Role of brainstem serotonin in analgesia produced by low-intensity exercise on neuropathic pain after sciatic nerve injury in mice. PAIN. 2015;156:2595-2606.
11. Stagg NJ, Mata HP, Ibrahim MM, et al. Regular exercise reverses sensory hypersensitivity in a rat neuropathic pain model of endogenous opioids. Anesthesiology. 2011;114:940-8.

Index

Note: Page numbers followed by *f* refer to figure, *t* refer to table and *fc* refer to flowchart.

A

Acetaminophen 135, 213, 269
Acidosis 70
Acupuncture 135
Acute coronary syndrome 22
Adenosine 291
   receptors, subtypes of 291
Adrenal insufficiency 153
Adrenoceptor agonists 210
Adult intensive care unit 210
Adult respiratory distress syndrome 144
Advance venous access catheter 273
Agitation 210, 213, 217
Airway 175
   device, placement of 93
   management 93t
   obstruction 93
Alagille syndrome 269t
Alfentanil 44
Allodynia 126
Alveolar
   arterial oxygen tension gradient 115
   oxygen, fraction of 93
American College of Physicians 134
American Heart Association 227
American Pain Society 134
American Society of Anesthesiologists 68, 228, 244
Amiodarone 232, 235
Amylase, serum 155
Amyloidosis 116, 195
Analgesia
   adequate 229
   epidural 43
Anaphylaxis 153
Anemia 93, 94
Anesthesia 154, 168, 174, 190, 196, 198, 267
   general 68
   induction of 174
   inhalation 148
   intravenous 148
   maintenance of 156, 175, 198
   medication template 246
   patient safety foundation 244
   preparation and premedication 272
   regional 175, 201
   total intravenous 199
Anesthesiology 1, 2, 7, 9, 10
   education 9
   research 8
   training 9
Anesthetic
   management 164, 173, 196
   technique 32, 273
Angiotensin converting enzyme inhibitor 228
Antegrade
   cardioplegia 293, 294, 294f
   warm blood cardioplegia 300
Antiadhesion 28, 29
Antiarrhythmics 64
Anticoagulants 32, 33t
Anticonvulsants 136
Antidepressants 136
Antifibrinolytic agents 280
Antihemophilic
   factor 20
   globulin 20
Anti-inflammatory cytokines 307
Antimicrobial therapy 155
Antiplatelet agents 22t
Antithrombin 20
Antitrypsin deficiency 269
Anxiety 217
Anxiolysis 198
Aorta, coarctation of 162
Aortic
   root cannula 294f
   valve replacement 295

Apnea 170
  duration of 93, 94
Apneic oxygenation 96
Arrhythmias, cardiac 147
Aspartate 299
Asthma, bronchial 113*f*
Atenolol 235
Atherogenesis 29
Atresia, esophageal 160
Atrial cardioplegia 295
Atrial fibrillation 30, 226, 228, 234
  classification of 227
  management of 233
  nonvalvular 33t
  pathophysiology of 228, 233*fc*
Atrial septal defect 162
Atropine prefilled syringes 245
Auditory evoked potentials 216

  hypoxic ischemic 252, 253, 254*f*
  ischemic 258
  relaxation 142, 144-146
  assessment of 145
  subcortical regions of 258*f*
Brassy cough 193
Breathing
  duration of 94
  system 54, 56
Bridging veins 143
Bronchial provocation test 105, 117
Bronchodilators 113*f*
Bronchoscopy 194
Budd-Chiari syndrome 269, 274
Bupivacaine 66
Burns 153
Burst-suppression 257
Byler's disease 269*t*

B

Back pain 131
Bacterial peritonitis, spontaneous 273
Bag valve mask 98
Barbiturates 148
Basal ganglia 258*f*
Baseline infusion 49
Behavior therapy 135
Behavioral pain scale 212
Benzodiazepines 148, 210
Beta blockers 64, 65, 231
Bispectral index 216
Blade curvature 79*f*
Bleeding tendencies, congenital 46
Blind spot 85
Blood 274
  cardioplegia 292, 300
  conservation strategies 280
  gas, arterial 106
  intraoperative transfusion of 279
  leuko-reduced 293
  pressure, systolic 67
  product 274, 279*fc*
    intraoperative transfusion of 279
  sugar 155
  vessels 20
Body plethysmography 114
Bone 20
  infection of 153
Brachial plexus 64
Brain
  beneath 260f
  computer tomography of 258
  injury

C

Calcium 20
  channel blockers 64, 70
  chloride 289
Carbon monoxide 116
Carcinoma, hepatocellular 269
Cardiac
  arrest 252, 255, 263*f*, 296
    pathophysiology of 253
  disease 64
  failure, congestive 233, 234
  life support, advanced 253
  malformations 170
  surgery 29, 104, 285
  tamponade 153
Cardiocerebral resuscitation 253
Cardiomyocytes 29
Cardioplegia 286
  perfluorocarbon-based 293
  second phase of 299
  solution 288, 289
    composition of 287
  vehicle 292
Cardiopulmonary
  bypass 22, 26, 200, 288
  exercise testing 116
Cardiotocography 45
Cardiovascular
  collapse 66
  disease 29
  safety 28
  support 171
  system 53, 170
  toxicity 65

Carpal tunnel syndrome 123
Cell
　adhesion molecules 16
　death 254
　saver 280, 280f
Central
　blood volume 271
　nervous system 66, 153
　　toxicity 65
　neuraxial analgesia 47
　pain syndrome 123
　pontine myelinolysis 147
　reorganization 124
　sensitization 124, 131
　venous
　　oxygen saturation 155
　　pressure 144, 155
Cerebral
　edema 258
　palsy 169
　performance category 255
　venous pressure 144
Cerebrospinal fluid 142
　drainage 147
Chemical neurolysis 127
Chemokine 307
Chemotherapy 123
Child-Turcotte-Pugh
　classification 268
　score 269
Cholangiocarcinoma 269
Christmas factor 20
Cirrhosis 269
Cisatracurium 273
Clichy's criteria 270
Cognitive behavioral therapy 135
Colchicine 233
Cold 297
　blood cardioplegia 298
　retrograde cardioplegia 299
Collagen vascular diseases 116
Combined spinal epidural technique 47
Comparative cardiovascular toxicity 66
Complete blood count 193
Complex regional pain syndrome 123
Compression myelopathy 123
Consciousness, altered level of 222
Continuous positive airway pressure 95, 169
Coronary
　artery
　　bypass graft 226, 243
　　disease 30, 295
　　left 295
　　ostial cannula 294f

sinus 295
　catheter 296f
　injury 296
Cortical veins draining 143
Corticosteroids 232
Cough test 106
Cranium and volume-pressure curve, components of 143f
Crigler-Najjar syndrome 269t
Critical illness myopathy 306
Cryoprecipitate 205, 207, 208
Crystalloid cardioplegia 292
Cyanosis 193
Cyclooxygenase 28
　inhibitors 213

D

De-Bono whistle blowing test 106
Deep breathing 95
Dehydration 172
Delirium 210, 216, 221
　prevention of 221
　treatment of 221
Delusion 222
Dense granules 21
Dermatan sulfate 18
Desflurane 148
Desipramine 126
Desmopressin 25
Diclofenac 212
Digoxin 235
Diltiazem 235
Direct oral anticoagulants 32
Disk herniation 133
Distal tracheal intubation 200
Distal tracheoesophageal fistula 160, 163f
Distension, abdominal 93
Diuresis 28, 147
Dorsal
　horn cells 124
　root ganglion 124
Drug 269
　errors, classification of 242
　interaction 64
　overdose 153
Duodenal atresia 162
Dynamic lung function tests 108
Dyselectrolytemia 278
Dysplasia, bronchopulmonary 169, 170

E

Echocardiogram 237
Ectopic neural activity 124

Electrical cardioversion 233
Electroencephalography 256, 257
Electrolytes
    balance 231
    serum 155
Embryology 160
Emergency airway management 98
Encephalitis 153
End stage liver disease 268
Endocarditis, infective 153
Endothelium 20, 28, 29
Endotracheal
    intubation 76
    neoplasm 114f
    tube 77, 197, 198, 200f
Enflurane 148
Epinephrine 30, 64, 68
Esmolol 235
Esophageal atresia, isolated 163f
Etomidate 148
European Society of Anesthesiology 208
European Society of Intensive Care
        Medicine 152
Euvolemia 230
Exercise therapy 134
Expired oxygen, fraction of 93
Extracellular fluid 142
Extracorporeal life support 179
    organization 181
Extracorporeal membrane oxygenation
        179, 180, 180f, 181, 182, 200
    cannulas, types of 185f
    monitoring of 185
    types of 181
    veno-arterial 182, 184
    veno-venous 182, 183f, 184
Extrinsic coagulation pathways 25
Extubation 198
Ex-utero intrapartum treatment
        procedures 50

F

Face mask seal 94
Facet joint 131
    dysfunctions 133
    interventions 137
Fatty infiltration 269
Femoroaortal inflow and outflow 188f
Fentanyl 44, 47, 212
Fever 93, 154
Fibrin
    genesis of 204
    stabilizing factor 20

Fibrinogen 20, 21, 204, 205
    concentrates 207, 208
        efficacy of 207
        safety of 208
    critical threshold value of 205
    dosing 206
    replacement therapy 205
    supplementation, perioperative 204
Fixed airway obstruction 114f
Flow volume loop 111, 113f, 115f
Fluid balance 278
Focal hypoxic brain insult 258f
Forced expiratory volume 105, 109, 109f
Fresh frozen plasma 206
Functional residual capacity 91, 108
Fundoplication 172

G

Gabapentin 126
Gas
    distribution tests 105
    exchange function 115
Gastroesophageal reflux 172, 191
    disease 194
Gastrointestinal
    disorders 171
    tract 153
Geriatric population 93
Global burden of disease study 129
Glottis 190
Glucose 289, 292
    management 171
Glutamate 299
Glycogen storage disease 269
Glycoprotein 16
Glycosaminoglycan 17
Glycosidases 21
Goiter 114f

H

Hageman factor 20
Hallucination 222
Headaches 217
Head-up tilt 148
Heart 292
    failure
        chronic 187
        congestive 147
    rate 67, 68
Heat 60

Helium dilution method 105, 112
Hemangioendothelioma, epithelioid 269
Hematology 171
Hemochromatosis, hereditary 269
Hemodiluted blood cardioplegia 293
Hemoglobin 155, 182
    optimization 230
Hemolysis 147
Hemophilia 25
Hemorrhage 153
    intraventricular 169, 171
Hemostasis 16, 17, 32
    physiology of 18
Heparan sulphate 17, 18
Heparin 32
    factor 18
    unfractionated 17
Hepatic
    artery thrombosis 282
    disease 64
Hepatitis
    A 269
    B 269
    C 269
    D 269
High molecular weight kininogen 25
High shear stress 30
Hoarseness 193
Humidity 60
Hydrothorax 272*f*
Hyperactive delirium 217
Hyperalgesia 126
Hyperkalemia 64, 147
Hyperkalemic normothermic blood cardioplegia 299
Hypernatremia 147
Hyperosmolar therapy 146
Hyperpathia 126
Hypertonic saline 146, 147, 147*t*
Hypertrophy, left ventricular 228
Hyperventilation 147
Hypofibrinogenemia, acquired 205
Hypoglycemia 171
Hypokalemia 147
Hypospadias 162
Hypotension 147, 152, 153
    arterial 154
Hypothermia 278, 297, 298
    systemic 299
    therapeutic 256, 257
Hypothesis 37, 38*f*
Hypoventilation 93

Hypovolemia 147
Hypoxemia 152, 211
    arterial 154
Hypoxia 64, 70

I

Iatrogenic neuralgias 123
Ibuprofen 212
Idiopathic pulmonary fibrosis 116
Idiopathic sensory neuropathy 123
Immunothrombosis 23, 31
Imperforate anus 162
Incremental shuttle walk test 117
Induction 156, 197-199
Inferior vena cava 276
Inflammatory demyelinating polyradiculoneuropathy 123
Infra-red spectroscopy 260
Inguinal hernia repair 172
Injection
    epidural 137
    rate of 64
Injury, ischemic 298
Insomnia 217
Inspiratory capacity 108
Intensive care
    delirium screening 222
    unit 83, 152, 201, 210, 306
        acquired weakness 306
Internal jugular vein, dual-lumen single cannulation of 185*f*
Interstitial fibrosis 115*f*
Intra-aortic balloon pump 179, 237
Intracranial pressure 142, 145, 149
    dynamic components of 143
Intrathoracic obstruction 114*f*
Intravenous fluid 17
    replacement 176
Intrinsic
    coagulation pathways 25
    vasoconstrictor action 64
Intubation 156, 175, 197, 199
Ionotropic theory 69
Islet cell tumor 269
Isoflurane 148

J

Jet ventilation 200
Joints, infection of 153
Jugular venous pressure 143

K

Ketamine 148, 213, 212
Ketoacidosis, diabetic 153
Kidney 28
　collecting ducts of 28
King's college criteria 270
Kovacs' sign 84*f*

L

Labor analgesia 43, 44, 48*t*, 49
Lam's KCL solution 287
Laparotomy 172
　decompressive 144
Laryngeal mask airways 197
Laryngoscopy, direct 194
Laryngotracheal stenosis 190, 195*t*, 196*t*
　classification systems for 192*t*
　surgery 201
Laser
　surgery 173
　therapy 196
Leukocytosis 154
Levobupivacaine 66
Ligaments 133
Lignocaine 65, 148
　patch 126
Lipid sink, theory of 69
Lipophilicity 64
Live donor liver transplant 268
Liver 20
　disease
　　alcoholic 269
　　chronic 269
　　cryptogenic 269
　　severity 268
　failure, acute 269, 270
　function tests 155
　malignant diseases of 269
　transplant 267, 269
　　indications 268
Local anesthetic
　drugs 63
　systemic toxicity 63
　　management 70*t*
Low axial pain 129, 130*t*, 131
Low back pain, chronic 129, 131
Low birth weight 169, 170
Low flow
　anesthesia 52, 53, 59, 60
　　advantages of 59
　　phases of 54
　technique 58

Low molecular weight heparin 17
Lower abdominal surgery 104
Lower limb defects 162
Lumbar canal stenosis 131
Lung
　capacities 108, 108*t*
　disease
　　chronic 169
　　obstructive 111, 113*f*
　function tests 107
　injury, acute 206
　pathologies 93
　resection surgeries 104, 117
　volume 108, 108*t*
Lysosomal granules 21

M

MacIntosh blade 77
MacIntosh laryngoscope 79*f*, 80*f*
MacIntosh type 77
Macula densa 29
Magnesium 232, 288, 289
　sulphate 288
Magnetic resonance imaging 258
Manual muscle strength testing 307
Mask ventilation 93
Massage therapy 212
Maternofetal transference 45
Maximal expiratory flow 112*f*
Maximal inspiratory flow 112*f*
Maximum breathing capacity 105, 110, 111
Maximum mid expiratory flow rate 111
Maximum voluntary ventilation 110
McCaffrey classification 192
McCaffrey system 192
Mean arterial pressure 143, 155
Medial branch block 137
Medullary interstitium 29
Membrane oxygenator pump 180*f*, 291
Meningitis 153
Meperidine 44, 47
Mesangial cells 28
Metabolic
　acidosis 64, 277
　flow 53
　liver disease 269
　status 231
　theory 69
Metastatic malignancy 261
Methadone 212
Metoprolol 235
Meyer cotton classification 192
Microplegia 293

Microspirometer 106
Minimally invasive interventions 136
Minnesota sedation assessment tool 214
Mixed venous oxygen saturation 155
Modified Oswestry low back pain
    disability questionnaires 132
Monocytes 30
Mononuclear cells 311
Mood 222
Morphine 212
Multiplanar reformations 194
Multiple breath N2 test 105
Muscle
    cramps 217
    mass, breakdown of 211
    relaxants 136
Music therapy 212
Myasthenia gravis 116
Myelopathy, ischemic 123
Myocardial
    infarction 29, 39, 153
    oxygen consumption 286
    protection 285
        adjuncts for 292
Myoclonus 217

N

Narcotics 210
Narcotrend index 216
National audit project 81
National Institute of Health 217
Native pulmonary function 182
Natriuresis 28
Nausea 217
    postoperative 37
Near infrared spectroscopy 259, 260*f*
Necrotizing enterocolitis 168, 169, 172
Neonatal brain 44, 45
Nephrotoxicity 59
Nerve compression 123
Neuralgia
    herpetic 123
    post-herpetic 123
    trigeminal 123
Neuraxial drug 242
Neurogenic inflammation 124
Neuromuscular disease 115*f*, 116
Neuron specific serum enolase 256
Neuropathic pain 122, 126*t*, 131
    assessment of 125
    mechanism of 124
    questionnaire 132
    treatment of 126

Neuropathy 123
    diabetic 123
    entrapment 123
Neutrophil
    extracellular traps 32
    phagocytic activity 211
New direct oral anticoagulants 236
New Sheffield sedation scale 214
Nitrogen
    alveolar 93
    washout technique 112
Nitrous oxide 47, 148
    use of 58
Nonalcoholic fatty liver disease 269
Noncardiac surgery 29, 234*fc*
Nondihydropyridine calcium channel
    blockers 232
Noninvasive positive pressure ventilation
    95, 98
Non-metastatic malignancy 261
Nonsteroidal anti-inflammatory drugs
    135, 156, 232
Normal flow volume loop 112*f*
Nortriptyline 126
Null hypothesis significance testing 36
Number counting test 106
Nutritional deficiency 123

O

Obese 93, 97, 115*f*, 116, 130
Obstructive pulmonary disease, chronic
    97, 228, 230
Obstructive sleep apnea syndrome 228
Omphalocele 162
Opioid 44, 148, 176
    analgesics 126, 135
    intravenous 44, 212
Optimal oxygenation 230
Organ dysfunction 153, 154
Oxidative stress 312
Oxygen demand 94
Oxygenation 92, 171

P

Pain 123, 132, 210, 211
    chronic 166
    diabetic neuropathic 123
    disorders, chronic 123
    generators 131
    intensity 125
    leg 131
    management 166

neuropathic 122, 123*t*
nociceptive 131
relief, postoperative 29
Pancreatitis, acute 153
Parkinson disease 123
Patent ductus arteriosus 162, 168, 170
Patrick or Faber test 133
Peak expiratory flow rate 111*f*
Pediatric cardiovascular system 68
Percutaneous coronary intervention 23*t*
Peritonitis 153
Phantom limb pain 123
Pharmacotherapy 126
Phenylephrine 64
Phenytoin 65
Plasma
    coagulation factors 20*t*
    factors regulating coagulation 26
    fibrinogen, level of 207
    thromboplastin
        antecedent 20
        component 20
Platelet 20
    activation 28
    adhesion 16
    aggregation 16
    inhibition 28
    microvesicles 21
Pneumonia 153, 261
Pneumonitis, recurrent 193
Polycystic kidney 162
Polydactyly 162
Polyneuropathy, alcoholic 123
Polyunsaturated fatty acids 230
Positive end expiratory pressure 95, 144
Positive pressure ventilation 200
Post-mastectomy 123
Postoperative atrial fibrillation,
    management of 234*f*
Post-reperfusion syndrome 277
Potassium 285, 287
    chloride 287
Pregnancy 64, 93, 96
    acute fatty liver of 269
Premature infants 168, 169
Prematurity, retinopathy of 168, 172
Preoxygenation 90, 94t, 96, 197
    markers of 92
    techniques of 94
Pressure
    intrathoracic 114*f*
    support ventilation 95, 97
Procaine 291
    hydrochloride 289

Proconvertin 20
Prognosis after resuscitation score 261
Prognostication, multimodal paradigm
    of 255
Propofol 70, 148, 176, 210
Prostaglandins 124
Protamine 32
Proteases 21
Protection against oxidative injury 28, 29
Prothrombin 20
    complex concentrates 17
Psychomotor agitation 222
Psychosis 222
Pudendal neuralgia 123
Pulmonary diseases, types of 104
Pulmonary function test 103-105, 194
    contraindications 104
    types of 104
Pulse oximetry 106
Pupillary reaction 256
Pure esophageal atresia 160
Pyloric stenosis 162

Q

Quantitative sensory testing 126

R

Radiation myelopathy 123
Radicular pain 131
Radiculopathy 123
Radio xenon scintigram 105
Radiotherapy 123
Ramsay sedation scale 214
Rankin scale score 255
Rate control drugs 235
Red blood cells 254*f*
Regional oxygen saturation 259, 260*f*
Relaxation techniques 212
Remifentanil 43, 44, 47, 212
    infusion regimens 48
Renal
    agenesis 162
    disease 64
    failure 147
    function 171, 278
    test 155
Residual volume 108, 111
Respiration, control of 170
Respiratory
    acidosis 64
    distress syndrome 153, 168, 181

mechanics, assessment of 105
rate 105
system 153, 169
Restrictive lung disease 111, 115*f*
Resuscitation, cardiopulmonary 252
Retrograde cardioplegia 295, 296*f*, 297
    disadvantages of 296
Reye's syndrome 269
Richmond agitation-sedation scale 215
Riker sedation-agitation scale 214
Rocuronium 273

S

Sabrasez breath holding test 105
Sacroiliac joint
    arthropathy 131
    injections 137
Sarcoidosis 116
Schneider's match blowing test 105
Sciatic nerve block 64
Sciatica 123, 133
Sclerosis, multiple 116, 123
Scoliosis 115*f*, 116, 162
Sedation intensive care score 214
Sensory neurons 125f
Sentinel event evaluation 247
Sepsis 93, 152, 153*t*, 154t, 261
    etiology of 153*t*
Septic shock 153
Sequential organ failure assessment 153, 308
Serine 16
Sevoflurane 59, 148
Single breath
    counting 106
    nitrogen test 105
Six minute walk test 117
Skin, infection of 153
Sleep-wake cycle disturbance 222
Smooth muscles 28, 29
Society of Critical Care Medicine 152
Sodium
    channel
        abnormal 124
        blockers 65
    chloride 289
Soft molecule 43
Soft tissues 133
    infection of 153
Somatosensory evoked potentials 256, 257
Sorbitol 289
Sotalol 232

Spinal
    abnormalities 46
    canal stenosis 123
    cord injury 123
    nerve injury 125, 125*f*
Spitz classification 161t
Split-lung function tests 105, 117
Spontaneous neural discharge ectopic sensitivity 125
Statins 232
Status epilepticus 257
Stenosis 196
    bronchial 114*f*
    post-intubation 195
    subglottic 190
    tracheal 190
Steroids 148
Stimulation techniques 127
Stress, psychological 310
Stridor 193
Stroke 123
Stuart-Prower factor 20
Superior vena cava 276
Supraglottic airways 8
Supraventricular tachyarrhythmias 230
Sweating 217
Sympathetic dysfunction 124
Syringomyelia 123
Systemic inflammatory response syndrome 152, 234

T

Target controlled infusions 49
Targeted temperature management 253, 259
Temperature regulation 172
Tetralogy of Fallot 162
Thebesian veins 295
Therapeutic temperature management 257
Thiobarbituric acid reactive substance 311
Thomas Starzl initiated liver transplant 267
Thoracic surgery 104
Thoracotomy pain 123
Thrombocytopenia, heparin induced 22
Thromboelastography 205, 274
Thromboelastometry 205, 274
Thrombomodulin 18
Thromboplastin 20
Thrombosis 29, 30
    arterial 30

Tidal volume 108
    breathing 94
Tissue factor 20
Total lung
    capacity 108, 111
    volume 112
Trace gases, accumulation of 59
Tracheal resection 198
Tracheobronchial manipulation 96
Tracheoesophageal fistula 162*t*
    classification of 160*t*, 161*f*
    congenital 159, 160
Tracheomalacia 196
Tramadol hydrochloride 126
Transcutaneous electrical nerve
    stimulation 124, 127
Transnasal
    high flow insufflation 96
    humidified rapid insufflation
    ventilatory exchange 96
Transplant procedure, complications of 277
Trauma, severe 153
Traumatic neuropathy 122, 123
Tricyclic antidepressants 126, 136
Trigger point injections 136
Tuberculosis 195
Tumors
    bronchial 114*f*
    carcinoid 269

U

Upper abdominal surgery 104
Urethral abnormalities 162
Urinary tract infection 153

V

Vascular endothelium 18, 28
Vasoconstrictor, addition of 64
Vasopressin 70
    synthetic analogue of 25
Venous thromboembolism 17, 31
Ventilation 171
    alveolar 94
    intraoperative 175
    spontaneous 200
Ventricular
    assist devices 179
    septal defect 162
Vertebral defects 162
Very low birth weight 169
Videolaryngoscope 76, 77, 83, 84
    complications of 84
    role of 83
    safety of 85
    scope of 81
    taxonomy of 78
Videolaryngoscopy
    advantages of 80
    disadvantages of 80
Vital capacity 108, 111
Vitamin 20, 32, 130, 136, 236
Vitrectomy 173
Vitronectin 21
Vocal cord 84*f*, 190
Vomiting 217
von Willebrand disease 25
von Willebrand factor 20, 23

W

Warm terminal reperfusion 300
Wegener granulomatosis 195
White blood cells 254*f*
Wilson's disease 269
Wright's peak flowmeter 106
Wright's respirometer 106

Z

Zymogen 20, 16, 23

EU GSPR Authorised Reprsentative
Logos Europe, 9 rue Nicolas Poussin
1700, La Rochelle, France
Phone: +33 (0) 6 67 93 73 78
E-mail: contact@logoseurope.eu

www.ingramcontent.com/pod-product-compliance
Ingram Content Group UK Ltd.
Pitfield, Milton Keynes, MK11 3LW, UK
UKHW051848210426
5322IPUK00024B/601